Risk Management in Emergency Medicine

Editors

LAUREN M. NENTWICH
JONATHAN S. OLSHAKER

EMERGENCY MEDICINE CLINICS OF NORTH AMERICA

www.emed.theclinics.com

Consulting Editor
AMAL MATTU

May 2020 • Volume 38 • Number 2

ELSEVIER

1600 John F. Kennedy Boulevard • Suite 1800 • Philadelphia, Pennsylvania, 19103-2899

http://www.theclinics.com

EMERGENCY MEDICINE CLINICS OF NORTH AMERICA Volume 38, Number 2
May 2020 ISSN 0733-8627, ISBN-13: 978-0-323-78949-3

Editor: Colleen Dietzler
Developmental Editor: Casey Potter

Emergency Medicine Clinics of North America (ISSN 0733-8627) is published quarterly by Elsevier Inc., 360 Park Avenue South, New York, NY, 10010-1710. Months of issue are February, May, August, and November. Business and Editorial Offices: 1600 John F. Kennedy Boulevard, Suite 1800, Philadelphia, PA 19103-2899. Customer Service Office: 6277 Sea Harbor Drive, Orlando, FL 32887-4800. Periodicals postage paid at New York, NY, and additional mailing offices. Subscription prices are $100.00 per year (US students), $352.00 per year (US individuals), $716.00 per year (US institutions), $220.00 per year (international students), $462.00 per year (international individuals), $882.00 per year (international institutions), $100.00 per year (Canadian students), $411.00 per year (Canadian individuals), and $882.00 per year (Canadian institutions). International air speed delivery is included in all *Clinics'* subscription prices. All prices are subject to change without notice. **POSTMASTER:** Send address changes to *Emergency Medicine Clinics of North America*, Elsevier Periodicals Customer Service, 11830 Westline Industrial Drive, St. Louis, MO 63146. Customer Service (orders, claims, online, change of address): Elsevier Periodicals **Customer Service, 11830 Westline Industrial Drive, St. Louis, MO 63146. Tel: 1-800-654-2452 (U.S. and Canada); 314-453-7041 (outside U.S. and Canada). Fax: 314-453-5170. E-mail: journalscustomerservice-usa@elsevier.com (for print support); journalsonlinesupport-usa@elsevier.com (for online support).**

Reprints. For copies of 100 or more of articles in this publication, please contact the Commercial Reprints Department, Elsevier Inc., 360 Park Avenue South, New York, NY 10010-1710. Tel.: 212-633-3874; Fax: 212-633-3820; E-mail: reprints@elsevier.com.

Emergency Medicine Clinics of North America is covered in *MEDLINE/PubMed (Index Medicus)*, *Current Contents/Clinical Medicine*, *EMBASE/Excerpta Medica*, *BIOSIS*, *SciSearch*, *CINAHL*, *ISI/BIOMED*, and *Research Alert*.

Contributors

CONSULTING EDITOR

AMAL MATTU, MD
Professor and Vice Chair of Academic Affairs, Department of Emergency Medicine, University of Maryland School of Medicine, Baltimore, Maryland

EDITORS

LAUREN M. NENTWICH, MD, FACEP
Assistant Professor, Department of Emergency Medicine, Medical Director of Quality and Patient Safety, Emergency Department, Boston Medical Center, Boston University School of Medicine, Boston, Massachusetts

JONATHAN S. OLSHAKER, MD, FACEP, FAAEM
Chief, Boston Medical Center, Professor and Chair, Department of Emergency Medicine, Boston University School of Medicine, Boston, Massachusetts

AUTHORS

CRISTOPHER AMANTI, MD
Medical Director, Department of Emergency Medicine, Boston Medical Center, Boston, Massachusetts

JONATHAN S. AUERBACH, MD
Assistant Professor of Clinical Medicine, University of Miami Miller School of Medicine, Miami, Florida

BENJAMIN BAUTZ, MD
Department of Emergency Medicine, Boston Medical Center, Boston, Massachusetts

GERALD (WOOK) BELTRAN, DO, MPH, MSIS, MSCJA, FACEP, FAEMS
Associate Professor, Department of Emergency Medicine, University of Massachusetts Medical School-Baystate, Baystate Health, Springfield, Massachusetts

SUZANNE BENTLEY, MD, MPH
Departments of Emergency Medicine and Medical Education, Icahn School of Medicine at Mount Sinai, NYC Health + Hospitals/Elmhurst, Elmhurst, New York

EVAN BERG, MD
Assistant Professor, Department of Emergency Medicine, Boston University School of Medicine, Boston, Massachusetts

KELLY BOOKMAN, MD, FACEP
Emergency Medicine, University of Colorado, Denver, Colorado

SHARON BORD, MD, FACEP
Assistant Professor, Department of Emergency Medicine, Johns Hopkins School of Medicine, Baltimore

JORGE L. CABRERA, DO
Assistant Professor of Clinical Medicine, University of Miami Miller School of Medicine, Miami, Florida

AVERY CLARK, MD
Chief Resident, Department of Emergency Medicine, Boston Medical Center, Boston, Massachusetts

DAVID DORFMAN, MD
Associate Professor, Department of Pediatrics, Division of Pediatric Emergency Medicine, Boston University School of Medicine, Boston, Massachusetts

DAVID A. DRUGA, MD
Department of Emergency Medicine, Boston University Medical Center, Boston, Massachusetts

B. LORRIE EDWARDS, MD
Instructor of Pediatrics, Department of Pediatrics, Division of Pediatric Emergency Medicine, Boston University School of Medicine, Boston, Massachusetts, USA

CHRISTOPHER EL KHURI, MD
Department of Emergency Medicine, Johns Hopkins School of Medicine, Baltimore, Maryland

ALISE FRALLICCIARDI, MD, MBA, MS
Emergency Department, University of Connecticut School of Medicine, University of Connecticut Emergency Department, Farmington, Connecticut

LUCAS GROVER, MD
Department of Emergency Medicine, Baystate Health, Springfield, Massachusetts

PILAR GUERRERO, MD
Attending Physician, Department of Emergency Medicine, Cook County Health, Assistant Professor, Emergency Department, Rush Medical College, Chicago, Illinois

JOSEPH H. KAHN, MD, FACEP
Associate Professor, Department of Emergency Medicine, Boston University School of Medicine, Boston Medical Center, Boston, Massachusetts

KENNETH KNOWLES, MD
Department of Emergency Medicine, Division of Prehospital and Disaster Medicine, Baystate Health, Springfield, Massachusetts

RICHARD M. LEVITAN, MD
Department of Medicine, Dartmouth Geisel School of Medicine, Dartmouth-Hitchcock Medical Center, Lebanon, New Hampshire

OMAR Z. MANIYA, MD, MBA
Department of Emergency Medicine, The Mount Sinai Hospital, Resident Physician, Icahn School of Medicine at Mount Sinai, New York, New York, USA

JOLION McGREEVY, MD, MBE, MPH
Medical Director, Department of Emergency Medicine, The Mount Sinai Hospital, Icahn School of Medicine at Mount Sinai, New York, New York, USA

RON MEDZON, MD
Department of Emergency Medicine, Boston University School of Medicine, Boston Medical Center, Boston, Massachusetts

ANDREW H. MERELMAN, BS
Rocky Vista University College of Osteopathic Medicine, Parker, Colorado

MARK B. MYCYK, MD
Research Director, Department of Emergency Medicine, Cook County Health, Associate Professor, Department of Emergency Medicine, Northwestern University Feinberg School of Medicine, Chicago, Illinois

LAUREN M. NENTWICH, MD, FACEP
Assistant Professor, Department of Emergency Medicine, Medical Director of Quality and Patient Safety, Emergency Department, Boston Medical Center, Boston University School of Medicine, Boston, Massachusetts, USA

THOMAS NOWICKI, MD
Department of Emergency Medicine, University of Connecticut School of Medicine, Hartford Hospital, Hartford, Connecticut, USA

JESSICA M. RAY, PhD
Department of Emergency Medicine, Yale School of Medicine, New Haven, Connecticut, USA

LEON D. SANCHEZ, MD, MPH
Associate Professor of Emergency Medicine, Harvard Medical School, Vice Chair for Operations, Department of Emergency Medicine, Beth Israel Deaconess Medical Center, Boston, Massachusetts

JEFFREY I. SCHNEIDER, MD
Associate Professor, Department of Emergency Medicine, Boston Medical Center, Assistant Dean for Graduate Medical Education, Boston University School of Medicine, Boston, Massachusetts

ALEXANDER Y. SHENG, MD, MHPE
Associate Residency Program Director, Department of Emergency Medicine, Boston Medical Center, Massachusetts

MATTHEW S. SIKET, MD, MS
Assistant Professor, Surgery, The Robert Larner, M.D. College of Medicine at the University of Vermont, Burlington, Vermont

DANIELLE E. SMITH, MS4
The Robert Larner, M.D. College of Medicine of the University of Vermont, Burlington, Vermont

STEPHANIE STAPLETON, MD
Department of Emergency Medicine, Boston University School of Medicine, Boston Medical Center, Boston, Massachusetts

BARBARA M. WALSH, MD
Division of Pediatric Emergency Medicine, Boston University School of Medicine, Boston Medical Center, Boston, Massachusetts

ADAM T. WEIGHTMAN, MD, MBA
Department of Emergency Medicine, Boston University Medical Center, Boston, Massachusetts

CURTIS W. WITTMANN, MD
Instructor, Department of Psychiatry, Massachusetts General Hospital, Boston, Massachusetts

RICHARD E. WOLFE, MD
Chair, Associate Professor, Department of Emergency Medicine, Harvard Medical School, Beth Israel Deaconess Medical Center, Boston, Massachusetts

AMBROSE H. WONG, MD, MSEd
Department of Emergency Medicine, Yale School of Medicine, New Haven, Connecticut

RICHARD D. ZANE, MD, FAAEM
Department of Emergency Medicine, University of Colorado School of Medicine, Aurora, Colorado

Contents

proactive in the culture of risk reduction and improved patient safety. Literature has demonstrated improved patient outcomes, improved team based skills, systems testing and mitigation of latent safety threats. Simulation may be incorporated into practice via different modalities. The simulation lab is helpful for individual procedures, in situ simulation (ISS) for system testing and teamwork, community outreach ISS for sharing of best practices and content resource experts. Serious medical gaming is developing into a useful training adjunct for the future.

More than half of pediatric malpractice cases arise from emergency departments, primarily due to missed or delayed diagnoses. All providers who take care of children in emergency departments should be aware of this risk and the most common diagnoses associated with medicolegal liability. This article focuses on diagnosis and management of high-risk diagnoses in pediatric patients presenting to emergency departments, including meningitis, pneumonia, appendicitis, testicular torsion, and fracture. It highlights challenges and pitfalls that may increase risk of liability. It concludes with a discussion on recognition and management of abuse in children, including when to report and decisions on disposition.

 Video content accompanies this article at http://www.emed. theclinics.com

The high-risk airway is a common presentation and a frequent cause of anxiety for emergency physicians. Preparation and planning are essential to ensure that these challenging situations are managed successfully. Difficult airways typically present as either physiologic or anatomic, each type requiring a specialized approach. Primary physiologic considerations are oxygenation, hemodynamics, and acid-base, whereas anatomic difficulty is overcome using proper positioning and skilled laryngoscopy to ensure success. It is essential to be comfortable performing alternative techniques to address varying presentations. Ultimately, competence in airway management hinges on consistent training, deliberate practice, and a dedication to excellence.

Many patients with acute behavioral or mental health emergencies use the emergency department for their care. Psychiatric patients have a higher incidence of chronic medical conditions and are at greater risk for injury than the general population. Patients with acute behavioral emergencies may stress already overcrowded emergency departments. This article addresses high-risk areas of the treatment and management of emergency department patients presenting with behavioral emergencies. This article identifies methods successful in determining whether the patient's behavioral emergency is the result of an organic disease process, as well as recognizing other potential acute medical emergencies in this high-risk population.

Violent, combative and intoxicated patients are a common problem in the emergency department, and the emergency physician must be prepared to control the situation safely and effectively when a patient begins to exhibit dangerous behavior. This article reviews initial de-escalation techniques to reduce the need for patient restraint. It then details the 2 types of restraints (physical and chemical) and the clear indications for each type. The high-risk nature of utilization of restraints is reviewed, as well as the means by which to ensure patient and staff safety and decrease adverse outcomes.

Nontraumatic chest pain is a frequent concern of emergency department patients, with causes that range from benign to immediately life threatening. Identifying those patients who require immediate/urgent intervention remains challenging and is a high-risk area for emergency medicine physicians where incorrect or delayed diagnosis may lead to significant morbidity and mortality. This article focuses on the 3 most prevalent diagnoses associated with adverse outcomes in patients presenting with nontraumatic chest pain, acute coronary syndrome, thoracic aortic dissection, and pulmonary embolism. Important aspects of clinical evaluation, diagnostic testing, treatment, and disposition and other less common causes of lethal chest pain are also discussed.

Abdominal and extremity complaints are common in the emergency department (ED) and, because of their frequency, clinical vigilance is vital in order not to miss the timely diagnosis of occult or delayed emergencies. Such emergencies, if not timely managed, are sources of significant patient morbidity and mortality and may expose ED physicians to possible litigation. Each patient complaint yields to a nuanced approach in diagnostics and therapeutics that can lead physicians toward the ruling in or out of the correct high-risk diagnosis. This article discusses the approach and risk management of this high-risk subset of abdominal and extremity diagnoses.

A careful history and thorough physical examination are necessary in patients presenting with acute neurologic dysfunction. Patients presenting with headache should be screened for red-flag criteria that suggest a dangerous secondary cause warranting imaging and further diagnostic workup. Dizziness is a vague complaint; focusing on timing, triggers, and examination findings can help reduce diagnostic error. Most patients presenting with back pain do not require emergent imaging, but those with new neurologic deficits or signs/symptoms concerning for acute infection or cord compression warrant MRI. Delay to diagnosis and treatment of acute ischemic stroke is a frequent reason for medical malpractice claims.

Surviving a Medical Malpractice Lawsuit

Kelly Bookman and Richard D. Zane

Being named in a medical malpractice case is one of the most stressful events in a physician's career. This article reviews the legal system and the medical malpractice process. It details the steps a physician experiences during a medical malpractice case, from being served to the deposition and then to trial and appeals if the physician loses. This article also reviews necessary steps to take in order to proactively participate in one's own defense.

EMERGENCY MEDICINE
CLINICS OF NORTH AMERICA

SERIES OF RELATED INTEREST

Orthopedic Clinics
https://www.orthopedic.theclinics.com/

THE CLINICS ARE NOW AVAILABLE ONLINE!
Access your subscription at:
www.theclinics.com

Foreword

Risk Management in Emergency Medicine

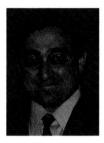

Amal Mattu, MD
Consulting Editor

There's no question that emergency medicine is a "high-risk" specialty. Patients present with undifferentiated and often multiple complaints, frequently with little information regarding past medical history and workups. Delirium and other causes of altered mental status limit our ability to obtain an adequate history. Nonclassic presentations are gradually becoming the norm in special populations, especially the elderly and the immunocompromised. Emergency department (ED) and hospital overcrowding are also common and cause already-limited resources to be further stretched. The overall result is that patients are at risk for misdiagnosis or delayed diagnosis of dangerous medical conditions and resultant poor outcomes.

But patients aren't the only ones at risk in the ED. Every interaction between an emergency health care provider and a patient represents not only health risk for the patient but also legal risk for the provider. The constant threat of malpractice is present in varying degrees in most regions of country, and it affects physician workups, practice patterns, and dispositions on a daily basis. It also serves as a major source of stress for all emergency health care personnel.

In this issue of *Emergency Medicine Clinics of North America*, Drs Lauren Nentwich and Jonathan Olshaker have assembled an outstanding group of physicians to educate us about managing risk in emergency medicine. These contributors have surveyed the legal landscape in our specialty and provide outstanding advice about how to provide optimal care to our patients while avoiding those legal landmines that we all fear. One of the first articles of the text is probably the most important one in terms of minimizing risk, "Communication and Documentation." This article should be mandatory reading for everyone in our specialty. Subsequent articles focus on practical matters, such as managing patients when they arrive via ambulance, patient flow, confidentiality and capacity, and proper supervision (of residents and advance practice providers). They also provide an article on the use of simulation programs that

Emerg Med Clin N Am 38 (2020) xiii–xiv
https://doi.org/10.1016/j.emc.2020.03.002
0733-8627/20/© 2020 Published by Elsevier Inc.

are helpful at mitigating clinical risk. For the unfortunate occurrence of a lawsuit, articles are provided on how to survive the litigation process and maintaining "wellness" in our high-risk environment. The authors conclude with a series of articles focusing on particularly high-risk groups of patients and high-risk chief complaints.

While most issues of *Emergency Medicine Clinics of North America* focus on how to improve patient care, this issue goes beyond patient care and also focuses on how to save our teams and how to save ourselves from a common danger in emergency medicine, malpractice. The reader is certain to gain a better understanding of legal risk and how to avoid it. Our thanks to Dr Nentwich, Dr Olshaker, and the contributors for providing an immensely important educational contribution to us all.

Amal Mattu, MD
Department of Emergency Medicine
University of Maryland School of Medicine
110 South Paca Street
6th Floor, Suite 200
Baltimore, MD 21201, USA

E-mail address:
amattu@som.umaryland.edu

Preface

Mitigating Risk in Emergency Medicine

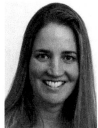

Lauren M. Nentwich, MD, FACEP   Jonathan S. Olshaker, MD, FACEP, FAAEM
Editors

Emergency physicians care for a high volume of patients who are critically ill or injured, and many times that number of patients appear well but signs or symptoms may represent less obvious life or limb threats. The practice conditions are challenging with increasing crowding and boarding, higher patient volumes, lack of ongoing relationships with patients, and extremely high expectations for zero errors. These challenges are coupled with increasing pressure to decrease use of costly imaging and other testing while simultaneously lowering admission rates.

The vast majority of emergency physicians are well trained, highly skilled, competent, and compassionate. Nevertheless, litigation is a constant threat. The very nature of the practice of emergency medicine makes adverse outcomes unavoidable and 100% diagnostic accuracy impossible.

Large studies of emergency department (ED) malpractice claims describe consistent trends. Four of 100,000 ED visits result in an allegation of malpractice. Eight percent of all medical practice cases involved patients seeking treatment in the ED. Plaintiffs' most common allegations were missed or delayed diagnosis (47%), improper management of medical treatment (28%), and medication errors (7%).[1] Another large review showed similar findings, with 56% of claims diagnosis related, 20% related to medical treatment, and 9% medication related. [2]

There are certainly no simple formulas for avoiding both bad outcomes and malpractice allegations, but there are basic principles and approaches that can help strengthen patient care and avoid litigation.

1. Priorities:
    When evaluating a patient, the clinician should try to thoughtfully consider all threats to life, organ, and limb and systematically rule them in or out to a high degree of certainty. Many diagnoses can be either made or excluded

Emerg Med Clin N Am 38 (2020) xv–xvii
https://doi.org/10.1016/j.emc.2020.03.001
0733-8627/20/© 2020 Published by Elsevier Inc.

via history and physical examination alone. Some will require testing or even hospital admission.

2. High-risk areas:

Keeping in mind the pitfalls from certain high-risk areas can be helpful. High-risk areas include change of shift, repeat visits, private patients, admitted patients with long ED stays prior to transfer to inpatient units, leaving against medical advice, and resident consultations.

3. Red flags:

It is extremely important to recognize red flags when they appear. This is especially relevant to many of life threats, including myocardial ischemia, thoracic aortic dissection, subarachnoid hemorrhage, abdominal aortic aneurysm, mesenteric ischemia, pulmonary embolism, and meningitis. Many of the articles in this issue will expand on this and highlight specific high-risk clinical presentations.

4. Communication:

Excellent communication is a priority. The clinician should always attempt to clearly communicate his or her thoughts and plan with the patient, the patient's family, consultants, and the patient's primary care provider when appropriate.

5. Documentation:

Careful documentation of history, physical examination results, and planned interventions is essential. Documentation of the thought process behind why the patient does or does not have a certain diagnosis is extremely beneficial from a medical-legal point of view. Inconsistencies in other parts of the chart should be addressed and not ignored. Repeat notes, even if they are brief, updating a patient's condition are essential.

6. Discharge instructions:

Careful and thorough documentation of treatment, new prescriptions, medication reconciliation, follow-up needed, and specific discharge instructions improves patient care and mitigates risk. It should be clear to all patients discharged from the ED that they should return to the ED immediately if they worsen.

The articles of this issue of the *Emergency Medicine Clinics of North America* will expand on the general principles of emergency medicine practice with a particular focus on high-risk areas and chief complaints. We hope this will provide valuable information to help emergency physicians avoid litigation, but more importantly, will be of value in helping improve care and avoid bad outcomes.

In appreciation for the work associated with this issue, we would like to thank all of the authors who contributed their time and knowledge to make this issue of risk management possible. Special thanks to Casey Potter, Nicholas Henderson, and the staff at Elsevier for their patience and support. Finally, a large thank you to you, the reader, who made the time to read this issue of *Emergency Medicine Clinics of North America*.

We hope that this issue provides you with additional knowledge and insights to allow you to continue to mitigate risk and provide excellent patient care.

Lauren M. Nentwich, MD, FACEP
Boston Medical Center
Department of Emergency Medicine
Boston University School of Medicine
1 Boston Medical Center Place
Boston, MA 02118, USA

Jonathan S. Olshaker, MD, FACEP, FAAEM
Boston Medical Center
Department of Emergency Medicine
Boston University School of Medicine
1 Boston Medical Center Place
Boston, MA 02118, USA

E-mail addresses:
lauren.nentwich@bmc.org (L.M. Nentwich)
jonathan.olshaker@bmc.org (J.S. Olshaker)

REFERENCES

1. 2011 Annual benchmarking report. Malpractice risk in emergency medicine. Crico Strategies; 2011. Available at:https://www.rmf.harvard.edu/Malpractice-Data/Annual-Benchmark-Reports/Risks-in-Emergency-Medicine, Accessed March 24, 2020.
2. A dose of insight. Emergency department risks: through the lens of liability claims. Coverys ED claims analysis 2014-2018. Available at: https://www.coverys.com/Knowledge-Center/a-dose-of-insight-emergency-department-risks, Accessed March 24, 2020.

Managing Emergency Department Risk Through Communication and Documentation

Omar Z. Maniya, MD, MBA*, Jolion McGreevy, MD, MBE, MPH

KEYWORDS

• Risk • Documentation • Communication

KEY POINTS

- Excellence in clinical care, as well as in communication and documentation, is critical for managing risk in the emergency department.
- High-risk areas for communication and documentation include (1) handoffs and transitions of care, (2) discharge and follow-up, and (3) consultation.
- Emergency physicians should use good communication and documentation practice to reduce not only malpractice risk but also financial, regulatory, and legal risk.

INTRODUCTION

The job description of the emergency physician (EP) contains many responsibilities, including identifying and managing life-threatening illness, providing symptomatic relief, determining safe and efficient disposition, managing department flow, providing customer service, improving public health, and ensuring wise resource utilization.[1] EPs must communicate effectively with patients, interdisciplinary clinical teams, and consultants both orally and through the medical record. Excellence in clinical care, as well as in communication and documentation, is critical for managing risk in the emergency department (ED).

Emergency Department Risk

EDs historically have focused on managing malpractice risk, although they also must consider additional risks, including regulatory, financial, and legal. Although risk never can be eliminated, it can be managed and reduced. Before examining approaches to risk management in detail, it is important to first put ED risk in context. Although some investigators have touted emergency medicine (EM) as one of the most litigious

Department of Emergency Medicine, The Mount Sinai Hospital, Icahn School of Medicine at Mount Sinai, One Gustave Levy Place, New York, NY 10029, USA
* Corresponding author.
E-mail address: omarmaniya@gmail.com

Emerg Med Clin N Am 38 (2020) 267–281
https://doi.org/10.1016/j.emc.2020.01.007
0733-8627/20/© 2020 Elsevier Inc. All rights reserved.

emed.theclinics.com

specialties, recent data show those fears to be exaggerated. A 2011 study of 25 specialties in *The New England Journal of Medicine* found that EPs are below the median and slightly above the mean for percentage of physicians with a malpractice claim annually, and payments to plaintiffs were far below average across specialties.[2] A *JAMA Internal Medicine* study showed the rate of paid malpractice claims for EPs decreased 47% between 1992 and 2014.[3] Mean malpractice payments increased 26% during the study period, however, and these data may underestimate the total dollar amounts because they represent only payments from physicians, not from hospitals.[4]

Communication

The landmark 1999 Institute of Medicine report *To Err is Human* estimated that 98,000 patients die annually through medical errors and hypothesized that poor communication was a leading cause of error.[5] Communication breakdowns have been cited in 80% of malpractice lawsuits, and the Joint Commission identified improving handoff communication as a prime safety goal in 2016.[6,7] Effective communication among the clinical team in the ED, during handoffs between providers, and with consultants is vital to safe patient care and risk management in the ED.

Documentation

Documentation in the ED serves the following purposes:

1. Communicating subjective and objective clinical data and medical decision making, as well as clinical status updates, to downstream providers
2. Supporting appropriate reimbursement
3. Ensuring care complies with hospital policies, regulatory rules, and legislative statutes
4. Shielding providers from malpractice risk

A detailed discussion of the first 3 purposes of ED documentation is beyond the scope of this article, but 2 points merit mention. First, ED documentation is most helpful to downstream providers when it is available before they assume care of a patient. This time frame ranges from minutes to hours for consultants and inpatient providers to days to weeks for outpatient providers. Second, most of the current documentation standards—such as the need to record a 4-point history of present illness, 10-point review of systems (ROS), and 2-point to 3-point past medical, family, or social history to support a level 5 professional fee—derive from arguably arbitrary Centers for Medicare and Medicaid Services (CMS) reimbursement requirements published in 1995 and 1997.[8] In 2019, CMS proposed dramatically streamlining these requirements for ambulatory visits. It remains to be seen whether these changes will be extended to the ED.[9] Nevertheless, future changes have the potential to drastically alter the requirements for ED documentation.

ED documentation, along with objective diagnostic laboratory and imaging data, often is the only contemporaneous exhibit that makes up the material facts of a regulatory review or malpractice case. Therefore, clear, concise, and accurate ED documentation is critical to managing risk in the ED.

TYPES OF COMMUNICATION
Communication with Patients and Family Members

It is well known that communication is critical to patient satisfaction. Communication may be more important than the quality of care provided in improving patients' perception of their care.[10] Compared with physicians in the top third of patient satisfaction scores, those in the middle third had a 26% higher rate of malpractice lawsuits, and those in the lowest third had a 110% higher rate.[11]

Patient communication in the ED is threatened by time constraints, operational variation, crowding and boarding, excessive ambient noise, and other factors. EPs who have achieved excellence in provider-patient communication, however, strive to answer questions, allay fears, enable trust, and perform shared decision making. The Studer Group AIDET framework is one widely recognized approach to effective patient communication[12]:

A: Acknowledge: greet the patient and family warmly, by name, and with eye contact.

I: Introduce: introduce yourself clearly by name, profession, and role on the ED team.

D: Duration: set generous expectations, particularly around timeliness of diagnostics. Then, try to beat them.

E: Explanation: give clear expectations, particularly around diagnostic uncertainty for nonemergent complaints, and negotiate and agree on plans of care.

T: Thank you: express gratitude for the patient placing his or her trust in you and your ED.

Other tools to improve ED patient communication include[13]

- Scripting common conversations, such as computed tomography (CT) wait times and magnetic resonance imaging availability, to ensure that physicians, nurses, and technicians send consistent messages[14]
- Purposefully and frequently rounding to update patients on their diagnostic workup, treatment, and disposition. Studies show that patients prefer multiple shorter interactions to single, longer ones.[15–17]
- Actively listening, while sitting down, when possible, which studies show results in patients perceiving encounters to last 3-times to 5-times longer[18]
- Creating visible communication whiteboards or patient care cards that summarize the care team, pending and resulted tests, and time expectations[19]

Disclosing Errors

A particularly critical and sensitive instance of patient communication is the disclosure of medical errors. Historically, physicians and health care organizations believed that disclosing errors increased risk exposure by drawing attention to errors that otherwise may have gone unnoticed. Today, approximately 40 states have passed laws to prevent apologies from being used against medical professionals in court. Lawsuits over disclosed errors that caused no harm rarely are successful.[20,21]

Most patients appreciate participating in and learning about their care, and prompt, sincere disclosures and apologies actually may decrease risk when a medical error has occurred.[22] One study found that 98% of patients desired acknowledgment of errors, even minor ones, and reported a 40% relative risk reduction in the likelihood of a lawsuit when a physician disclosed the error.[23] Other studies have shown, however, that routinely disclosing medical errors may increase risk exposure.[20] Therefore, it is important that EDs consult with their risk management department to establish a consistent institutional approach to disclosure of medical errors. It is important that EDs manage disclosures deliberately as opposed to haphazardly. Best practices include[24,25]

1. Disclosing in a timely manner, before a patient or family member discovers the error
2. Explicitly stating that an error has occurred

3. Describing the error in clear and concise language
4. Explaining potential harms, even if unlikely
5. Expressing regret and/or formally apologizing
6. Explaining steps that will be taken to prevent recurrences

TYPES OF DOCUMENTATION

Since the passage of the Health Information Technology for Economics and Clinical Health (HITECH) Act, part of the American Recovery and Reinvestment Act of 2009, which devoted more than $13 billion in incentives to drive adoption of electronic health records (EHRs), electronic documentation has been a practice-defining force in acute care hospitals.[26,27] Although this has improved accuracy, availability, and legibility of records, studies have shown mixed results in terms of provider efficiency and patient flow, and EHRs have created a new set of problems.[28–30]

Templates

Many EMRs have integrated templates for a wide variety of chief complaints, which cover common history, ROS, and physical examination elements necessary to support high-complexity professional fee coding. Although some investigators have argued that EHRs allow EDs to more effectively up-code visits to higher-intensity codes through documentation, a recent study showed that this hypothesis may explain only some of the variations in charges.[31,32] Although these templates may increase provider efficiency and increase quality of care (eg, prompt providers to consider red flag symptoms for headache), they suffer from charting ambiguity (eg, boxes left blank), lack of specificity to patients, and multiple opportunities for discrepancies (eg, an unresponsive patient who has normal behavior checked on ROS). These factors may increase malpractice risk.

Dictation

Although some providers prefer to type notes, many use automated speech recognition software, in-person scribes, or virtual scribes to facilitate documentation. Automated speech recognition, although originally hyped as a way to increase provider efficiency and satisfaction, has faced problems regarding accuracy, particularly for physicians with accents.[33] In-person scribes may increase patients seen per hour by up to 15% and may save up to $30/h but involve a cultural adjustment of including a second person in the room and require providers to carefully review charts for inaccuracies.[34] Virtual or remote scribes use secure video feeds to assist in real-time documentation and recently have emerged as a more cost-effective option that requires further study.[35]

MALPRACTICE RISK

In a malpractice suit, the plaintiff must prove that

1. A professional duty existed
2. The duty was breached
3. The breach caused an injury
4. The injury resulted in damages[36]

A recent national study of 11,500 claims over 2 decades showed that EPs were the primary defendant in only 19% of ED claims. The top determinations in the claims were errors in diagnosis, no errors identified, improper performance, failure to supervise, failure to perform, delays, and medication errors. The study found that 64% of claims were withdrawn, dropped, or dismissed, and 29% were settled with a payment to the plaintiff. Only 7% of claims were resolved by verdict, 6% in favor of the defendant and 1% in favor of the plaintiff.[37] This study, as well as a recent systematic review, identified chest pain and acute myocardial infarction as the most common diagnoses associated with a claim, followed by abdominal pain and appendicitis, fractures and wounds, aortic aneurysms, intracranial hemorrhage, and pediatric fever and meningitis.[37,38] Another recent study of 10 million ED visits showed that although years in practice and higher patient volumes were associated with increased malpractice claims, other physician factors, such as board certification, night practice, Press Ganey scores, relative value units per hour, admission rates, working at multiple facilities, and practicing in less favorable jurisdictions, were not.[39]

Current Controversies

Two areas of controversy exist with regard to malpractice risk in the ED. The first involves real-time charting. Best practice is to chart contemporaneously, while a patient is in the ED. Although this may not always be possible, given the volume and acuity of patients in the department, EPs should prioritize real-time charting on critically ill patients, patients with high-risk chief complaints who are being discharged, and patients whose clinical status or mental status is rapidly improving or deteriorating (eg, asthmatics and intoxicated patients). Many EPs intuitively believe that real-time charting with timestamped interventions, decisions, and consultations decreases malpractice risk. Real-time documentation holds EPs to a higher standard of documentation, however, than physicians in other high-acuity practice settings, such as intensive care units. Other EPs believe that charting just prior to dispositioning a patient and incorporating diagnoses, results, interventions, and consultations into the chart with the benefit of hindsight vision decrease malpractice risk. There is a dearth of high-quality data on this topic, and a need for further study remains.

There is controversy among EPs regarding documenting thought processes and mentioning differential diagnoses, such as pulmonary embolus, for which a patient has not been worked-up. Some EPs believe that documenting why they considered a diagnosis and did not pursue it results in less malpractice risk, whereas other EPs believe that mentioning a diagnosis that is not worked-up increases malpractice risk. Again, there are few high-quality data to answer this question, and further research is needed.

High-Risk Area 1: Handoffs and Transitions of Care

Sign-out, although unavoidable given the nature of ED shift work, has been referred to as "the most dangerous procedure in the emergency department."[40] Communication breakdowns are cited in 80% of malpractice claims, with those occurring during sign-out involved in 24% of ED malpractice claims.[41,42] One study found that 14% of ED handoffs omitted abnormal vital signs.[43] Therefore, improving handoffs of care is critical to managing risk in the ED. Specific potential barriers to high-quality handoffs include[44]

1. Signal-to-noise ratio: disorganized handoffs with extraneous or irrelevant information, taking place in the context of elevated ambient noise and interruptions, can decrease the effectiveness of the information transfer.
2. Conciseness versus completeness: every patient is unique, and physicians must implicitly decide how thorough their sign-outs should be, weighing the signal-to-noise ratio and time constraints.
3. No standard approach: physicians often personalize sign-outs, given local culture and experience, rather than following scripts. The lack of high-quality peer-reviewed sign-out scripts exacerbates this barrier.

4. Ambiguous transitions: EPs often remain in the department and may continue to care for patient after sign-out, which can confuse nurses, ancillary staff, and oncoming providers. Admitting teams located upstairs may comanage ED patients, which can create confusion.

Potential solutions to improving the quality of ED handoffs include[44]

1. Reducing the number of handoffs through shift buffering, resisting the temptation to sign up for patients close to the end of a shift, and creating overlapping shifts
2. Limiting interruptions during sign-out, which may be accomplished by moving to a quieter location
3. Headlining the sign-out with a succinct overview of the patient to provide the oncoming physician with a framework to organize details, for example, "This is a 64-year-old woman with chest pain awaiting her second troponin."
4. Anticipating results and communicating a clear plan for dealing with them, for example, "If the CT scan is positive, consult surgery; if negative and she tolerates liquids, discharge."

Current areas of controversy among EPs exist regarding the utility of bedside rounding, the use of standardized mnemonics for handoffs, and the use of multidisciplinary rounds.[44]

High-Risk Area 2: Discharge and Follow-up

More than 100 million Americans will be discharged from an ED this year, but studies have shown that 78% of patients lack an understanding of their discharge instructions and recognize that deficiency in understanding only 20% of the time.[45] Improving discharge communication and documentation is critical to ED risk management.

Critical aspects of discharge communication and documentation include

1. Reevaluation and consent: reviewing a patients' vital signs and results and reevaluating patients. Ask if they are comfortable being discharged and if there are any barriers that would prevent a safe discharge (eg, inability to ambulate). Then, document these findings in the chart.[46]
2. Clear verbal instructions: verbal instructions are critical to safe discharges. Providers should sit down with patients, explain their instructions, solicit questions, check for understanding, and document that these discussions have occurred. Case law has shown that verbal instructions can supplement deficient written instructions.[47,48] If an interpreter is used, that should be documented as well.
3. Individualized written instructions: written instructions should be simple, specific, individualized, in the patient's preferred language, and include[49]
   a. Diagnosis, with care to not be overly specific and lead to downstream diagnostic anchoring
   b. Prescriptions, with clear instructions on how and when to take medications
   c. Specific postdischarge care instructions
   d. Follow-up instructions, including the time frame, provider, and, if possible, patient contact information
   e. Specific, open-ended return precautions, which include a general statement to return to the ED if symptoms worsen[50]
   f. Patient signature: up to half of patients do not recall receiving discharge instructions. Some states mandate that patients sign a copy of their discharge instructions for inclusion in the chart.[51]

g. Incidentalomas and pending results: incidental laboratory and imaging abnormalities should be clearly flagged in the discharge instructions and documented in the chart.

Specific areas of controversy pertaining to discharge instructions include the use of diagnosis-specific computerized discharge instructions, post-ED interventions, patients who leave against medical advice (AMA), and novel dispositions.

Diagnosis-specific computerized discharge instructions
Many standardized discharge instructions for common conditions exist, which can decrease the time burden on the EP and ensure common follow-up and return precautions are conveyed.[52] They also may miss critical nuances of an individual patient, however, and at least 1 study has shown that they do not effect 72-hour return rates or the rates of medically inappropriate repeat ED visits.[53] Therefore, it is best practice to select a standardized diagnosis-specific discharge instruction if available, and then individualize it to patients with additional narrative text, while highlighting the important elements in the verbal instructions and documenting that this was performed.

Leaving against medical advice
Although a discussion of decisional capacity, particularly as it relates to intoxicated patients, is beyond the scope of this article, there are a few critical communication and documentation issues EPs should consider. Many EPs incorrectly believe that it is a requirement to have a patient sign an AMA form, that a patient signing an AMA form provides immunity from malpractice risk, or that a patient's insurance does not cover the visit if the patient leaves AMA.[54–56] None of these is true. Having a patient sign an AMA form may create an adversarial dynamic, and many hospital-provided AMA forms lack the specificity to mitigate risk adequately. Therefore, it is critical for EPs to document the following in the record of all patients who leave AMA[57]:

1. A statement that the patient has decisional capacity
2. Conversation informing the patient of the risks of refusal of care and alternatives to the refused treatment
3. The patient's understanding of the risks and alternatives
4. Discharge instructions, including follow-up care
5. An invitation to return at any time to continue care

Documenting witnesses, such as friends or family members, and avoiding a distrustful and divisive interaction also may mitigate risk during AMA conversations.

Novel dispositions
EDs increasingly discharge more and more patients.[58] Many of these increased discharges utilize novel dispositions, including rapid follow-up protocols (eg, for low-risk chest pain), observation, admission to home, and transfers to affiliated institutions.[59] In addition, although the rate of direct admissions to the hospital that bypass the ED overall is shrinking, some hospitals have used rapid admission protocols for patients to specialized units.[60] Data on documentation standards for these novel dispositions are lacking; therefore, EPs should carefully identify their institutions protocols and document that patients meet the established guidelines.

High-Risk Area 3: Consultations

Consultations are requested for 20% to 40% of all ED patients. Consultations have been cited in one-third of malpractice claims and, therefore, are a major opportunity to improving communication and documentation and to mitigating risk.[42,61] One best practice consultation technique, specific to EPs, is outlined by the 5 Cs[62]:

1. Contact: introduce yourself to the consultant and build a relationship.
2. Communication: present a concise patient presentation, incorporating relevant data and identifying information (e.g. medical record number and location)
3. Core question: articulate the specific question the consultant is being asked (eg, "Is this patient a surgical candidate?").
4. Collaboration: ask if there is anything you can do to help the consultant answer the core question (eg, additional laboratory or imaging studies).
5. Closing the loop: decide on a time frame and method of follow-up with the consultant.

Additional factors to be wary of include[63]:

1. Timeliness: institutions should create clear expectations for the timeliness of consultants to examine patients in the ED and develop recommendations. Best practices involve automatically timestamping consultation requests in the EHR and monitoring various consulting services' timeliness to ensure compliance.
2. Supervision: residents, fellows, and advanced practice providers often evaluate patients initially, particularly in academic settings. Although this may be appropriate for certain conditions, such as common fractures, consulting services should document clearly what level of oversight was provided (attending evaluation, phone call or conversation, or no interaction). Best practice is for institutions to create and adhere to policies regarding the level of attending supervision required for various complaints based on the provider's experience and experience with the particular condition as well as provide clear protocols for attending consultations in high-risk cases or where diagnostic or therapeutic uncertainty exists.
3. Information consultations: it is best to avoid informal consultations, also known as curbside consults, except for specific areas in which a hospital has clearly defined parameters (eg, discussing an electrocardiogram with the cardiac catheterization team). This is because informal consultations may include substandard evaluations and recommendations, which expose the ED to risk.
4. On-call physicians: the Emergency Medical Treatment and Active Labor Act (EMTALA) mandates the hospital to provide a list of on-call physicians. These physicians are expected not only to consult on cases in the ED but also to manage the follow-up care related to the acute presentation.

An emerging area regarding consultation to the ED is telemedicine (eg, telestroke). Although there is little evidence to guide risk management in this area, EPs should follow institutional policies regarding the levels of evaluation and documentation required for this modality and strive to meet the same standard as with entirely in-person care.

REGULATORY AND COMPLIANCE RISK
Emergency Medical Treatment and Active Labor Act

EMTALA, passed in 1986, establishes 3 requirements for EDs that accept Medicare funding.
These include

1. Performing a medical screening examination on all patients to determine if an emergency medical condition exists
2. Stabilizing emergency medical conditions (or transferring to a higher level of care if the facility does not have the necessary resources for stabilization)

3. Accepting transfers of patients with an emergency medical condition from facilities that do not have the capabilities to stabilize[64]

It is essential that EPs document thorough medical screening examinations for discharged patients and medical necessity for transferred patients. The average fine for an EMTALA violation is $104,000. Only 8% of violations investigated by the CMS, however, result in fines, of which 97% are levied against hospitals rather than against providers.

Health Insurance Portability and Accessibility Act

The Health Insurance Portability and Accessibility Act (HIPAA), passed in 1996, governs the confidentiality of protected health information (PHI).

First, the organizational imperative to comply with HIPAA was underscored in 2009 when the HITECH Act, part of the American Recovery and Reinvestment Act, increased penalties for HIPAA violations to up to $1.5 million per institution for repeated disclosures of PHI.[65]

Second, communication with patients must be performed in a confidential manner. Providers should make every effort to minimize inadvertent disclosures of PHI, such as human immunodeficiency status, by speaking in private areas, speaking in hushed voices, and avoiding discussing patients in public areas of the hospital. Additionally, providers should ask all patients whether they would like to excuse family members and visitors before discussing sensitive information.

Third, when inadvertent disclosures are possible, it is important to document the extra measures taken, such as asking parents or family members to leave the room when interviewing patients.

FINANCIAL RISK

One purpose of ED documentation is to support adequate reimbursement. The quality of EP documentation can have a large financial impact on both the ED and hospital. Specific areas in which documentation is critically important are discussed.

Billing and Revenue Cycle

Once a physician completes a chart, the ED coders can code the visit (both professional physician fee and facility fee) for a biller to submit for reimbursement. All ED billing originates with the documentation in the chart. Therefore, many hospitals have implemented clinical documentation improvement programs, often with retrospective chart feedback and prospective electronic tools, such as templates and coding predictors, to remind EPs to include required elements and to help assess what level of billing the chart supports.[66] Although some have cited EHRs as the driving force behind increasingly higher-complexity ED billing patterns, a recent study showed that much of this growth in billing is explained by the increasing intensity of services provided.[32]

Justifying Admissions

EP documentation is necessary for inpatient reimbursement.
    Currently, CMS requires 3 criteria for inpatient admission:

1. An admission order
2. A certification that the patient requires inpatient admission with supporting diagnoses and rationale

3. An expectation that the patient requires a hospitalization for at least 2 midnights. The 2-midnight rule includes time spent in the ED once care is initiated (excluding time in the waiting room and triage time). In general, CMS considers exceptions to the 2-midnight rule to be rare and limited to deaths, transfers, patients who leave AMA, and dramatic clinical improvements that were unexpected.[67]

Medicare Recovery Audit Contractors

Recovery audit contractors were created with the Medicare Modernization Act of 2003 to identify Medicare overpayments and underpayments within both Medicare Part A (hospitals) and Medicare Part B (physicians). In 2018, these programs recovered $73 million in improper payments.[68] Because all hospitals and physicians accepting Medicare fee-for-service dollars are subject to these unannounced audits, continuous compliance with documentation standards is vital.

LEGAL RISK
Criminal Liability

Although many of the risks discussed thus far involve civil or monetary penalties, the potential for criminal liability exists, particularly when providers alter a medical record after the fact. Such changes may invalidate a provider's malpractice insurance.[69,70] Furthermore, knowingly falsifying a medical record may constitute a felony.[71] Therefore, best practices include not altering a medical record after a certain period of time—never after an adverse outcome or malpractice or regulatory inquiry—and having a zero-tolerance policy for falsifying a chart. Studies have shown that up to 90% of clinicians routinely copy and paste prior notes and that copying and pasting contribute to 3% of diagnostic errors. Although the routine practice of copying and pasting prior notes has generally been regarded as an inpatient dilemma, with limited risk to EPs, further study is needed to elucidate the risks of this practice in the ED.[72]

Law Enforcement Requests

Per HIPAA, PHI must not be disclosed to law enforcement without a compelling reason, such as a court order or an imminent danger to self or others. Inadvertent disclosures to law enforcement may bring legal and regulatory risk on an ED. Given the myriad local, state, and federal laws and regulations as well as the complexity of various enforcement actions, it is best practice for EDs to

1. Avoid casual and inadvertent hallway disclosures of PHI to law enforcement
2. Create policies, in conjunction with the hospital attorney, to address common law enforcement inquiries
3. Have a low threshold for consulting the hospital attorney for any nonstandard requests

SUMMARY

EPs face a moderate amount of malpractice risk relative to other specialties and also are exposed to other kinds of risk, including regulatory and financial. These risks can be managed through effective communication and documentation. Specifically, physician-patient communication strongly influences patient perceptions of care, and sensitive areas of communication include disclosure of errors. High-risk areas for EP documentation include handoffs of care, dispositions, and consultations. EPs should develop a structured approach to managing and mitigating the various risks of practicing emergency medicine.

DISCLOSURE

The authors have nothing to disclose.

REFERENCES

1. Strayer R. EM Mindset: 8 Responsibilities of the EM Doc. emDOCs.net - Emergency Medicine Education. 2017. Available at: http://www.emdocs.net/em-mindset-reuben-strayer-8-responsibilities-of-the-em-doc/. Accessed August 10, 2019.
2. Jena AB, Seabury S, Lakdawalla D, et al. Malpractice risk according to physician specialty. N Engl J Med 2011;365(7):629–36.
3. Schaffer AC, Jena AB, Seabury SA, et al. Rates and characteristics of paid malpractice claims among US physicians by specialty, 1992-2014. JAMA Intern Med 2017;177(5):710–8.
4. Raja AS. Emergency medicine malpractice claim rates are decreasing, but payment amounts are increasing. NEJM Journal Watch Emergency Medicine 2017. Available at: https://www.jwatch.org/na43850/2017/04/04/emergency-medicine-malpractice-claim-rates-are-decreasing.
5. Kohn LT, Corrigan JM, Donaldson MS, editors. Committee on Quality of Health Care in America. To err is human: building a safer health system. Washington (DC): Institute of Medicine; 2000.
6. Burrell M. Shift report: Improving a complex process to enhance patient safety. J Healthc Risk Manag 2006;26:9–13.
7. Wears RL, Perry SJ, Shapiro M, et al. Shift changes among emergency physicians: best of times, worst of times. In: Proceedings of the human factors and Ergonomics Society 47th annual meeting. Denver (CO): Human Factors and Ergonomics Society; 2003. p. 1420–3.
8. Edelberg C, Strauss R, Mayer T. Introduction to Coding. In: Strauss R, Mayer T, editors. Emergency department management. New York: McGraw Hill Education; 2017. p. 524–35.
9. Robeznieks A. Medicare E/M proposal will slash physicians' documentation load. American Medical Association; 2019. Available at: https://www.ama-assn.org/practice-management/medicare/medicare-em-proposal-will-slash-physicians-documentation-load. Accessed August 10, 2019.
10. Chang JT, Hays RD, Shekelle PG, et al. Patients' global ratings of their health care are not associated with the technical quality of their care. Ann Intern Med 2006; 144:665–72.
11. Stelfox H, Gandhi T, Orav E, et al. The relation of patient satisfaction with complaints against physicians and malpractice lawsuits. Am J Med 2005;118(10): 1126–33.
12. AIDET Patient Communication. Studer Group A Huron Solution. Available at: https://www.studergroup.com/aidet. Accessed August 10, 2019.
13. Mayer T, Kaplan J, Strauss R, et al. Customer service in emergency medicine. In: Strauss R, Mayer T, editors. Emergency department management. New York: McGraw Hill Education; 2017. p. 60–73.
14. Mayer T. Putting it all together: education and the right tools establish a culture of service. Healthc Exec 2011;26:56–9.
15. Mayer T, Cates RJ. Leadership for great customer service: satisfied patients, satisfied employees. Chicago: Health Administration Press; 2004.
16. Bujak JS. Inside the physician mind: finding common ground with doctors. Chicago: Health Administration Press; 2008.

17. Baker SJ. Hourly rounding in the emergency department: how to accelerate results. J Emerg Nurs 2012;38(1):69–72.
18. Sqayden KJ, Anderson KK, Connelly LM. Effect of sitting vs standing on perception of provider time at bedside: a pilot study. Patient Educ Couns 2012;86: 166–71.
19. Morris BJ, Richards JE, Archer KR, et al. Improving patient satisfaction in the orthopaedic trauma population. J Orthop Trauma 2014;28(4):e80–4.
20. McMichael BJ, Van Horn RL, Viscusi WK. Sorry is never enough: The effect of state apology laws on medical malpractice liability risk. Stanford Law Rev 2016;71(2):341.
21. Thurman AE. Institutional responses to medical mistakes: ethical and legal perspectives. Kennedy Inst Ethics J 2001;11(2):147–56.
22. Cleopas A, Villaveces A, Charvet A, et al. Patient assessments of a hypothetical medical error: effects of health outcome, disclosure, and staff responsiveness. Qual Saf Health Care 2006;15(2):136–41.
23. Witman AB, Park DM, Hardin SB. How do patients want physicians to handle mistakes? A survey of internal medicine patients in an academic setting. Arch Intern Med 1996;156(22):2565–9.
24. Chamberlain CJ, Koniaris LG, Wu AW, et al. Disclosure of "nonharmful" medical errors and other events: duty to disclose. Arch Surg 2012;147(3):282–6.
25. Gallagher TH, Studdert D, Levinson W. Disclosing harmful medical errors to patients. N Engl J Med 2007;356(26):2713–9.
26. Cohen MF. Impact of the HITECH financial incentives on HER adoption in small, physician-owned practices. J Med Inform 2016;94:143–54.
27. Health IT Quick Stats. Health IT Dashboard. Office of the National Coordinator for Health Information Technology. Available at: https://dashboard.healthit.gov/quickstats/quickstats.php. Accessed August 10, 2019.
28. Feblowitz J, Takhar S, Ward M, et al. A Custom Developed Emergency Department Provider Electronic Documentation System Reduces Operational Efficiency. Ann Emerg Med 2017;70(5):674–82.
29. Baumlin KM, Shapiro JS, Weiner C, et al. Clinical information system and process redesign improves emergency department efficiency. Jt Comm J Qual Patient Saf 2010;36:179–85.
30. Ward MJ, Froehle CM, Hart KW, et al. Transient and sustained changes in operational performance, patient evaluation, and medication administration during electronic health record implementation in the emergency department. Ann Emerg Med 2014;63:320–8.
31. Alltucker K. Really astonishing': Average cost of hospital ER visit surges 176% in a decade, report says. USA Today. 2019. Available at: https://www.usatoday.com/story/news/health/2019/06/04/hospital-billing-code-changes-help-explain-176-surge-er-costs/1336321001/. Accessed August 10, 2019.
32. Burke L, Wild Rb, Orav E, et al. Are trends in billing for high-intensity emergency care explaiend by changes ins ervices provided in the emergency department? An observational study among US Medicare beneficiaries. BMJ Open 2018;8(1): e019357.
33. Geesbreght J, Baine R, Ruben J, et al. Scribes. In: Strauss R, Mayer T, editors. Emergency department management. New York: McGraw Hill Education; 2017. p. 151–6.
34. Walker K, Ben-Meir M, William D, et al. Impact of scribes on emergency medicine doctors' productivity and patient throughput: multicentre randomised trial. BMJ 2019;364:l121.

35. Caliri A. The case for virtual scribes: more and more physicians are employing medical scribes to decrease their clerical burden. Becker's Hospital Review. 2019. Available at: https://www.beckershospitalreview.com/hospital-physician-relationships/the-case-for-virtual-scribes.html. Accessed August 10, 2019.
36. Aya I, Cedric D, Schlicher N, et al. Medical liability reform. In: Schlicher N, Haddock A, editors. Emergency medicine advocacy handbook. 5th edition. Dallas (TX).p.123-128: EMRA; 2019. p. 123–8.
37. Brown T, McCarthy M, Kelen G, et al. An epidemiologic study of closed emergency department malpractice claims in a national database of physician malpractice insurers. Acad Emerg Med 2010;17:553–60.
38. Ferguson B, Geralds J, Petrey J, et al. Malpractice in emergency medicine – a review of risk and mitigation practices for the emergency medicine provider. J Emerg Med 2018;55(5):659–65.
39. Carlson J, Foster K, Pines J, et al. Provider and practice factors associated with emergency physicians' being named in a malpractice claim. Ann Emerg Med 2018;71(2):157–64.
40. Safer Sign Out Protocol. American College of Emergency Physicians. Available at: https://www.acep.org/how-we-serve/sections/quality-improvement–patient-safety/toolbox/safer-sign-out-protocol/. Accessed August 10, 2019.
41. Levinson W. Physician-patient communication: a key to malpractice prevention. JAMA 1994;272:1619–20.
42. Kachalia A, Gandhi TK, Puopolo AL, et al. Missed and delayed diagnoses in the emergency department: a study of closed malpractice claims from 4 liability insurers. Ann Emerg Med 2007;49:196–205.
43. Venkatesh A, Curley D, Chang Y, et al. Communication of vital signs at emergency department handoff: opportunities for improvement. Ann Emerg Med 2015;66(2):125–30.
44. Cheung D, Kelly J, Beqch C, et al. Improving handoffs in the emergency department. Ann Emerg Med 2010;55(2):171–80.
45. Engel K, Heisler M, Smith D, et al. Patient comprehension of emergency department care and instructions: are patients aware of when they do not understand? Ann Emerg Med 2009;53(4):454–61.
46. Betz A. Maximizing the "safe" discharge. emDOCs.net - emergency medicine education. 2015. Available at: http://www.emdocs.net/maximizing-the-safe-discharge/. Accessed August 10, 2019.
47. Samuels-Kalow M, Stack A, Porter S. Effective discharge communication in the emergency department. Ann Emerg Med 2012;60(2):152–9.
48. Carter C. Clelland v. Haas. (Louisiana Court of Appeal 2000). Available at https://www.aliem.com/erem-pitfalls-and-perils-of-emergency-department-discharge-instructions/.
49. McCarthy D, Engel K, Buckley B, et al. Emergency department discharge instructions: lessons learned through developing new patient education materials. Emerg Med Int 2012;2012:306859.
50. DeLaney M. EREM: pitfalls and perils of emergency department discharge instructions. ALiEM. 2015. Available at: https://www.aliem.com/2015/07/erem-pitfalls-and-perils-of-emergency-department-discharge-instructions/. Accessed August 10, 2019.
51. Grover G, Berkowitz CD, Lewis RJ. Parental recall after a visit to the emergency department. Clin Pediatr (Phila) 1994;33:194–201.
52. Taylor D, Cameorn P. Discharge instructions for emergency department patients: what should we provide? J Accid Emerg Med 2000;17:86–90.

53. Lawrence L, Zhou J, Givens T. The effect of diagnosis-specific computerized discharge instructions on 72-hour return visits to the pediatric emergency department. Pediatr Emerg Care 2009;25(11):733–8.
54. Alfandre D, Schumann J. What is wrong with discharges against medical advice (and how to fix them). JAMA 2013;310:2393–4.
55. Devitt PJ, Devitt AC, Dewan M. Does identifying a discharge as "against medical advice" confer legal protection? J Fam Pract 2000;49(3):224–7.
56. Schaefer GR, Matus H, Schumann JH, et al. Financial responsibility of hospitalized patients who left against medical advice: medical urban legend? J Gen Intern Med 2012;27(7):825–30.
57. Marco C, Brenner J, Krauss C, et al. Refusal of emergency medical treatment" case studies and ethical foundations. Ann Emerg Med 2017;70(5):696–703.
58. Lin MP, Baker O, Richardson LD, et al. Trends in emergency department visits and admission rates among US acute care hospitals. JAMA Intern Med 2018;178(12):1708–10.
59. Katz MH. Decreased admission rate from the emergency department with increased emergency department visits—the good and the bad. JAMA Intern Med 2018;178(12):1710–1.
60. Schuur JD, Venkatesh AK. The growing role of emergency departments in hospital admissions. N Engl J Med 2012;367(5):391–3.
61. Lee RS, Woods R, Bullard M, et al. Consultations in the emergency department: a systematic review of the literature. Emerg Med J 2008;25:4–9.
62. Kessler C, Afshar Y, Sardar G, et al. A propsective, randomized, controlled study demonstrating a novel, effective model of transfer of care between physicians: the 5 Cs of consultation. Acad Emerg Med 2012;19(8):968–74.
63. Schurr J, Tibbles C. Risks associated with specialty consultation in the ED. In: Debbie LaValley, editor. Consults and patient safety, vol. 27. CRICO FORUM; 2009 (2). Available at: https://www.rmf.harvard.edu/Clinician-Resources/Article/2009/September-2009-Forum-Consults-and-Patient-Safety.
64. TenBrink W, O'Sullivan E, Dhaliwal R, et al. The impact of EMTALA. In: Schlicher N, Haddock A, editors. Emergency medicine advocacy handbook. 5th edition. Dallas (TX).p.21-28: EMRA; 2019. p. 21–8.
65. Peth H. Reporting requirements, confidentiality, and HIPAA. In: Strauss R, Mayer T, editors. Emergency department management. New York: McGraw Hill Education; 2017. p. 637–42.
66. Fuller K. 6 tips for using clinical documentation to drive revenue cycle management. Healthcare Finance News. 2013. Available at: https://www.healthcarefinancenews.com/news/clinical-documentation-driving-rcm. Accessed August 10, 2019.
67. Reviewing Hospital claims for patient status: admissions on or after October 1, 2013. Center for Medicare & Medicaid Services. 2013. Available at: https://www.cms.gov/Research-Statistics-Data-and-Systems/Monitoring-Programs/Medical- Review/Downloads/ReviewingHospitalClaimsforAdmissionFINAL.pdf. Accessed August 10, 2019.
68. La Pointe J. Recovery audit contractor reform eases provider Burden, CMS Says. RevCycleIntelligence. 2019. Available at: https://revcycleintelligence.com/news/recovery-audit-contractor-reform-eases-provider-burden-cms-says. Accessed August 10, 2019.
69. What's the verdict: a case of changing medical records. Medical Economics. 2015. Available at: https://www.medicaleconomics.com/practice-management/whats-verdict-case-changing-medical-records. Accessed August 10, 2019.

70. Alteration of a Medical Record Carries Serious Consequences. MLMIC Insurance Company. 2016. Available at: https://www.mlmic.com/blog/hospitals/alteration-of-a-medical-record-carries-serious-consequences. Accessed August 10, 2019.
71. Becker M. Falsification of Medical Records. The Becker Law Firm. 2017. Available at: https://www.beckerjustice.com/blog/2017/october/falsification-of-medical-records. Accessed August 10, 2019.
72. Tsou A, Lehmann C, Michel J, et al. Safe practice for copy and paste in the EHR: systematic review, recommendations, and novel model for health IT collaboration. Appl Clin Inform 2017;8(1):12–34.

Confidentiality and Capacity

Joseph H. Kahn, MD

KEYWORDS

- Confidentiality • HIPAA • Protected health information • Capacity
- Informed consent • Refusal of care • Against medical advice

KEY POINTS

- Patient confidentiality is not only an ethical imperative, it is a legally protected right.
- There are situations when clinicians are legally required to reveal protected health information to protect the public or specific individuals.
- Capacity is the term used to determine whether patients have the mental ability to make informed decisions regarding their medical care.
- Emergency physicians are expected to provide life-sustaining treatment to patients who present with acute life-threatening illnesses/injuries but are unable to give informed consent due to the acuity of their conditions.
- Discharging a patient against medical advice is a high-risk process which involves more than simply having a patient sign a standard form.

CONFIDENTIALITY

Patient confidentiality sits at the center of the doctor-patient relationship. Because an accurate history is usually essential in establishing a medical diagnosis, doctors often ask patients probing and personal questions that would not be appropriate in another setting. Patients will generally answer these questions in the medical setting, with the understanding that their personal information will not be released to other persons or entities without their permission. Patient confidentiality is not only an ethical imperative, it is a legally protected right.

Health Insurance Portability and Accountability Act and Related Regulations

The Health Insurance Portability and Accountability Act (HIPAA) went into effect in 1996 and addresses the privacy and security of patients' health care information.[1] Although practitioners and health care facilities have always had a duty to protect patients' medical information, HIPAA established national standards regarding protected health information (PHI).[1] As most health care facilities and practitioners are shifting to electronic health records, the privacy and security regulations of HIPAA have become even more important.[2]

Department of Emergency Medicine, Boston University School of Medicine, Boston Medical Center, 1 Boston Medical Center Place, Boston, MA 02118, USA
E-mail address: jkahn@bu.edu

Emerg Med Clin N Am 38 (2020) 283–296
https://doi.org/10.1016/j.emc.2020.01.003   emed.theclinics.com
0733-8627/20/© 2020 Elsevier Inc. All rights reserved.

HIPAA mandates that all health care facilities and providers give patients the "Notice of Privacy Practices," which describes the patient's rights and health care provider's responsibilities regarding PHI, which the patient or proxy must sign and date.[2] An exception to this rule occurs when a patient is incapacitated or in need of emergency services.[2] The American College of Emergency Physicians states that all physicians have a legal and ethical duty regarding PHI, outlined in "Confidentiality of Patient Information," which was revised in 2017, 2008, 2002, and 1998, and first was published as "Patient Confidentiality" in 1994.[3]

"Privacy" refers to physical seclusion, protection of personal information, protection of personal identity, and the ability to make decisions autonomously.[4] "Confidentiality" refers to not disclosing personal information without the person's permission.[4]

Protecting PHI may be more important and more difficult in the emergency department (ED) than in most practice settings.[5] Semi-open wards with overflow of patients into hallways, combined with the sensitive nature of many ED visits, as well as the multiple staff members involved in a patient's care, makes patient confidentiality particularly challenging in the emergency setting.[5] To preserve privacy and confidentiality, use of "status boards" in the ED that are in plain sight of passersby are obviously unacceptable, but it is also important not to have computer screens with PHI visible to unauthorized persons in the vicinity, and not to discuss PHI within earshot of the public.[5] There are times, however, when the need to protect PHI may be overridden by other duties.[5]

Avoiding Breaches of Confidentiality of Protected Health Information

The very design of most EDs poses difficulties in maintaining patient confidentiality. It has been reported in 1 university hospital ED that breaches of privacy and confidentiality are not infrequent.[6] Another study reported that unauthorized persons are more likely to see or overhear patients when they are in curtained bays than in rooms with walls.[6] ED crowding, often including patients cared for in hallway beds, further compromises patient privacy and confidentiality.[6]

Portable privacy screens may help maintain privacy when patients need to be examined or undergo procedures in open areas.[6] When possible, It is good practice to move hallway patients into rooms, even if only temporarily, while they undergo history and physical and procedures. Visitors should accompany patients into treatment areas only with the patient's or surrogate's permission, and should not wander into the space where other patients are being treated.[6]

Law enforcement officers are frequently present in the ED, either as in-house employees or outside law enforcement personnel. They often assist in caring for violent and uncooperative patients who may be a danger to themselves or staff.[7] Law enforcement officers may also bring in individuals who are in their custody and need medical treatment. Not infrequently, law enforcement officers are present in the ED to investigate a crime and collect evidence.[7] When possible, ED patients should be asked for permission to be visited by law enforcement officers.[6] It is important not to allow law enforcement activities to interfere with patient care.[6,8] Hospital policies can help guide interactions between patients, staff, and law enforcement personnel.[8]

When students or other observers are present in the ED, it is best to ask the patient's or surrogate's permission for them to be present during a medical evaluation, although there is some controversy regarding this issue.[6] In addition to asking permission to be present, observers who "shadow" clinicians during patient encounters should first complete HIPAA training.[9] Clinicians should be aware that even when patients consent to the presence of observers, they may not reveal sensitive information to the clinician with an observer present.[9]

Computerized screens must not reveal medical information that unauthorized persons can see. They should be situated out of the view of unauthorized persons, should be password protected, and should be set to time out to a screen saver in a short period of time when not in use.[6] Clinicians should be aware that they will be held accountable for use and misuse of patient's PHI in the electronic medical record and must never share their passwords and should log-out of the medical record when leaving their computer unattended.

Each hospital should have a policy guiding telephone inquiries about patients in the ED, so that PHI is not released without the patient's or surrogate's permission.[6]

Facsimile

Facsimile transmission (fax) provides for rapid exchange of information between professionals.[10] Confidential medical information is often transmitted via fax, whether from hospital to hospital, medical office to hospital, hospital to medical office, and hospital to consultant. Faxing is thought to improve communication between medical practitioners and the ED.[11] Faxing may allow unauthorized individuals to see confidential information.[10] Information may be faxed to the wrong recipient by entering an incorrect number, especially in the situation where speed-dial buttons are used.[10] Some techniques for avoiding breaches of information when using fax transmission include avoiding the use of fax for highly sensitive information, placement of fax machines away from areas where unauthorized persons may be present, the use of fax cover sheets addressed to a specific individual, and checking that the correct number has been entered before sending.[10,12]

Electronic Mail

Medical practitioners use e-mail (electronic mail) communication with patients and other providers, but guidelines for use are limited.[13] E-mails between providers regarding patients should be on devices which are encrypted and secure.[13] HIPAA ensures that PHI remain confidential, but does not give clear guidelines regarding what is considered adequate security of e-mail communication.[13] The American Medical Informatics Association (AMIA) recommends that practices have printed guidelines describing the security measures to be taken, including labeling the e-mail as confidential in the subject line or at the top of the message, and not forwarding e-mails containing patient information without the written permission of the patient.[13] Whether to incorporate confidential e-mails into the medical record is another unclear question, especially when the communication is involved in clinical management decisions.[13]

AMIA recommends the following guidelines for e-mail communication regarding patients: "proof-read each e-mail for proper spelling, grammar, and punctuation; use meaningful subject line that is descriptive of e-mail content; avoid background colors, patterns, all capitals, and unusual fonts; avoid humor that may be misinterpreted; do not send an e-mail to the wrong person—be especially careful with reply all and mass forwarding; do not send emotionally charged e-mails—consider a direct conversation for complex or sensitive topics; transmit protected data cautiously using a private or secured computer or handheld device via an encrypted, secured network—avoid sending such data to or from a public e-mail service, such as Gmail, Yahoo, or Hotmail."[13]

Smartphones

Smartphone use in medical practice is a growing trend, with increasing dependence on smartphone applications, as well as capturing, storing, and transmitting images with a smartphone.[14,15] Emergency physicians not infrequently use smartphones to transmit EKG images to cardiologists, skin lesion images to dermatologists, and sometimes transmit images to other specialists, such as ophthalmologists.

It is essential to safeguard patient privacy when using smartphone technology. The Australian Medical Association released guidelines for use of medical imaging with smartphone devices: "make sure the patient understands why the image is being taken and with whom it will be shared; obtain informed consent from the patient before taking the image; document consent in the medical record; have security controls on the mobile device to prevent unauthorized access to the images; delete clinical images from smartphones after saving them in the medical record."[15]

According to Stevenson, "failing to use appropriate security precautions poses an emerging medico-legal risk for practitioners."[15] Medical practitioners should take reasonable measures to protect PHI, as outlined above.[15]

Social Media

The use of social media platforms by clinicians to rapidly disseminate medical information is a growing trend.[16] It is essential that information exchanged on social media sites is monitored for accuracy, and confidentiality and privacy must be maintained.[17] The use of social media for education, patient care, and dissemination of clinical information has been endorsed by the Society of American Gastrointestinal and Endoscopic Surgeons and other professional societies.[16] Many professional societies have released documents guiding the use of social media in clinical practice, including the American Medical Association, the American College of Physicians, the Federation of State Medical Boards, the Canadian Medical Association, and others.[18]

Social media sharing sites are used for many purposes from clinicians sharing medical images with one another to sharing of medical education presentations to rapid notification of patients regarding health warnings.[19] Limitations of social media platforms include possible lack of reliability of information, and lack of confidentiality regarding PHI.[17] The various types of social media, including but not limited to, blogs (Web logs), microblogs, such as Twitter, social networking sites, such as Facebook, wiki sites, such as Wikipedia, professional networking sites, such as LinkedIn, all are subject to these limitations.[19]

Social media creates many risks for physicians in terms of patient confidentiality. Fayyaz[20] suggests the following guidelines for physicians in the use of social media: "maintain strict control on privacy settings of platform in use; thoroughly understand 'Terms of Use' for professional accounts on social media; maintain professional and personal accounts separately; apply the same standards of physician-patient interactions on social media as in physical encounters; maintain confidentiality of health data to the utmost unless extremely necessary, where a direct patient benefit or harm is clearly involved, and apply discretion on sharing identifiers unless extremely necessary; disclose Conflict of Interest in 'about' or 'profile' section or whichever way it gets easy visibility; complete disclosure of intent and extent of sharing information followed by written consent; no sharing of data including images and visuals of patients on any social media platform for branding or practice promotion."[20]

Required Breaks in Confidentiality

There are times when a clinician is required to reveal PHI to protect the health of the general public or specific individuals.

The Tarasoff case has established that physicians have a duty to warn third parties of a danger of harm by a patient.[5] If a physician becomes aware that their patient is intending to harm another individual, then that physician has the duty to breach confidentiality and warn the targeted individual and notify law enforcement authorities of the threat.[4–6]

Reporting of suspected child abuse is mandated in all 50 states, and elder abuse is mandated in most states.[4,5] Reporting of domestic violence is mandated in several states, but in most states requires permission from the victim.[4,5]

Injuries suspected to be gunshot and/or stab wounds must be reported to law enforcement agencies.[5]

There are multiple infections that must be reported to public health agencies.[4–6] The list of nationally reportable conditions can be found on the Centers for Disease Control web site.[21] Some diseases need to be reported to state health departments. The list of mandated reporting of infectious diseases to the Department of Public Health in Massachusetts includes anthrax, measles, meningitis, mumps, pertussis, rubella, tuberculosis, typhoid fever, viral hemorrhagic fevers, and many others.[22] Other states may have different disease-reporting requirements that can be found in the statutes and health department regulations of each respective state.

Another possibly required breach in confidentiality is reporting of a seizure to the motor vehicle department. The reporting laws vary from state to state, with some states mandating that physicians report the condition, even if the patient objects. Even if physician reporting is not required in your state, it is advisable to tell the patient to report the condition to the motor vehicle department and not to drive until cleared to do so by the patient's doctor. This conversation should be clearly documented in the medical record. The length of the seizure-free interval before a physician can certify that a patient is cleared to drive again also varies from state to state. The Epilepsy Foundation maintains a database of each state's regulations regarding driving and reporting of epilepsy.[23]

Clinicians failing to report can lead to serious disciplinary actions, including lawsuits or criminal prosecution, and all practicing clinicians should know their states guidelines and reporting laws.

CAPACITY

Emergency physicians generally accept the axiom that patients arriving in the ED want to be treated, but this is not always the case. Deciding whether a patient has the mental capacity to refuse care is one of the most anxiety-provoking situations that emergency physicians are confronted with. What makes this situation particularly challenging in the ED, as opposed to other health care settings, is that the need for treatment is often urgent. This places emergency physicians in a conflict between doing everything within their ability to preserve the life and well-being of the patient while respecting the patient's autonomy and wishes.

Determining Patient's Capacity/Capability/Competency to Make Clinical Decisions

Patients must have the capacity to make medical decisions to consent to or refuse medical care.[24] The ethical principle of autonomy, or right to self-determination, generally supports the concept that patients are assumed to have the capacity to make medical decisions until proven otherwise.[25] Capacity is the term generally used in the medical arena to determine whether a patient has the mental ability to make an informed decision regarding their evaluation and treatment.[26] Competence is a legal term and refers to whether a person has the legal right to make their own decisions, including managing finances, living independently, and other life choices.[25,26]

Capacity is largely determined by a patient's cognitive ability.[26] There are 4 primary components of the capacity to make decisions: (1) the ability to receive information, (2) the ability to understand and process the information received, (3) the ability to deliberate, and (4) the ability to make, articulate, and defend choices[24,27] (**Table 1**). In most clinical encounters of lucid patients, the patient's decision-making capacity is determined to be intact based on the answers given while obtaining the medical history.[24] Goldfrank and Wittman[28] describe capacity determination as a "complex calculation involving a patient's mental status, cognitive ability, culture, education, health literacy, and ability to articulate the issues of concern." In addition, capacity is always attached to a particular medical decision at a particular time, and patients lacking capacity for one specific medical decision may have capacity for other decisions.

It may be more difficult to determine capacity, or lack of capacity, in patients with limited English proficiency. According to 2013 data, 25 million people, or approximately 8% of the US population older than 5 years, have limited English proficiency, and this number continues to grow.[29,30] Federal law requires all hospitals and their EDs who receive federal financial assistance to provide interpretive services to their patients with limited English proficiency.[29] Although an emergency physician may begin evaluation and treatment of a patient with an emergency condition using an ad hoc interpreter, such as a family member, the use of a medically trained interpreter is superior in the medical assessment and in the determination of capacity.[29] Furthermore, deaf patients may need an American Sign Language (ASL) interpreter to assist in determining their medical needs and in determining their capacity to make medical decisions. Written communication may help start the evaluation and treatment process, but may not be an acceptable substitute for ASL when communicating with the patient about sensitive issues.[29]

Cognition may be permanently impaired due to a chronic medical condition, such as dementia, or temporarily altered by an acute factor, such as illness, injury, delirium, psychosis, intoxication, or other acute situational issues.[24] Emergency nurses may be the first to recognize that a patient does not seem to understand the planned testing and/or treatment, and will often notify the practitioner of their concerns, which may lead to further assessment of decision-making capacity before proceeding.[25] Decision-making capacity is preserved in most psychiatric patients, and it is not appropriate to allow a previous or current psychiatric diagnosis determine a patient's capacity. In situations of current mood disorder, severe psychosis, or suicidality, a psychiatrist may need to be consulted to assist in determining capacity.[31]

Determining whether a patient has the capacity to consent to or refuse care is challenging. Different standardized tools have been developed to aid in this determination, including the DECISION approach,[24] the University of California San Diego Brief Assessment of Capacity to Consent Tool (UBACC),[32] and mental status examination questions, which assess memory, judgment, understanding, and attention.[24]

Generally the emergency physician makes the determination of decision-making capacity, often with the help of the patient's family, sometimes with the help of a psychiatric consultation if that service is available and the issue is less time-sensitive, based on whether the patient is able to understand, process, deliberate over the information, and make an informed decision.[24]

When a patient presents with life-threatening illness or injury, and refuses treatment, and there is doubt regarding the patient's capacity to refuse treatment, it is generally

Table 1
Legally relevant criteria for decision-making capacity and approaches to assessment of the patient

Criterion	Patient's Task	Physician's Assessment Approach	Questions for Clinical Assessment[a]	Comments
Communicate a choice	Clearly indicate preferred treatment option	Ask patient to indicate a treatment choice	Have you decided whether to follow your doctor's [or my] recommendation for treatment? Can you tell me what that decision is? [If no decision] What is making it hard for you to decide?	Frequent reversals of choice because of psychiatric or neurologic conditions may indicate lack of capacity
Understand the relevant information	Grasp the fundamental meaning of information communicated by physician	Encourage patient to paraphrase disclosed information regarding medical condition and treatment	Please tell me in your own words what your doctor [or I] told you about: The problem with your health now The recommended treatment The possible benefits and risks (or discomforts) of the treatment Any alternative treatments and their risks and benefits The risks and benefits of no treatment	Information to be understood includes nature of patient's condition, nature and purpose of proposed treatment, possible benefits and risks of that treatment, and alternative approaches (including no treatment) and their benefits and risks
Appreciate the situation and its consequences	Acknowledge medical condition and likely consequences of treatment options	Ask patient to describe views of medical condition, proposed treatment, and likely outcomes	What do you believe is wrong with your health now? Do you believe that you need some kind of treatment? What is treatment likely to do for you? What makes you believe that it will have that effect? What do you believe will happen if you are not treated? Why do you think your doctor has [or I have] recommended this treatment?	Courts have recognized that patients who do not acknowledge their illnesses (often referred to as "lack of insight") cannot make valid decisions about treatment. Delusions of pathologic levels of distortion or denial are the most common causes of impairment

(continued on next page)

Table 1
(continued)

Criterion	Patient's Task	Physician's Assessment Approach	Questions for Clinical Assessment[a]	Comments
Reason about treatment options	Engage in rational process of manipulating relevant information	Ask patient to compare treatment options and consequences and to offer reasons for selection of option	How did you decide to accept or reject the recommended treatment? What makes [chosen option] better than [alternative option]?	This criterion focuses on the process by which a decision is reached, not the outcome of the patient's choice, since patients have the right to make "unreasonable" choices

[a] Questions are adapted from Grisso and Applebaum. Patients' responses to these questions need not be verbal.
Adapted from Magauran BG. "Risk management for the emergency physician: competency and decision-making capacity, informed consent, and refusal of care against medical advice." Emerg Med Clin N Am 2009;27:605–614 and Appelbaum PS. "Assessment of patients' competence to consent to treatment." N Engl J Med 2007;357(18):1834-1840.

appropriate to proceed with life-saving treatment, or at least not to allow the patient to leave, even if it requires some form of well-thought out sedation or restraint.[33,34]

Informed Consent

Informed consent is a legal as well as a medical term.[35] For informed consent to treatment to be valid, appropriate information should be disclosed to a patient who is capable of making a choice as to whether to proceed with treatment.[36] The elements of informed consent include describing the following to the patient or surrogate: the nature of the treatment; reasonable alternatives; the risks, benefits, and uncertainties related to the treatment and the alternatives; patient understanding of the conversation; and voluntary acceptance of the treatment by the patient without coercion.[35,37]

Informed consent before medical treatment is an essential component of the concept of autonomy. With autonomy, the patient can determine the correct treatment option consistent with their own goals and values.[35] In the ED setting, the patient does not get to choose which physician treats them, and may not have been able to choose which ED to be taken to, so autonomous decision-making is limited to treatment decisions, making informed consent especially important when it can be obtained.[35]

Informed consent is not valid if manipulation, coercion, or duress was used to persuade the patient to consent to a treatment.[35] It is reasonable, however, for the emergency physician to recommend a course of treatment to the patient or proxy based on their knowledge and expertise of the subject.[35]

Generally, a patient signs a consent for treatment form as part of the registration process on arrival to the ED. This does not obviate the need for the emergency physician to document their conversations with the patient regarding informed consent or attempts at informed consent for specific risky tests or treatments.[35]

An exemption to informed consent occurs when a patient arrives to the ED with a life-threatening illness or injury and is acutely unable to make medical decisions because of their acute condition. In this situation, the emergency physician is expected to act in the best interest of the patient and provide life-sustaining treatment without informed consent.[35] In this situation, it is assumed that the patient would consent to the treatment if they were capable of doing so.[27,35]

Barriers to Consent

Emergency physicians frequently treat patients who cannot consent for treatment. It is often not possible to obtain written or even verbal consent before instituting evaluation and treatment in the ED or prehospital setting. Frequent barriers to obtaining informed consent for treatment include language proficiency, impaired level of consciousness or other mental status changes, age less than 18 years, psychiatric illness, limited reasoning ability, intoxication, and time urgency of the intervention.[36,37] The legal principle of implied consent includes the situation in which a patient who may be unconscious or otherwise impaired, but has an acute medical issue requiring urgent treatment, to which the patient would consent if they were able.

In acute medical situations, the ED may need to proceed to treatment without informed consent.[35,37] If there is time, it is appropriate to attempt to call the patient's health care proxy, next of kin, or other family member before initiating treatment. If it is necessary to treat without waiting for consent, then notification of the patient's family should be attempted as soon as possible after the treatment has started. Withholding emergency care due to lack of consent is not appropriate if the patient is likely to deteriorate due to the delay. Again, if consent cannot be obtained, and in the clinician's judgment the patient or family would give consent if they were able, then the clinician should proceed with emergency care.[35] It is the medical principle of beneficence that requires a physician to carry out life-saving treatment when informed consent cannot be obtained.[37] If the patient arrives in the ED with a valid, signed advance directive form, this may help guide the physician regarding treatment decisions.

Refusal of Care

When patients choose to refuse medical treatment, the emergency physician should try to determine whether the patient is making an informed decision, and whether the patient has the capacity to make that decision.[38] Dickens states that the clinician should "...ensure that the patient really understands the nature of the proposed treatment, the reason why it is recommended, and implications for the patient's health and future if the treatment is not undertaken."[39]

If a patient refuses the recommended test, procedure, treatment, or admission, disclosure of the risks of refusing care should be emphasized by the clinician, without taking away the patient's autonomy by pressuring the patient.[39] Alternative treatment plans should be discussed with the patient, if any exist.[39] However, a physician is not under obligation to try a scientifically unproven therapy which they think is not appropriate in this situation.[39] A reasonable alternative is to admit a patient (if they are willing to stay in the hospital) who is refusing a procedure or other aspect(s) of care, to continue to provide medical care for the patient, after careful documentation of the refusal of the recommended test or treatment.

Patient's wishes regarding end-of-life care have evolved dramatically in recent years, with the use of advance directives, palliative care services, and hospice care. Discussion of life-sustaining treatment for this very important subset of patients is beyond the scope of this article.

Substitute Judgment

If a patient is not capable of consenting to or refusing treatment, another person (usually a health care proxy or next of kin) may make a decision on behalf of the patient that is in line with the patient's values and goals.[35] If a patient has signed a power of attorney document, then the person named in the power of attorney may legally make medical decisions for an incapacitated patient.[39]

Patients transferred to the ED from skilled nursing facilities usually arrive with paperwork giving phone numbers of family members and the patients' physicians, so that the discussion of medical decisions with family members and physicians who know the patient can sometimes proceed in timely fashion if the patient is incapacitated or defers decisions to next of kin.[35] Patients often arrive with advance directives, such as medical orders for life-sustaining treatment, physician orders for life-sustaining treatment, do-not-resuscitate orders, do-not-intubate orders, or comfort-care-only orders. These forms may help guide the physician in the treatment of ED patients, but not infrequently the situation at hand may not be covered by the existing forms, or the orders may be confusing, so communication with the designated family member or the patient's doctor may help guide the treatment course.

When confronted with patients who are acutely incapable of making medical decisions due to a life-threatening illness or injury, and no substitute judgment is available, the emergency physician should act in the patient's best interest and render life-sustaining treatment.[35]

Discharging Against Medical Advice

The number of patients who leave the ED against medical advice (AMA) is significant, estimated at 1% to 3% of ED visits.[27] As many as 6% of hospital/ED discharges serving urban patients in the United States may be AMA.[40,41] One study at an academic medical center reports an AMA rate of 2.7% from the ED.[40] The number of AMA discharges seems to be growing, as Kaiser Health News reports that the number of AMA discharges from California EDs rose from 1.8% in 2012 to 2.4% in 2017.[42] For the purpose of this discussion, AMA discharges include those patients who leave the ED after being seen by the emergency practitioner, but left before the recommended treatment was completed, whether they informed the staff before their departure or not. AMA discharges generally do not include patients who elope from the waiting room without being seen by a practitioner.

Patients who leave AMA have a higher rate of return ED visits, higher rate of hospital admission, and higher 30-day mortality, than patients who do not leave AMA.[27,40,41]

If the patient notifies the ED staff of their intention to leave without completing the recommended testing, treatment, observation, and/or admission to the hospital, it is incumbent on the emergency physician to take the time to communicate with the patient (and family) precisely why they think the recommended plan is important for the patient's well-being, outline the risks of leaving, answer the patient's questions, and try to ascertain why the patient wants to leave.[28] Goldfrank and Wittman[28] advocate for increasing communication, satisfaction, and efficiency to help reduce the number of patients who leave AMA, thereby reducing harm to patients. If the patient insists on leaving AMA despite the emergency physician's best efforts, it is important to assess the patient's capacity to make this decision, to carefully review with the patient the risks associated with leaving prematurely, and to document these discussions in the medical record.[40] This documentation in the medical record should be accomplished promptly, even before the patient leaves the ED, if possible. This documentation not only helps protect the provider against liability, but also notifies the next provider of what treatment was recommended, if and when the patient returns. It is also essential to give the patient careful discharge instructions, both verbally and in writing, in a language that they understand, prescriptions for recommended treatments, instructions on urgent follow-up care, and clearly inform the patient that they are not only welcome but actually encouraged to return to the ED to complete the recommended testing, treatment, observation, and/or admission at any time.

The AMA form itself may offer limited legal protection for the practitioner and hospital.[40] The standard boilerplate hospital AMA form with a single sentence stating that the patient is being discharged AMA is not as useful as the more detailed AMA forms that are now available. More detailed AMA forms may include documentation of capacity, medical risks, and possible outcomes resulting from the AMA decision.[40] Even a signed AMA form, although helpful, does not necessarily provide total protection from a malpractice lawsuit.[40] It is important to also document these factors in the medical record itself, as stated above. Some patients will refuse to sign the AMA form. In this case, the form should be filled out as above, and then documented that the patient refused to sign it. The physician should proceed with giving the patient discharge instructions as outlined above. The emergency physician should not make signing the AMA form a condition for receiving discharge instructions, necessary prescriptions, and follow-up care. In addition to the AMA form, the clinician should always document the patient's capacity and full discussions on alternative treatments and recommendations of care in the patient's chart in real time.

A more difficult situation arises when the patient leaves the ED without informing anyone, after the emergency physician's evaluation/treatment has been initiated, but is not complete. This premature departure from the ED should be carefully documented in the medical record, including what the plan was, what results may have come back, what results may be pending, and what attempts were made to find or reach out to the patient to complete their care.

SUMMARY

Issues of patient confidentiality and capacity are high-risk areas for emergency physicians. It is important for emergency physicians to have an understanding of confidentiality issues surrounding PHI, including HIPAA compliance, and when breaks in confidentiality are required. Furthermore, basic knowledge of patients' capacity to consent or refuse medical care is essential to the practice of emergency medicine.

DISCLOSURE

The author has nothing to disclose.

REFERENCES

1. Murray TL, Calhoun M, Philipsen NC. Privacy, confidentiality, HIPAA, and HITECH: implications for the health care practitioner. JNP 2011;7(9):747–52.
2. Huang HF, Liu KC. Efficient key management for preserving HIPAA regulations. J Syst Softw 2011;84:113–9.
3. Confidentiality of patient information. Ann Emerg Med 2017;70(1):117.
4. Geiderman JM, Moskop JC, Derse AR. Privacy and confidentiality in emergency medicine: obligations and challenges. Emerg Med Clin North Am 2006;24: 633–56.
5. Moskop JC, Marco CA, Larkin GL, et al. From Hippocrates to HIPAA: privacy and confidentiality in emergency medicine - Part I: conceptual, moral and legal foundations. Ann Emerg Med 2005;45(1):53–9.
6. Moskop JC, Marco CA, Larkin GL, et al. From Hippocrates to HIPAA: privacy and confidentiality in emergency medicine - Part II: challenges in the emergency department. Ann Emerg Med 2005;45(1):60–7.
7. Baker EF, Moskop JC, Geiderman JM. Law enforcement and emergency medicine: an ethical analysis. Ann Emerg Med 2016;68(5):599–607.
8. Tahouni MR, Liscord E, Mowafi H. Managing law enforcement presence in the emergency department: highlighting the need for new policy recommendations. J Emerg Med 2015;49(4):523–9.
9. Geiderman JM. Observers in the medical setting. Ann Emerg Med 2017;70(1): 86–92.
10. Dodek DY, Dodek A. From Hippocrates to facsimile: protecting patient confidentiality is more difficult and more important than ever before. Can Med Assoc J 1997;156:847–52.
11. Taylor DMCD, Graham IS, Chappell-Lawrence J. "Facsimile communication between emergency departments and GP's, and patient data confidentiality. Med J Aust 1997;167:575–8.
12. Spath P. Here is what you can do to protect patient privacy. Hosp Case Manag 1999;7:136–8.
13. Malka ST, Kessler CS, Abraham J, et al. Professional e-mail communication among health care providers: proposing evidence-based guidelines. Acad Med 2015;90:25–9.
14. Thomairy NA, Mummaneni M, Alsalamah S, et al. Use of smartphones in hospitals. Health Care Manag 2015;34:297–307.
15. Stevenson P, Finnane AR, Soyer HP. Teledermatology and clinical photography: safeguarding patient privacy and mitigating medicao-oegal risk. Med J Aust 2016;204:198–201.

16. Bittner JG, Logghe HJ, Kane ED, et al. A Society of Gastrointestinal and Endo-scopic Surgeons (SAGES) statement on closed social media (FacebookR) groups for clinical education and consultation: issues of informed consent, patient privacy, and surgeon protection. Surg Endosc 2019;33:1–7.

17. Moorhead SA, Hazlett DE, Harrison L, et al. A new dimension of health care: systematic review of the uses, benefits, and limitations of social media for health communication. J Med Internet Res 2013;15:1–16.

18. Hennessy CM, Smith CF, Greener S, et al. Social media guidelines: a review for health professionals and faculty members. Clin Teach 2019;16:1–6.

19. Grajales FJ III, Sheps S, Kendall H, et al. Social media: a review and tutorial of applications in medicine and health care. J Med Internet Res 2014;16:1–23.

20. Fayyaz M. Social media and ethos of clinical practice. J Pak Med Assoc 2019;69: 541–4.

21. National notifiable conditions (Historical). 2018. Available at: https://wwwn.cdc.gov/nndss/conditions/notifiable/2018/. Accessed May 24, 2019.

22. Diseases reportable to the Massachusetts Department of Public Health and local boards of health. Available at: https://www.mass.gov/lists/infectious-disease-reporting-and-regulations-for-health-care-providers-and-laboratories#diseases-reportable-to-the-massachusetts-department-of-public-health-and-local-boards-of-health-. Accessed May 24, 2019.

23. State driving laws database. Available at: https://www.epilepsy.com/driving-laws. Accessed May 24, 2019.

24. Larkin GL, Marco CA, Abbott JT. Emergency determiantion of decision-making capacity: balancing autonomy and benificence in the emergency department. Acad Emerg Med 2001;8:282–4.

25. Mitchell MA. Assessing patient decision-making capacity: it's about the thought process. J Emerg Nurs 2015;41(4):307–12.

26. Karlawish J. Assessment of decision-making capacity in adults. UpToDate. Accessed April 16, 2019. Available at: https://www.uptodate.com/contents/assessment-of-decision-making-capacity-in-adults?search=assessment%20of%20decision-making%20capacity%20in%20adults&source=search_result&selectedTitle=1~150&usage_type=default&display_rank=1.

27. Marco CA, Brenner JM, Kraus CK, et al. Refusal of emergency medical treatment: case studies and ethical foundations. Ann Emerg Med 2017;70:696–703.

28. Goldfrank LR, Wittman I. Capacity? Informed discharge? Uncertainty! Ann Emerg Med 2017;70(5):704–6.

29. Brenner JM, Baker EF, Iserson KV, et al. Use of interpreter services in the Emergency Department. Ann Emerg Med 2018;72:432–7.

30. Available at: https://www.migrationpolicy.org/article/limited-english-proficient-population-united-states. Accessed June 9, 2019.

31. Baruth JM, Lapid MI. Influence of psychiatric symptoms on decisional capacity in treatment refusal. AMA J Ethics 2017;19(5):416–25.

32. Martel ML, Klein LR, Miner JR. A brief assessment of capacity to consent instrument in acutely intoxicated emergency department patients. Am J Emerg Med 2018;36:18–23.

33. Eagle K, Ryan CJ. "Potentially incapable patients objecting to treatment: doctors' powers and duties. Med J Aust 2014;200(6):352–4.

34. Cheung EH, Heldt J, Strouse T, et al. The medical incapacity hold: a policy on the involuntary medical hospitalization of patients who lack decisional capacity. Psychosomatics 2018;59(2):169–76.

35. Magauran BG. Risk management for the emergency physician: competency and decision-making capacity, informed consent, and refusal of care against medical advice. Emerg Med Clin North Am 2009;27:605–14.
36. Appelbaum PS. Assessment of patients' competence to consent to treatment. N Engl J Med 2007;357(18):1834–40.
37. De Bord J. "Informed consent." Ethics in medicine, University of Washington School of Medicine. Available at: https://depts.washington.edu/bioethx/topics/consent.html#ref1. Accessed May 26, 2019.
38. Derse AR. What part of "no" don't you understand? Patient refusal of recommended treatment in the emergency department. Mt Sinai J Med 2005;72(4):221–7.
39. Dickens BM, Cook RJ. Patients' refusal of recommended treatment. Int J Gynaecol Obstetrics 2015;131:105–8.
40. Levy F, Mareiniss DP, Iacovelli C. The importance of a proper against-medical-advice (AMA) discharge: how signing out AMA may create significant liability protection for providers. J Emerg Med 2012;43(3):516–20.
41. Brenner J, Joslin J, Goulette A, et al. Against medical advice: a survey of ED clinicans' rationale for use. J Emerg Nurs 2016;42(5):408–11.
42. Reese P. As ER wait times grow, more patients leave against medical advice. Kaiser Health News 2019. Available at: https://www.medscape.com/viewarticle/913489. Accessed May 27, 2019.

Physician Well-Being

Leon D. Sanchez, MD, MPH*, Richard E. Wolfe, MD

KEYWORDS

- Stress • Burnout • Maslach inventory • Agency • Work environment • Wellness

KEY POINTS

- Burnout is a work-related condition characterized by feelings of energy depletion or exhaustion, increased mental distance from one's job, and reduced professional efficacy.
- The worsening conditions of the work environment contribute to fatigue, depression, and depersonalization. These system issues are not amenable to individual wellness solutions.
- Studies are needed to determine the relationship between burnout scores and the degree of patient and provider harm that it causes.
- New measurement tools of burnout need to be developed using biological markers or assessment by unbiased observers, supervisors, colleagues, or patients.

INTRODUCTION

Burnout is emerging as a serious threat to the practice of emergency medicine (EM). Emergency physicians (EPs) are often exposed to high levels of stress because of the severity of emergency patient illness, crowding of emergency departments (EDs), imposition of computerized records, and inadequate staff and space resources to optimally fulfill professional responsibilities. The work schedule of EPs is disruptive to the circadian rhythm, as well as social and family life. Thus, it is not surprising that, despite shorter hours than other specialties, EPs have one of the highest incidences of burnout in terms of exhaustion and cynicism.[1]

Burnout is an affliction that can affect providers in any medical discipline based on exposure to stress in the workplace. It is now viewed as a serious, widespread problem for all types of health care providers. The prevalence of burnout among US physicians has increased rapidly to epidemic proportions.[2] There is a pressing need to understand the causes of burnout and develop preventive interventions to ensure the health and well-being of the EM workforce and our health care system.

The authors have no financial or commercial conflicts of interest with regards to the material presented.
Department of Emergency Medicine, Beth Israel Deaconess Medical Center, WCC-2, Boston, MA 02215, USA
* Corresponding author.
E-mail address: Lsanche1@bidmc.harvard.edu

BACKGROUND

The first landmark study on burnout, done on flight controllers, was published in 1969. Triggered by a series of fatal midair collisions linked to human error and at the request of the Federal Aviation Institute, a prospective cohort study followed 416 air traffic controllers for more than 3 years. At a time of rapid increase in air traffic, they reported poor training environments, inadequate equipment, changing shift patterns, long shifts without breaks, monotony, and challenges arising from human–machine interfaces. The report defined the resulting professional fatigue as burnout. They also showed that this burnout was associated with an increased incidence of hypertension and the development of psychiatric problems.[3-5]

Burnout was first described in health care providers in1974 by Herbert J. Freudeberger.[6] While working intensively as a psychiatrist in the free clinic movement, he observed and personally experienced a number of psychological findings: exhaustion, excessive involvement with bodily functions, and poor emotional control. Borrowing a term from the drug addict slang of his patients in New York's East Village, he wrote about "staff burn-out": a syndrome defined as failure or exhaustion because of excessive demands on energy, strength, or resources.[6,7] Besides exhaustion, he characterized the syndrome with physical findings (eg, frequent headaches gastrointestinal disorders, insomnia, and shortness of breath), and behavioral symptoms (eg, frustration, anger, paranoia, overconfidence, cynicism, depression, and use of sedatives). He felt that predisposing personality characteristics such as dedication and organizational interventions were risk factors. To prevent burnout, he felt that shorter working hours, regular job rotations, frequent supervision, and staff training would be helpful. Simultaneously, Christina Maslach, a psychologist at the University of Berkeley, showed that nurses had an increased risk for post-traumatic stress disorder factors characterized by negative behavior toward the patient, increased workload, excessive ambiguity, and role conflict.[8]

Maslach broke down burnout into 3 dimensions—emotional exhaustion, depersonalization (ie, cynicism), and a low sense of personal accomplishment—and developed the first survey to measure the incidence and severity of the syndrome. The Maslach Burnout Index (MBI) has been used extensively and is the basis for most measures of burnout[9] and is discussed in detail later in this article. The categorization of burnout as a clinical syndrome has led to a large number of studies over the past 40 years. The initial focus of investigations was in the service industry. It then spread to all professional activities that experience chronic stress.

In 2019, the World Health Organization (WHO) added burnout to its International Classification of Diseases as a syndrome resulting from chronic workplace stress that has not been successfully managed. The WHO characterized burnout by 3 dimensions: (1) feelings of energy depletion or exhaustion, (2) increased mental distance from one's job, or feelings of negativism or cynicism related to one's job, and (3) decreased professional efficacy. According to the WHO, burnout refers specifically to phenomena in the occupational context and should not be applied to describe experiences in other areas of life.[10] Although other life or social stressors can contribute to the general sense of well-being experienced by an individual, burnout refers specifically to the work environment and experience. The chronic nature of burnout is evidence by its stability over time, regardless of the cultural context or length of follow-up surveys.[11]

EPIDEMIOLOGY

With the professional challenges and increasing workload associated with modern practice, more than one-half of US physicians have experienced symptoms of burnout. Those affected have decreased effectiveness and a shortening of their professional lifespan.[12] The adverse effect of the practice of EM on providers begins early in one's professional career as the majority of US EM residents report symptoms consistent with burnout.[13] In one study, EM resident burnout correlated with having a significant other, low job satisfaction, and a lack of clinical and administrative autonomy.[14] Multiple studies have shown that women are disproportionately affected in EM, as in all types of professions.[15,16]

Because burnout impedes cognitive performance by exacerbating negative emotions, it also leads to biased decision making, exacerbating problems such as the disparities in care.[17] The end result is that burnout is contributing to a shortfall of physician manpower and may be causing a deterioration of the quality and equity of care delivered in the emergency setting.

Burnout seems to be worsening over time. The American Board of Emergency Medicine longitudinal study in 2008 showed very high levels of satisfaction with the practice of EM and only one-third of EPs citing burnout as a significant problem.[18] By 2017, the Medscape nationwide survey showed that EPs in North America placed at the top of the burnout risk list, with 59% of providers experiencing symptoms associated with burnout.[1] The 2017 survey also showed that the incidence of burnout had steadily increased over the past years. Juggling multiple patients limits the time needed to provide comfort and maintain emotional equilibrium in upsetting situations. The deterioration of the workplace caused by worsening ED crowding and rising complaints adds to the stress of practicing of EM.[19]

In 2019, the incidence of burnout in EPs has decreased to 48%, although it is unclear whether this decrease is due to improvements in the workplace, interventions with providers to prevent burnout, or insensitivity of the measuring tools. Many of the suspected causes of the increase in burnout, such as implementation of electronic health records and ED crowding, have worsened since 2017. Despite the high incidence of burnout, severity for EPs was below average for medical specialties.[2]

STRESS, BURNOUT PSYCHOLOGY, AND PHYSIOLOGY

Stress can be described as a reaction to particular physiologic stimuli with a range of physiologic and psychological responses. Stress triggers a physiologic response with increased catecholamine levels. Although a certain amount of arousal and stimulation is beneficial to promote learning, cognition, and decision making, stress, for the purposes of our discussion, denotes a level of stimulation or a response that is deleterious or maladaptive. Chronic stress can lead to decreased performance and can negatively impact health. The same stimulus level or situation may yield varying responses in different individuals or in the same individual at different points in time.

Burnout is defined as physical, mental, and emotional exhaustion secondary to stress. This state goes beyond the experience of work-related stress and is defined as a separate psychological state secondary to chronic stress. A similar level of demands (stress) with different levels of perceived control (agency) can lead to a greater likelihood of burnout. Karasek's job demands–control model is the model used for a wide range of research into this topic.[20] In brief, the model postulates that the ability to have control at work can mitigate the strain of work demands. It is not a phenomenon specific to EM, but has been described in detail in many settings. Similar levels of demand can lead to more stress if the individual feels less ability to have control over aspects of the situation. In the ED, many factors can contribute to this loss of control. External mandates, electronic medical records, and physician order entry force physicians to enter data that may not have a direct patient care function, but must still be performed. ED boarding increases the EP's work burden with a set of patients that are better served in the hospital. There are also a myriad of other impositions that have become part of EP's work routine that add to this burden.

The Yerkes-Dodson Law

The Yerkes-Dodson law, sometimes referred to the inverted U theory owing to its graphical representation, outlines the relationship between pressure (ie, stress) and performance.[21] It postulates that both very low and very high levels of stress will lead to lower performance and that moderate levels of stress or demand can result in peak performance. Peak performance, sometimes referred to as a flow state, is something that many individuals experience while performing demanding tasks under moderate levels of stress. Although the theory is most popular in sports psychology, it is illustrative that stress is not always a negative entity; stimulus, stress, or arousal at some level is necessary for a number of physiologic functions and for peak performance.

Health Effects of Burnout and Chronic Stress

Specific emotions caused by stress and fatigue can lead to specific biological changes that may provide independent measures defining burnout. One example was demonstrated in a recent study showing telomere attrition in residents exposed to long work hours.[22] The relationship between burnout and cardiovascular disease may be explained by the enhanced inflammatory response and oxidative injury caused by repeated stress-induced triggering of the active phase response. This response to emotional states is suggested by heighten concentration of C-reactive protein and fibrinogen in women with burnout. In men, this increased was not noted with burnout, but rather with depression.[23] Stress effects of chronic stress and burnout as a risk factor for diabetes, cardiovascular disease, and hypercholesterolemia have all been described.[24–26] Burnout has also been implicated in the development of depression, increased substance abuse, and increased potential for suicide.[1,2,27–29]

CAUSES OF BURNOUT

Maslach has defined 6 dimensions that contribute to burnout:

1. Workload overload
2. Lack of control
3. Insufficient reward
4. Workplace community
5. Absence of fairness
6. Conflicting values

Providers have been surveyed to try to identify and measure the incidence of specific causes of burnout. An excessive number of bureaucratic tasks has been identified as the leading cause. Mandated work not involving patient care is identified as a problem. Specifically, the problems created by increasing computerization of practice, work to ensure optimal payment, and maintenance of certificate requirements are seen as contributing factors.[30] The overall working conditions in terms of too many hours spent at work or reimbursement are also a leading driver when surveying all medical disciplines. Stress and fatigue experienced in the workplace, the threat of malpractice, overexposure to death, violence, and adverse outcomes with patients contribute as well. The lack of professional fulfillment, the inability to keep up with the expansion of new medical knowledge, and the lack of respect from administration, colleagues, and patients are also identified as potential causes. EPs are the least likely physicians to work long hours, suggesting that administrative tasks, lack of respect, and lack of control are the primary drivers of burnout.[1,2] However, the assessment of the work hours of EPs fail to take into account the time spent charting and the fact that hours worked include a much greater proportion of evenings, nights, and weekends when compared with other specialties.[31]

The worsening conditions of the work environment contribute to fatigue, depression, and depersonalization. The aging of the population, the dramatic increase in copays, and the expansion of urgent care centers have resulted in an increase in the acuity and complexity of the average ED patient. Financial pressures and lack of inpatient capacity have led to progressive worsening of ED crowding and a shift of inpatient care from hospitalists and intensivists to EPs. Responsibilities for the care of boarding patients is ill-suited to the environment and the expertise of EPs, with patient waiting time acting as an independent predictor of physician burnout.[32]

SIGNS AND SYMPTOMS

The earliest reports note that fatigue and cynicism are the hallmarks of burnout. The individual reports feeling tired and drained most of the time, and this condition does not respond to adequate rest. Sarcasm, negativism, and worsening interpersonal relations reflect increasing depersonalization. Poor emotional control with outbursts of anger after minimal provocation, frequent crying for no apparent reason, and a lack of empathy with indifference to patients' problems can be observed. The EP will also develop a sense of failure and self-doubt, feelings of helplessness, and a decreased sense of accomplishment. Changes in appetite, sleep habits, and a decrease in libido may occur. Ultimately, clinical depression and suicidal ideation may develop. Freudenberger in his hallmark article described increased somatization and obsession with minor medical complaints such as frequent headaches, back pain, or myalgias.[6] Lowered immunity from stress may increase the risk of viral illness and other infectious disease.[33,34]

MEASUREMENTS OF BURNOUT
The Maslach Burnout Inventory

The MBI is a survey tool designed to assess burnout. It consists of 22 questions using a ranking from 0 to 7 ranging from never to every day.[8,9] The survey measures 3 subscales: emotional exhaustion, depersonalization, and reduced personal accomplishments. It can be self-administered and takes about 15 minutes to complete. It has been widely used and reported in the literature.

The MBI can be administered multiple times and is designed to assess the participant's state of mind at that point in time. As such, it can be used in a longitudinal fashion to assess the well-being of individuals or groups over time. The MBI is the most commonly used tool for measuring burnout in physicians in general and EPs in particular. As designed, the tool has been well-validated for the identification of burnout, but may not be predictive of earlier stages that can result in burnout.

Copenhagen Burnout Inventory

The Copenhagen Burnout Inventory was developed by Danish researchers in response to perceived limitations of the MBI.[35] At the time, the MBI was widely adopted but without validation by a gold standard. The MBI restricts measurements to workers in fields where human interaction is a large component of the work, such as social work and nursing. The MBI assumes that burnout is a single entity with 3 dimensions, yet other studies have not found that personal accomplishment contributes significantly to the syndrome.[36] Emotional exhaustion and depersonalization may also be independent precursors, each with their own consequences rather than connected as a single entity. Finally, the questionnaire developed for American participants confused or angered many of the Danish participants when taking the survey, showing that cultural differences might limit the effectiveness of the MBI.

The Copenhagen Burnout Inventory consists of 3 scales measuring personal burnout, work-related burnout, and client-related burnout. The questions were formulated so that they would apply to workers in all types of industries and cultures. Personal burnout measures the degree of fatigue experienced by the participant, irrespective of work experience or occupational status. Work-related burnout is the degree of fatigue related to the participant's work and explores the participant's perception of how work contributes to the fatigue. These 2 scales help to distinguish fatigue owing to nonwork factors from that caused by work-related stress. Client-related burnout is the degree of fatigue perceived to be related to work with clients. This scale measures the extent to which participants attribute their fatigue to their work with clients (or the appropriate term based on the study group), rather than objectively measuring levels of exhaustion from working with people.

After the initial study, the Copenhagen Burnout Inventory has been validated in Italian teachers with the limitation that it did not specifically measure the effect of the relationship with colleagues and supervisors.[35–39]

Perceived Stress Scale

The Perceived Stress Scale (PSS) is a self-reported survey scale that is used in psychology research to assess an individual's perception of their level of stress.[40] There has been limited use of the PSS as a measure of stress in EM, but preliminary studies exist.[41] The PSS may be useful to identify individuals who may have greater difficulty managing stress, which may help to target early interventions to prevent burnout.

The PSS consists of 10 questions rated in a 0 to 4 scale. It is not a static measurement and changes over time, reflective of an individual's current and recent situation. Higher levels of perceived stress have been shown to have a physiologic effect, such as glycemic control in diabetics.[42]

State Trait Anxiety Inventory

The State Trait Anxiety Inventory (STAI) is a survey test aimed at assessing an individual's propensity to experience anxiety when faced with stress.[43] It was first described in 1976 and has been widely used in a variety of settings. The STAI is meant to describe an individual's general propensity to experience stress and is interpreted as a relatively stable personality trait rather than a variable day-to-day assessment of general stress level, which is what the PSS attempts to measure. There is a close correlation identified between the STAI and the PSS in EPs.[41]

Grit Scale

The Grit Scale is a recently developed measurement of the ability of individuals to maintain focus on long-term goals.[44] It was found to be predictive of long-term goal success in areas such as college GPA and improved success in West Point cadets. Grit is an independent character trait from what the STAI measures and was not found to be correlated with STAI in EPs.[41] Grit was also not found to correlate with cortisol levels, which were used as a surrogate marker for stress.[45]

Physiologic Measurements

To date, stress and burnout measurement tools are mostly reliant on surveys or questionnaires. The advantage of these is the ease of administration. More physiologic measurements, such as cortisol, telomere aging, and heart rate variability, may be better markers of physiologic injury, but are significantly more difficult to perform and may be logistically prohibitive to do in a broad and recurrent fashion. The MBI has become the default measurement tool in the medical field, with the majority of physician studies in the literature using it as the measurement tool.[46] This situation is limiting, because the MBI is not helpful in predicting burnout. Better tools to assess predisposition to maladaptive responses to stress would be of value to identify individuals at earlier stages of the process.

CONSEQUENCES OF BURNOUT

Burnout leads to a series of changes in attitude, job performance, and, ultimately, mental health disorders. Chronic stress also has a number of deleterious physiologic and health consequences, as discussed elsewhere in this article. Depression can be severe occasionally resulting in suicide, which is much higher in the physician population.[27,29]

Burnout has widespread consequences that reach beyond the individual provider. Provider dissatisfaction and attrition from medical practice can all be downstream effects of individual burnout.[27] Physician performance is also diminished.[47] By decreasing professional longevity and effectiveness, burnout exacerbates the shortage of EPs. Burned out physicians are unlikely to seek professional treatment and may attempt to deal with their substance abuse, depression, and suicidal thoughts alone.

Another consequence of provider burnout is the adverse effect it has on patient care. A large number of studies over the past 20 years have shown that physician burnout worsens clinical care and causes medical errors. These findings have relied on physician self-assessment and more objective measures of preventable adverse events or errors are needed to measure the actual harm that occurs.[48–50] In a meta-analysis in 2018, burnout was found to be associated with twice the odds of involvement in patient safety incidents. This finding was also true for symptoms of depression and emotional distress in physicians.[51]

As expected, patient satisfaction is also negatively affected by burnout.[52] In particular, depersonalization was associated with 4.5-fold increased odds for low patient-reported satisfaction.[51]

Cynicism and loss of empathy can lead to greater explicit and implicit racial biases, worsening racial disparities in health care.[17] There are no good estimates quantifying the systemwide effects of shortened careers, increased errors, and decreased efficiency and productivity, all of which can result from chronic stress and burnout.

Moral Injury

Recently, there has been a movement to reframe the burnout epidemic not as something that can be remedied by wellness programs, but as an issue resulting from moral injury.[53] Moral injury is a term first used to describe experiences in war veterans.[54] The moral injury paradigm can be useful to reframe the burnout conversation in a way that recognizes that providers are at the mercy of institutional factors that have significant effects on their practice, work environment, and experience that are outside of their control but have significant effects on their ability to provide quality patient care. This may be in part a reaction to the perception that burnout is often regarded as an individual problem and to shift the focus to the systemic work environment barriers to patient care.[55] The WHO definition of burnout recognizes the large role the work environment plays in individual burnout, and it may not be necessary to compare the stress of working in an ED, even when faced with all the daily frustrations and barriers to care, with the experience of soldiers in battle.

PREVENTION AND INTERVENTIONS

A number of studies have reported on interventions to decrease or prevent burnout. These interventions can be broken down into 2 types of strategies: those that help individuals to decrease stress through different types of meditation, stress management training programs, or discussion groups, and those that act by altering the working environment.[56–61] Both interventions targeting individual practitioners' ability to cope with stress and those modifying the organization of the workplace resulted in statistically significant reduction in burnout scores in emotional exhaustion and depersonalization.[46] Only 1 study from Ireland has looked at interventions in EPs.[57] Using an attention-based training program, based on Mantra meditation, the investigators were able to decrease the emotional exhaustion component of the MBI as well as improve in biological markers of well-being such as proinflammatory cytokines.

There is very little published with regards to system interventions aimed at decreasing nonprovider sources of stress. The electronic medical record has been shown to be an added source of stress for physician practice.[30] Interventions aimed at decreasing the burden of health information technology could help to decrease the overall daily work-related stress. Issues that affect the ED disproportionately, but are outside of direct ED control, such as boarding and crowding, should also be targets for intervention if the goal is to decrease burnout and improve the work environment.

Cognitive–Behavioral Techniques

Although there is no published literature in EM showing that older physicians underperform on overnight shifts or suffer from greater physiologic stress after working an overnight, many EM groups transition their more senior providers out of overnights. This strategy recognizes the fact that these are shifts that require greater time to recover from than a comparable day shift. Circadian solutions to decrease the physiologic burden of overnight shifts have been proposed, such as the concept of anchor sleep. When possible, circadian considerations should be part of the creation of provider schedules in an attempt to manage this source of physiologic stress.

The American College of Emergency Physicians has published recommendations with regards to shift length, frequency, and circadian progression[62,63] (**Box 1**). The guidelines recommend shifts being scheduled in a forward rotating circadian pattern when possible. Although there is no specific recommendation with regard to the number of consecutive shifts worked, there is a recognition that working many shifts in a row can be damaging. The recommendations addressing night shifts is to either minimize the number of night shifts done in a row (ideally only one) or to do blocks of nights a limited number of times a year. Depending on other constraints, shorter shifts are preferable to longer shifts (8 hours vs 12 hours). There are several published articles showing decreasing numbers of new patients for every subsequent hour on shift.[64–66]

Many factors will affect how ED groups schedule their shifts with regards to length and nights. In EDs with low volume during night shifts, several hours of sleep may be possible. This allows for different solutions with shift length and overnight work when compared with higher volume EDs, which may require more than a single physician for

---

Box 1
American College of Emergency Physicians shift recommendations regarding circadian rhythms and shift work

Isolated night shifts or long sequences of nights

Avoid long stretches of shifts

Shifts should last 12 hours or less

Rotating shifts in a clockwise manner

Regularly scheduled periods of at least 24 hours off work

Data from American College of Emergency Physicians. Emergency Physician Shift Work [Internet]. 2017. Available at: https://www.acep.org/patient-care/policy-statements/emergency-physician-shift-work/#sm.00001fag7md9wf4x1199q1z4gowni. Accessed 1 August 2019.

---

coverage during all or parts of the day. In general, 8-hour shifts are preferable to 12-hour shifts and forward rotating circadian patterns are less physiologically difficult.

LIMITATIONS AND FUTURE DIRECTIONS OF BURNOUT RESEARCH

Despite considerable productivity and scholarly work over the past 40 years, there remains serious concerns about burnout research and the validity of the findings.[35,67] Burnout is measured by self-assessment surveys. These are based on an empiric definition and rising scores have not been shown to predict that the full spectrum of burnout will occur. The method of measuring burnout causes a circular validation of the empiric definition, because there is yet to be a gold standard for burnout in terms of a biological profile. Psychologically, burnout itself may not be a single clinical entity, but simply a combination of mental health disorders, each resulting from stress at the workplace and independent of the others. The potential for missing major depression by mislabeling individuals as burned out exists.[68] Methods of measurement to predict the development of burnout in a person and to measure the effectiveness of preventive interventions are still needed. Further studies are also needed to determine the relationship between burnout scores and the degree of patient harm that it causes. In addition to self-assessment surveys, new measurement tools of burnout need to be developed using biological markers or assessment by unbiased observers, supervisors, colleagues, or patients. This is needed to validate that burnout is indeed an independent clinical entity, to determine the true underlying drivers of the syndrome, and to develop effective preventing measures.

EM is by nature a stressful profession. The risk of adverse outcomes and errors is constantly present from having to make split second decisions in critical patients with minimal background information. Distractions and interruptions are common in busy EDs. Because there is no prior patient–physician relationship, patient hostility and even violence targeted against providers are common occurrences. The choice of a specialty is a critical decision and is often made with misconceptions about the reality of routine practice. Different individuals have different personalities, skill sets, and talents that may either help or detract from the ability to perform as needed and to deal with stress. Optimizing the environment and training providers in stress management may certainly mitigate the development of burnout. However, the risk of provider burnout may be associated with longstanding, maladaptive personality tendencies that predate entrance into medical training.[69] If true, there is an opportunity to intervene before training starts or even during residency training by redirecting the candidate to a more suitable specialty. Ensuring that an EM candidate has the right personality for the job could be incorporated into the matching process. Tailoring interventions to the trainee's personality might also enhance the effectiveness of stress management programs. Screening criteria for risk of burnout could be used as a part of the selection process to prevent putting someone through the rigors of specialty training that will lead to a personal psychic damage and patient harm. Personality traits present before training as a practicing physician found to correlate with burnout included low self-esteem, feelings of inadequacy, dysphoria and obsessive worry, passivity, social anxiety, and withdrawal from others.[69]

The importance of personality in the development of burnout has been described in a number of reports.[70–72] Determining the specific personality traits best suited to avoid burnout in the practice of EM appear to be a yet uncovered but potentially fruitful area for research.

SUMMARY

Burnout in the practice of EM presents a growing risk to patient care and effectiveness of the EM workforce. A greater understanding of the underlying causes and interventions needed to ensure wellness is a worthwhile goal. Work should not be harmful to your health. Although this is an obvious statement for individuals, it should also be a clear priority from an institutional perspective. At the most basic transactional level, happier employees tend to be more productive and have greater longevity at their job, which translates into a higher institutional yield per provider. EPs, when advocating for their groups, need to be able to argue these priorities in ways that are effective for enacting meaningful change. At the administrative and institutional levels, return on investment arguments often carry more weight.

Wellness programs need to go beyond providing healthy snacks and exercise programs to truly have a meaningful impact. At the individual level, helping people with resilience techniques, stress management resources, and mechanisms for early identification and intervention are a good starting point and should be within reach of even small provider groups.

At the system level, highlighting areas that are outside the control of the individual but may be amenable to group or institutional intervention is key. Within EM groups, evaluation of patient loads, hours worked, and time spent outside of scheduled hours documenting or engaging in other administrative duties can help to decrease the level of stress to a level that is manageable and less likely to lead to burnout.

Institution-level interventions and commitment to decrease issues such as boarding, difficulty obtaining consults, or having adequate resources to care for patients can lead to greater perceptions of agency at work and improve job satisfaction and longevity. It is also better patient care.

Stress in EM is multifactorial. Although some of the stress experienced is part and parcel of the profession, a lot of it can be mitigated even when not able to be fully eliminated. A number of interventions will likely be necessary to address the different sources of stress at work.

REFERENCES

1. Peckham C. Medscape national physician burnout and depression report 2018. Available at: https://www.medscape.com/slideshow/2018-lifestyle-burnout-depression-6009235. Accessed August 1, 2019.

2. Kane L. Medscape national physician burnout and depression report 2019. Available at: https://www.medscape.com/slideshow/2019-lifestyle-burnout-depression-6011056. Accessed August 1, 2019.

3. Samra R. Brief history of burnout. We have much to learn from established countermeasures in aviation. BMJ 2018;363:k5268.

4. Controller Stress. The PATCO Journal 1969;36–9.

5. Rose RM, Jenkins CD, Hurst MW. Air traffic controller health change study. Report prepared by Boston University School of Medicine for US Dept of Transportation. FAA Office of Aviation Medicine; 1978. Report No. FAA AM-78/39.

6. Freudenberger H. Staff burn-out. J Soc Issues 1974;90(1):159–65.

7. Freudenberger HJ. The staff burn-out syndrome in alternative institutions. Psychother Theor Res Pract Train 1975;12(1):73–82.

8. Maslach C. Burned-out. Hum Behav 1976;5:16–22.

9. Maslach C, Jackson SE, Leiter MP. Maslach burnout inventory. 3rd edition. Palo Alto (CA): Consulting Psychologists Press; 1996.

10. WHO burnout classification. Available at: https://icd.who.int/browse11/l-m/en#/http://id.who.int/icd/entity/129180281. Accessed August 1, 2019.

11. Shirom A, Melamed S. Does burnout affect physical health? A review of the evidence. Chapter 39. In: Antoniou ASG, Cooper CL, editors. Research companion to organizational health psychology. Cheltenham (UK): Edward Elgar Publishing; 2005. p. 599–622.

12. Dyrbye LN, Varkey P, Boone SL, et al. Physician satisfaction and burnout at different career stages. Mayo Clin Proc 2013;88(12):1358–67.

13. Lin M, Battaglioli N, Melamed M, et al. High prevalence of burnout among us emergency medicine residents: results from the 2017 National Emergency Medicine Wellness Survey. Ann Emerg Med 2019. https://doi.org/10.1016/j.annemergmed.2019.01.037 [pii:S0196-0644(19)30064-2].

14. Takayesu JK, Ramoska EA, Clark TR, et al. Factors associated with burnout during emergency medicine residency. Acad Emerg Med 2014;21:1031–5.

15. Marchand A, Blanc ME, Beauregard N. Do age and gender contribute to workers' burnout symptoms? Occup Med 2018;68:405–11.

16. McMurray JE, Linzer M, Konrad TR, et al. The work lives of women physicians results from the physician work life study. The SGIM career satisfaction study group. J Gen Intern Med 2000;15(6):372–80.

17. Dyrbye L, Herin J, West CP, et al. Association of Racial Bias With Burnout Among Resident Physicians. JAMA Netw Open 2019;2(7):e197457.

18. Cydulka RK, Korte R. Career satisfaction in emergency medicine: the ABEM Longitudinal Study of Emergency Physicians. Ann Emerg Med 2008;51(6):714–22.

19. Atkinson P, Ducharme J, Campbell S. #Burnout - Burnout is inevitable in clinical emergency medicine practice. CJEM 2017;19(5):386–9.

20. Karasek RA. Job demands, job decision latitude, and mental strain: implications for job redesign. Admin Sci Q 1979;24(2):285–308.

21. Yerkes RM, Dodson JD. The relation of strength of stimulus to rapidity of habit-formation. Journal of Comparative Neurology and Psychology 1908;18(5):459–82.

22. Ridout KK, Ridout SJ, Guille C, et al. Physician training stress and accelerated cellular aging. Biol Psychol 2019;86(9):725–30.

23. Toker S, Shirom A, Shapira I, et al. The association between burnout, depression, anxiety, and inflammation biomarkers: C-reactive protein and fibrinogen in men and women. J Occup Health Psychol 2005;10(4):344–62.

24. Melamed S, Shirom A, Toker S, et al. Burnout and risk of cardiovascular disease: evidence, possible causal paths, and promising research directions. Psychol Bull 2006;132(3):327–53.
25. Shirom A, Toker S, Melamed S, et al. Life and job satisfaction as predictors of the incidence of diabetes. Appl Psychol Health Well Being 2012;4(1):31–48.
26. Shirom A, Toker S, Melamed S, et al. Burnout and vigor as predictors of the incidence of hyperlipidemia among healthy employees. Appl Psychol Health Well Being 2013;5(1):79–98.
27. Stehman CR, Testo Z, Gershaw RS, et al. Burnout, drop out, suicide: physician loss in Emergency Medicine, Part 1. West J Emerg Med 2019;20(3):485–94.
28. Shanafelt TD, Boone S, Tan L, et al. Burnout and satisfaction with work-life balance among US physicians relative to the general US population. Arch Intern Med 2012;172(18):1377–85.
29. Schernhammer ES, Colditz GA. Suicide rates among physicians: a quantitative and gender assessment (meta-analysis). Am J Psychiatry 2004;161(12): 2295–302.
30. Gardner RL, Cooper E, Haskell J, et al. Physician stress and burnout: the impact of health information technology. J Am Med Inform Assoc 2019;26(2):106–14.
31. Machi MS, Staum M, Callaway CW, et al. The relationship between shift work, sleep, and cognition in career emergency physicians. Acad Emerg Med 2012; 19(1):85–91.
32. De Stefano C, Phillipon AL, Krastinova E, et al. Effect of emergency physician burnout on patient waiting times. Intern Emerg Med 2018;13(3):421–8.
33. Cohen S, Williamson GM. Stress and infectious disease in humans. Psychol Bull 1991;109(1):5–24.
34. Cohen S, Tyrrell DA, Smith AP. Psychological stress and susceptibility to the common cold. N Engl J Med 1991;325:606–12.
35. Kristensen TS, Borritz M, Villadsen E, et al. The Copenhagen Burnout Inventory: a new tool for the assessment of burnout. Work Stress 2005;19(3):192–207.
36. Schutte N, Toppinen S, Kalimo R, et al. The factorial validity of the Maslach Burnout Inventory-General Survey (MBI-GS) across occupational groups and nations. Br J Educ Psychol 2000;73(1):53–66.
37. Fiorilli C, De Staso S, Benevene P, et al. Copenhagen Burnout Inventory (CBI): a validation study in an Italian Teacher Group. TPM 2015;22(4):537–51.
38. Milfont TL, Denny S, Ameratunga S, et al. Burnout and wellbeing: testing the Copenhagen Burnout Inventory in New Zealand teachers. Soc Ind Res 2008;89(1): 169–77.
39. Sestili C, Scalingi S, Cianfanelli S, et al. Reliability and use of Copenhagen Burnout Inventory in Italian sample of university professors. Int J Environ Res Public Health 2018;15:1708.
40. Cohen S, Kamarck T, Mermelstein R. A global measure of perceived stress. J Health Soc Behav 1983;24:385–96.
41. Wong ML, Anderson J, Knorr T, et al. Grit, anxiety, and stress in emergency physicians. Am J Emerg Med 2018;36:1036–9.
42. Vasanth R, Ganesh A, Shanker R. Impact of stress on type 2 diabetes mellitus management. Psychiatr Danub 2017;29(S3):416–21.
43. Kendall P, Finch A Jr, Auerbach S. The state-trait anxiety inventory: a systematic evaluation. J Consult Clin Psychol 1976;44:406–12.
44. Duckworth AL, Peterson C, Matthews MD, et al. Grit: perseverance and passion for long-term goals. J Pers Soc Psychol 2007;92:1087–101.

45. Wong ML, Peters G, Joseph JW, et al. Salivary cortisol concentrations, grit, and the effect of time. AEM Educ Train 2019 May 20;4(1):30–5.

46. West C, Dyrbye LN, Erwin PJ, et al. Interventions to prevent and reduce physician burnout: a systematic review and meta-analysis. Lancet 2016;388(10057): 2272–81.

47. Dewa CS, Loong D, Bonato S, et al. How does burnout affect physician productivity? A systematic literature review. BMC Health Serv Res 2014;14:325.

48. Firth-Cozens J, Greenhalgh J. Doctors' perceptions of the links between stress and lowered clinical care. Soc Sci Med 1997;44:1017–22.

49. Shanafelt T, Bradley K, Wipf J, et al. Burnout and selfreported patient care in an Internal Medicine residency program. Ann Intern Med 2002;136:358–67.

50. West C, Huschka M, Novotny P, et al. Association of perceived medical errors with resident distress and empathy: a prospective longitudinal study. JAMA 2006;296:1071–8.

51. Panagioti M, Geraghty K, Johnson J, et al. Association between physician burnout and patient safety, professionalism, and patient satisfaction: a systematic review and meta-analysis. JAMA Intern Med 2018;178(10):1317–31.

52. Haas J, Cook E, Puopolo A, et al. Is the professional satisfaction of general internist associated with patient satisfaction? J Gen Intern Med 2000;15:122–8.

53. Talbot SG, Dean W. Statnews.com. 2018. Available at: https://www.statnews.com/2018/07/26/physicians-not-burning-out-they-are-suffering-moral-injury/. Accessed August 1, 2019.

54. Litz BT, Stein N, Delaney E, et al. Moral injury and moral repair in war veterans: a preliminary model and intervention strategy. Clin Psychol Rev 2009;29(8): 695–706.

55. Dean W. Why Burnout is the wrong term for physician suffering. Medscape. Available at: https://www.medscape.com/viewarticle/915097?src=WNL_bom_190728_MSCPEDIT&uac=198976CY&impID=2040534&faf=1. Accessed August 1, 2019.

56. Oman D, Hedberg J, Thorensen CE. Passage meditation reduces perceived stress in health professionals: a randomized, controlled trial. J Consult Clin Psychol 2006;74(4):714–9.

57. Dunne PJ, Lynch J, Prihodova L, et al. Burnout in the emergency department: randomized controlled trial of an attention-based training program. J Integr Med 2019;17(3):173–80.

58. Butow P, Cockburn J, Girgis A, et al. Increasing oncologists' skills in eliciting and responding to emotional cues: evaluation of a communication skills training program. Psychooncology 2008;17:209–18.

59. Bragard I, Etienne A, Merckaert I, et al. Efficacy of a communication and stress management training on medical residents' self-efficacy, stress to communicate and burnout. J Health Psychol 2010;15:1075–81.

60. West CP, Dyrbye LN, Rabatin JT, et al. Intervention to promote physician well-being, job satisfaction, and professionalism: a randomized clinical trial. JAMA Intern Med 2014;174:527–33.

61. Lucas BP, Trick WE, Evans AT, et al. Effects of 2- vs 4-week attending physician inpatient rotations on unplanned patient revisits, evaluations by trainees, and attending physician burnout: a randomized trial. JAMA 2012;308:2199–207.

62. American College of Emergency Physicians. Emergency physician shift work 2017. Available at: https://www.acep.org/patient-care/policy-statements/emergency-physician-shift-work/#sm.00001fag7md9wf4x1199q1z4gowni. Accessed August 1, 2019.

63. Circadian rhythms and shift work: policy resource and education paper (PREP). Irving (TX): American College of Emergency Physicians; 2017.
64. Jeanmonod R, Jeanmonod D, Ngiam R. Resident productivity: does shift length matter? Am J Emerg Med 2008;26:789–91.
65. Joseph JW, Henning DJ, Strouse CS, et al. Modeling hourly resident productivity in the emergency department. Ann Emerg Med 2017;70(2):185–90.
66. Joseph JW, Davis S, Wilker EH, et al. Modeling attending physician productivity in the emergency department: a multi-center study. Emerg Med J 2018;35(5): 317–22.
67. Eckleberry-Hunt J, Kirkpatrick H, Barbera T. The Problems with Burnout Research. Acad Med 2018;93(3):367–70.
68. Oquendo MA, Bernstein CA, Mayer LES. A key differential diagnosis for physicians-major depression or burnout. JAMA Psychiatry 2019. https://doi.org/10.1001/jamapsychiatry.2019.1332. Accessed August 15, 2019.
69. McCranie EW, Brandsma JM. personality antecedents of burnout among middle-aged physicians. Behav Med 1988;14(1):30–6.
70. McManus IC, Keeling A, Paice E. Stress, burnout and doctors' attitudes to work are determined by personality and learning style: a twelve year longitudinal study of UK medical graduates. BMC Med 2004;2(29):1–12.
71. Mustafa OM. Health behaviors and personality in burnout: a third dimension. Med Educ Online 2015;20(1). https://doi.org/10.3402/meo.v20.28187.
72. Alarcon G, Eschleman KJ, Bowling NA. Relationships between personality variables and burnout: a meta-analysis. Work Stress 2009;23(3):244–63.

Emergency Department Operations I

Emergency Medical Services and Patient Arrival

Kenneth Knowles, MD[a],*,
Gerald (Wook) Beltran, DO, MPH, MSIS, MSCJA[a], Lucas Grover, MD[b]

KEYWORDS

- Risk mitigation • ETMALA • Hospital triage • Waiting room safety
- Left without being seen

KEY POINTS

- Mitigation of risk before patient arrival with the proper management of medical control for prehospital services.
- The Emergency Medical Treatment and Active Labor Act (EMTALA) is briefly reviewed, including the statutory obligations and liabilities.
- On patient arrival to the hospital, triage in the emergency department is reviewed with proposed best practices to minimize risk in triage, including the necessary requirements of a proper medical screening examination.
- For patients who are not brought directly back into the department, this article reviews techniques for decreasing risk in the waiting room patient.
- Responsibilities for patients who leave the emergency department without being seen.

INTRODUCTION

The emergency department (ED) is by its nature inherently an environment with the potential for chaos because of the high volume and varied types of patients cared for in an ED setting. This chaos can create a risk to the patients, the providers, and the health care system. This article discusses ED operations risk from the prehospital environment through patients' arrival before being placed in an ED bed.

MEDICAL CONTROL

According to the National Association of State EMS Officials, "Emergency Medical Services (EMS) is the integrated system of medical response established and

[a] Department of Emergency Medicine, Division of Prehospital and Disaster Medicine, Baystate Medical Center, 759 Chestnut Street, Springfield, MA 01199, USA; [b] Department of Emergency Medicine, Baystate Health, 759 Chestnut Street, Springfield, MA 01199, USA
* Corresponding author.
E-mail address: kenneth.knowlesMD@baystatehealth.org

Emerg Med Clin N Am 38 (2020) 311–321
https://doi.org/10.1016/j.emc.2020.01.001
0733-8627/20/© 2020 Elsevier Inc. All rights reserved.
emed.theclinics.com

designed to respond, assess, treat, monitor observe, and determine the disposition of patients with injury or illness and those in need of medically safe transportation."[1] The National Association of State EMS Officials document "The Definition of EMS" states that "EMS is the practice of medicine and as such, any of the activities that constitute EMS require oversight by a physician."[1]

The topic of proper management of medical control for prehospital services is vast and extremely nuanced. As such, it is recommended that those serving as an EMS medical director be board certified in EMS medicine.[2] Proper medical control starts with a close working relationship between the EMS services and the EMS medical director. It is important that the EMS medical director be available and visible to the providers in the service and to the service directors.

The EMS medical director should have authority for oversight of verification of provider competency and provider credentialing.[2] Furthermore, the EMS medical director must be intimately involved in the continuous quality improvement (CQI) process. This allows him or her to identify trends and opportunities within their region or a specific service. The involvement of the EMS medical director in CQI should come in the form of direct and indirect CQI. Direct CQI involves the EMS medical director participating in patient care in the field. This allows the EMS medical director to identify opportunities and address them in real time. Indirect CQI involves the review of patient care reports. Both forms of CQI have their own advantages and a combination of the two is vital to effective CQI. The role of the EMS medical director is vital but for it to be successful, the EMS medical director must also be empowered to "develop and implement education standards for all providers who work in the EMS service."[2]

EMS regulations vary in each state. Therefore, it is important for physicians responsible for medical control of prehospital services to be well versed in the state or local regulations for EMS. Most of what prehospital providers do in the field is based on the available protocols and standing orders, known as offline medical control. Therefore, the EMS medical director should actively review and improve current protocols and work to develop new ones. For those physicians who receive live requests from providers, known as online medical control, it is important that they are familiar with the protocols and the scope of practice of the provider.

Patient refusals are common for EMS but pose a patient and medical legal risk. In general, a patient who is refusing care needs to have capacity, clinical sobriety, be informed of the risks of refusing care in terms they can understand, and, if possible, have alternatives discussed. Online medical control can and should be used for guidance and assistance in high-risk situations. In some situations, it is appropriate for the online medical control physician to speak directly to the patient. There are many advantages to speaking directly to the patient. For one, it allows the online medical control physician to perform their own assessment of the patient's capacity. Each state is different regarding the regulations surrounding bringing a patient to the ED against their will. For example, in Massachusetts, a patient who is presenting for a complaint related to a psychiatric illness and lacks capacity for this reason can be brought to the ED on a Section 12A. However, a patient who lacks capacity because of drugs or alcohol intoxication cannot be brought on a Section 12A. In this situation, the police must be involved for assistance in bringing the patient to the ED under protective custody. Given the statutory and regulatory variation among states, it is important for the online medical control physician to be intimately familiar with their state statutory and regulatory requirements to be able to guide EMS.

The Emergency Medical Treatment and Active Labor Act

The Emergency Medical Treatment and Active Labor Act (EMTALA), which was signed into law on April 7, 1986, was in response to several high-profile incidents in which underinsured or uninsured patients were denied or delayed care at several private hospitals. The Federal Statutes, specifically 42 USC §1395dd(a),[3] states that a hospital must "provide for an appropriate medical screening examination within the capability of the hospital emergency department." This applies to "any individual" who "comes to the emergency department" and makes a request for examination and/or treatment. Specifically, examination and treatment cannot be delayed to enquire about insurance status or method of payment. In face 42 USC §489.24(d)(4) advises the following regarding delay in examination or treatment:

i. A participating hospital may not delay providing an appropriate medical screening examination required under paragraph (a) of this section or further medical examination and treatment required under paragraph (d)(1) of this section in order to inquire about the individual's method of payment or insurance status.

ii. A participating hospital may not seek, or direct an individual to seek, authorization from the individual's insurance company for screening or stabilization services to be furnished by a hospital, physician, or nonphysician practitioner to an individual until after the hospital has provided the appropriate medical screening examination required under paragraph (a) of this section, and initiated any further medical examination and treatment that may be required to stabilize the emergency medical condition under paragraph (d)(1) of this section.

iii. An emergency physician or nonphysician practitioner is not precluded from contacting the individual's physician at any time to seek advice regarding the individual's medical history and needs that may be relevant to the medical treatment and screening of the patient, as long as this consultation does not inappropriately delay services required under paragraph (a) or paragraphs (d)(1) and (d)(2) of this section.

iv. Hospitals may follow reasonable registration processes for individuals for whom examination or treatment is required by this section, including asking whether an individual is insured and, if so, what that insurance is, as long as that inquiry does not delay screening or treatment. Reasonable registration processes may not unduly discourage individuals from remaining for further evaluation.

Moreover, EDs must post signs notifying their patients and the public of their rights to a medical screening examination (MSE) and treatment and the hospital's EMTALA obligations.

EMTALA: Emergency condition: Emergency Medical Treatment and Active Labor Act

This statute further states that the purpose of screening examinations is to "determine whether or not an emergency medical condition....exists".[4] This statute (42 USC §1395dd [e][1]) defines that an emergency condition is:

A. A medical condition manifesting itself by acute symptoms of sufficient severity (including severe pain) such that the absence of immediate medical attention could reasonably be expected to result in:
   a. Placing the health of the individual (or, with respect to a pregnant woman, the health of the woman or her unborn child) in serious jeopardy,
   b. Serious impairment to bodily functions, or
   c. Serious dysfunction of any bodily organ or part; or

B. With respect to a pregnant woman who is having contractions -
   a. That there is inadequate time to effect a safe transfer to another hospital before delivery, or
   b. That transfer may pose a threat to the health or safety of the woman or the unborn child.

If the appropriate MSE identifies that the patient has an emergency medical condition, then the statute further advises that the hospital may provide "such further medical examination and such treatment as may be required to stabilize the medical condition,"[4] or the hospital may transfer the patient "to another medical facility...."[5] Stabilization or "to stabilize" is defined under this statute as, "with respect to an emergency medical condition described in paragraph (1)(A), to provide such medical treatment of the condition as may be necessary to assure, within reasonable medical probability, that no material deterioration of the condition is likely to result from or occur during the transfer of the individual from a facility, or, with respect to an emergency medical condition...."[6]

EMTALA: Enforcement
The US Department of Health and Human Services (HHS) is responsible for enforcing EMTALA. The Office of the Inspector General (OIG) is responsible for civil monetary penalties, whereas the Center for Medicare and Medicaid Services (CMS) is responsible for termination sanctions. Both of these agencies report up to HHS.

Action on EMTALA can occur in two ways. The first is by administrative enforcement action through OIG or CMS. Through the OIG, the hospital can receive a maximum monetary penalty of $104,826 per violation if the hospital has more than 100 beds or $52,414 per violation if the hospital has less than 100 beds. Additionally, CMS can take administrative enforcement actions by terminating a hospital from participating as a Medicare provider. In addition to the hospital, the involved provider can have enforcement action against him or her. The maximum financial penalty the OIG can give a physician is up to $104,826, although a recent ruling (Fed Regist. 2017;82:9129-9174) mentions a civil penalty of $52,414 but it is not clear if this was a policy statement or an inaccurate statement by HHS. As with the hospitals, CMS can terminate a medical provider's ability to participate as a Medicare provider.

The second way that EMTALA is enforced, is through civil lawsuits. The civil lawsuit is against the hospital. This suit is considered in addition to, and not a replacement for, state tort claims of medical malpractice. Additionally, punitive damages may be assessed if the law of the state in which the hospital is located permits such damages. Civil lawsuits for EMTALA violations can only be made against a hospital, and not the medical provider.[7]

EMTALA: Patient arriving at the emergency department
One of the elements that is important to consider under EMTALA is when a patient "comes to the ED." There are four ways in which a patient could be considered as coming to the ED. First, is if the patient presents to a hospital's dedicated ED and requests care for medical treatment or could reasonably be interpreted as a request for care. Second, is if the patient is outside of the dedicated ED, but is on hospital property within 250 yards of the main building and presents with a potential emergency condition. Third, is if a patient is in a hospital owned and operated ambulance for the express purpose of examination and/or treatment of a medical condition, even if the ambulance is not on hospital property. Fourth, is if the patient arrives at the hospital's dedicated ED in an ambulance not owned by the hospital.

Helipad and helicopter An interesting recognized exception to a patient "comes to the ED" is the hospital helipad. The hospital helipad by itself does not trigger EMTALA. If a service uses the helipad simply to obtain access for loading into the helicopter and there is not a specific request for an MSE, or the helicopter is owned by the hospital and is bringing a patient to the hospital for care, then this does not usually trigger an EMTALA obligation. In fact the State Operations Manual advises the following two circumstances will not trigger EMTALA[8]:

- The use of a hospital's helipad by local ambulance services or other hospitals for the transport of individuals to tertiary hospitals located throughout the State does not trigger an EMTALA obligation for the hospital that has the helipad on its property when the helipad is being used for the purpose of transit as long as the sending hospital conducted the Medical Screening Examination prior to transporting the individual to the helipad for medical helicopter transport to a designated recipient hospital. The sending hospital is responsible for conducting the Medical Screening Examination prior to transfer to determine if an emergency medical condition exists and implementing stabilizing treatment, or conducting an appropriate transfer. Therefore, if the helipad serves simply as a point of transit for individuals who have received a Medical Screening Examination performed prior to transfer to the helipad, the hospital with the helipad is not obligated to perform another Medical Screening Examination prior to the individual's continued travel to the recipient hospital. If, however, while at the helipad, the individual's condition deteriorates, the hospital at which the helipad is located must provide a Medical Screening Examination and stabilizing treatment within its capacity *if requested* by medical personnel accompanying the individual.
- If as part of the EMS protocol, EMS activates helicopter evacuation of an individual with a potential emergency medical condition, the hospital that has the helipad does not have an EMTALA obligation if they are not the recipient hospital, unless a request is made by EMS personnel, the individual, or a legally responsible person acting on the individual's behalf for the examination or treatment of an emergency medical condition.

EMTALA: Request for examination
Under EMTALA, there are two ways that an individual could be construed as requesting medical care[9]:

- If the individual makes a specific request (or a request is made on the individual's behalf) for examination or treatment of a medical condition; or
- The individual's appearance or behavior would cause (or not cause) a "prudent layperson observer" to believe that examination or treatment of a medical condition is needed and that the individual would request that examination or treatment for himself or herself if he or she were able to do so.

EMTALA: Inpatients
The EMTALA regulatory requirement ends once a patient is admitted as an inpatient. The Code of Federal Regulations advises that: "if an emergency medical condition is determined to exist, (the hospital) must provide any necessary stabilizing treatment, as defined in paragraph (d) of this section, or an appropriate transfer as defined in (e) of this section. If the hospital admits the individual as an inpatient for further treatment, the hospital's obligation under this section ends, as specified in paragraph (d)(2) of this section."[10]

In fact the Code of Federal Regulations defines what is considered "inpatient" as: "an individual who is admitted to a hospital for bed occupancy for purposes of receiving inpatient hospital services as described in Section 409.10(a) of this article with the expectation that he or she will remain at least overnight and occupy a bed even though the situation later develops that the individual can be discharged or transferred to another hospital and does not actually use a hospital bed overnight."[11]

Medical Screening Examination

CMS-1063-F, which discusses EMTALA requires "an appropriate medical screening examination for any individual who requests it (or has a request made on his [or her] behalf) to determine whether an emergency medical condition exists or if the patient is in active labor."[12] It is not well defined what constitutes an appropriate MSE. According to EMTALA, "a medical screening examination is the process required to reach, with reasonable clinical confidence, the point at which it can be determined whether the individual has an emergency medical condition or not. A medical screening examination is not an isolated event. It is an ongoing process that begins, but typically does not end, with triage."[13] An MSE is required even if the patient presents with a condition that the ED or hospital is not equipped to manage, such as a patient who presents via EMS for evaluation of a stroke but the hospital computed tomography scanner is down. This patient requires an MSE and any required stabilization before transfer even though they are presenting with a time sensitive emergency. A proper MSE depends on the nature of the presenting problem but at a minimum, an evaluation of the patient's airway, breathing, and circulation is required. If the presenting problem warrants a more detailed evaluation for the presence of an emergency medical condition, this should be completed as part of the MSE. Note that the MSE also includes evaluation for active labor. Obtaining a complete set of vital signs is up to the discretion of the provider.[12] One final piece of a proper MSE is documentation. It is imperative that the provider document the nature of the complaint and the MSE that was performed.

Of important note, fulfilling the MSE under EMTALA is not the same as meeting the standard of care for diagnosis and treatment of an ED patient. EMTALA may be satisfied by a qualified medical person providing an MSE and documenting that there is not an emergent medical condition, but this type of examination does not necessarily constitute standard care for the patient in front of the provider and unforeseen medical deterioration later may still create risk to the provider for malpractice claims.

Decreasing Risk in the Waiting Room

After EMS, the ED serves as the first point of contact for patients into the health care system. Total number of ED visits continues to climb and in 2016, there were more than 145 million visits.[14] Data from the same time period show that the percentage of patients who are seen in fewer than 15 minutes is 39%.[14] As the number of ED visits continues to rise, the length of time patients spend in the waiting room is likely to mirror this trend. In addition, hospital overcrowding and ED boarding add to the decreased throughput through the ED and increased volume and length of time ED patients spend in the waiting room. It is imperative that EDs develop ways to minimize the risk associated with prolonged waiting room stays.

Historically, the trend in EDs was to provide beds to patients arriving by EMS despite their chief complaint while patients in the waiting room continued to wait. More and more, however, patients arriving via EMS are being triaged to the waiting room.

Waiting room time is not dependent only on ED volume. The entire health system plays a role in the throughput of patients in the ED. The Cambridge Hospital ED exemplified this with a system-wide improvement project in which they focused on five major areas: (1) patient flow, (2) laboratory turnaround time, (3) ED to inpatient nurse report, (4) physician admitting orders, and (5) inpatient discharges.[15] As a result they were able to decrease time spent on diversion, length of stay, door-to-provider time, and "left without being seen" (LWBS) rates. They were also able to increase patient satisfaction and successfully achieve ED quality core measures.[15]

For patients who start their visit in the ED waiting room, there have been many ways suggested to help improve safety and ED throughput. One such way is to have a provider in triage. The triage provider would be able to treat low acuity patients and discharge them directly from the waiting room.[16] Additionally, they may perform an MSE and initiate any testing or management until the patient is able to get a bed in the ED.[16] If used, the provider in triage model must be customized to the department and hospital; the model that works most effectively is dependent on several personal factors, including volume, acuity, physical space, and staffing.

The concept of an ED waiting room nurse who is separate from the ED triage nurse has also been described in the literature.[17] The role of the waiting room nurse is to perform secondary triage responsibilities, allowing the triage nurse to perform the initial triage screening. Additionally, the waiting room nurse should assess and monitor the condition of patients in the waiting room, initiate interventions early, and monitor for clinical deterioration.[17] The waiting room nurse role relies on appropriate and approved standing orders.[17]

One such role is the clinical initiative nurse (CIN), specifically introduced to manage waiting room patients independent of triage and lower acuity designations, such as fast track. Although specific protocols vary based on institution, CIN responsibilities generally include initiating diagnostic evaluation and treatment beyond the initial triage assessment, and have been found to contribute to faster patient evaluation and intervention.[18] In one study comparing CIN patients with fast track or an expanded fast track treatment area, CIN-managed waiting room patients had shorter times to nursing care; higher incidence of electrocardiograms (ECGs), blood glucose measurements, and intravenous placement; more pathology testing and urinalysis obtained; and higher incidence of analgesic administration.[19]

Other studies have further explored additional nonphysician roles and their impact on various waiting room patient safety measures. One study identified the addition of clinical assistants responsible for facilitating patient flow, communicating waiting times, and helping to calm anxious patients to decrease waiting times and patients LWBS.[20] Another study used EMT-Basics to reassess patients based on their triage level and found they can effectively identify patients that needed additional intervention by a triage nurse including medication administration or uptriaging based on vital sign deterioration or change in symptoms.[21] For more immediate identification of potentially critically ill patients, implementing a dual-tiered rapid triage system and specifically a registered nurse greeter before registration lead to faster identification of Emergency Severity Index level 2 patients.[22]

The role of phlebotomists in the waiting room has also been explored. In a study in an Arizona ED, a technician was employed as a waiting room phlebotomist 8 hours per day, 4 days a week in conjunction with a physician in triage.[23] In their study, the presence of a phlebotomist led to a reduction in left before treatment completion despite an increased door-to-room time, time to primary physician evaluation, and disposition times.[23] Early point-of-care testing in triage has also been assessed to identify patients who may need more rapid invention. One such study evaluated stable walk-in patients with eight predefined chief complaints with protocol point-of-care testing (including but not limited to basic metabolic panel, troponin, lactate, hemoglobin, international normalized ratio, urinalysis) compared with traditional laboratory testing after ED provider assessment and found a decreased ED disposition time of approximately 1 hour.[24] Another study found that among patients with high-risk complaints presenting to triage, similar point-of-care testing resulted in 14% of patients having their Emergency Severity Index level increased or decreased, and 6% of patients being evaluated sooner by a physician.[25]

Care and safety of patients in the waiting room extends to nationally recognized core measures including ST-segment elevation myocardial infarction management, where time to diagnosis and subsequent treatment improves patient outcomes. When compared with patients who arrive by ambulance, patients who arrive as walk-ins to the ED experience significantly longer delays in management including door-to-ECG and door-to-balloon times.[26] This is especially noteworthy considering approximately 40% of patients with ST-segment elevation myocardial infarction present as walk-ins rather than transported by EMS, making rapidly obtained and interpreted ECGs from the waiting room the first critical step toward definitive treatment.[26] With current American Heart Association/American College of Cardiology guidelines recommending door-to-ECG time of less than 10 minutes, studies have assessed improvement strategies to meet this goal. One method used an ED greeter trained to enquire and perform an ECG on any patient with symptoms concerning for acute cardiac syndrome, and mean door-to-ECG time decreased from approximately 30 minutes to 9 minutes.[27] Another strategy used registration clerks to identify patients with chest pain and facilitate rapid ECGs by directly paging a technician, increasing patients receiving an ECG within 10 minutes from 16% to 64%.[28] Additionally, implementation of a specific cardiac triage designation, which included an immediate ECG by a technician physically in triage, significantly reduced door-to-ECG and door-to-balloon times.[29]

Automatic electronic medical record alerts are another innovation to help identify and prioritize potentially sicker patients, evidenced by applications to facilitate treatment of patients with sepsis. Since the introduction of early goal-directed therapy, early antibiotic administration is considered a key component of sepsis management.[30] Using automatic electronic medical record alerts based on vital signs and infectious sources, information gathered from triage intakes is used to prioritize ED beds or physician evaluation for patients presenting with concern for sepsis. In one study, an ED nursing alert system based on systemic inflammatory response syndrome criteria was applied to triaged waiting room patients, and door-to-antibiotic time was found to decrease by more than 30 minutes.[31] In a similar study using triage alerts based on systemic inflammatory response syndrome criteria, flagged patients falling into one of two sepsis severity categories prompted nursing and physician communication, additional resources, and a standardized sepsis order set including antibiotics and intravenous fluid for more immediate management. In this multidisciplinary approach, door-to-IVF time was decreased by 30 minutes, and door-to-antibiotic time by almost 1 hour.[32]

Responsibilities for Patients Who Leave the Emergency Department Without Being Seen

As waiting times continue to increase, hospitals are constantly striving to reduce the percentage of patients LWBS because they are associated with decreased safety and patient satisfaction.[33,34] Organizations, such as the CMS and the Joint Commission, are starting to use the LWBS as a measure of quality and potentially future reimbursement.[35] The national average rate of LWBS is 1.7% but individual institutions range from 0.84% to 15%.[34] Although most patients LWBS likely have low acuity complaints, there are still patients who leave despite requiring emergency care. In fact, a study from 1990 found that 11% of those patients LWBS required hospitalization or emergency surgery within 1 week.[36,37] The purpose of the triage process is to accurately sort patients and determine the order in which patients require evaluation. However, it does not take the place of an MSE.[12] If a patient decides to LWBS by the physician, they are no longer requesting an evaluation and EMTALA no longer applies. Even though EMTALA does not apply, there is still risk to the emergency physician from patients LWBS. The processes described earlier can help to mitigate risk. The most important thing to remember is that triage is a fluid process. As more information becomes available or patient condition changes, the order in which patients are seen may also change. It is important that there is good documentation by the entire team, even before evaluation by a physician. Documentation should include, but is not limited to, repeat vital signs, nursing reassessment, and patient events. One study even suggests the importance of subcategorization of the left against medical advice discharge option to include "left before triage, left before seeing the physician, left before treatment, or left AMA [against medical advice]."[33] The largest responsibility that an emergency physician likely has is prompt and efficient evaluation of the patients currently in beds. This allows for decreased time to disposition and ultimately for more patients to be seen. Unfortunately, waiting room times are not only an ED problem and reflect the strain of the hospital system as a whole. It is prudent that the emergency physician monitors the waiting room and at times it may be required that he or she performs a brief evaluation of a waiting room patient before they receive a bed. The success of a safe ED relies on teamwork with continuous communication from everyone who is providing patient care.

SUMMARY

There are many potential opportunities early in the ED visit for reducing risk. Addressing and reducing the patients LWBS improves patient care and experience. Similarly, implementing strategies to reduce risk in the waiting room can improve patient outcomes. Recognition that ED waiting room times are multifactorial, often beyond the control of the ED (including, but not limited to, inpatient flow and patient boarding), can assist in development of policy to mitigate risk. Recognition of the need for integration of the different departments can potentially reduce risk and improve outcomes. Using triage strategies with proven or expected increased safety to patients can also reduce risk. Understanding EMTALA with its regulatory obligations and liabilities permits development of strategies and policies to mitigate risk. Finally, development and support of strong medical control in the prehospital environment can substantially reduce risk to patients and the systems receiving these patients.

There are multiple risks to patients, providers, and health care systems given the environment and high patient volume in the ED. The ED is often the only place patients know where to go to be seen when acutely ill. The environment is extremely busy and chaotic, creating a risk to the patients, the providers, and the health care system. The points discussed here provide a starting point for executive leadership to develop and support systems and policies to reduce risk for patients during their prehospital encounter and the initial part of their ED visit.

DISCLOSURE

The authors have nothing to disclose.

REFERENCES

1. Council NMD. The definition of EMS 2012. Available at: https://nasemso.org/wp-content/uploads/Definition-of-EMS-2012.pdf.
2. Physician oversight of emergency medical services. Prehosp Emerg Care 2017; 21(2):281–2.
3. 42 U.S.C. § 1395dd(a).
4. 42 U.S.C. § 1395dd(b).
5. 42 U.S.C. § 1395dd(c).
6. 42 U.S.C. § 1395dd(e)(3)(a).
7. 42 U.S.C. § 1395dd(d)(2)(a).
8. United States Department of Health and Human Services, CMS. State operations manual, appendix v - interpretive guidelines - responsibility guidelines - responsibilities of Medicare participating hospitals in emergency cases 2019. Revision 191.
9. 68 Fed. Reg. 53,222 53,234 (2003).
10. 42 U.S.C. §489.24(a)(ii).
11. 42 U.S.C. § 489.24(b).
12. Clarifying policies related to the responsibilities of medicare-participating hospitals in treating individuals with emergency medical conditions2003Department of Health and Human Services, Centers for Medicare & Medicaid Services.Fed Regist. 2003 Sep 9;68(174):53222-64.
13. United States Department of Health and Human Services, CMS. State operations manual, appendix V - interpretive guidelines - responsibility guidelines - responsibilities of Medicare participating hospitals in emergency Cases 2010. Revision 60.
14. Rui P, Kang K, Ashman J. National hospital ambulatory medical care survey: 2016 emergency department summary tables 2016. Available at: https://www.cdc.gov/nchs/data/ahcd/nhamcs_emergency/2016_ed_web_tables.pdf.
15. Sayah A, Rogers L, Devarajan K, et al. Minimizing ED waiting times and improving patient flow and experience of care. Emerg Med Int 2014;2014: 981472.
16. Committee EMP. Emergency department crowding: high impact solutions 2016.
17. Innes K, Jackson D, Plummer V, et al. Emergency department waiting room nurse role: a key informant perspective. Australas Emerg Nurs J 2017;20(1):6–11.
18. Fry M, Jones K. The clinical initiative nurse: extending the role of the emergency nurse, who benefits? Australas Emerg Nurs J 2005;8(1–2):9–12.
19. Considine J, Lucas E, Payne R, et al. Analysis of three advanced practice roes in emergency nursing. Australas Emerg Nurs J 2012;15(4):219–28.
20. Huang E, Liu S, Fang C, et al. The impact of adding clinical assistants on patient waiting time in a crowded emergency department. Emerg Med J 2013;30(12): 1017–9.
21. Blank F, Santoro J, Maynard A, et al. Improving patient safety in the ED waiting room. J Emerg Nurs 2007;33(4):331–5.
22. Howard A, Brenner G, Drexler J. Improving the prompt identification of the emergency severity index level 2 patient in triage: rapid triage and the registered nurse greeter. J Emerg Nurs 2014;40(6):563–7.
23. Stowell JR, Pugsley P, Jordan H, et al. Impact of emergency department phlebotomists on left-before-treatment-completion rates. West J Emerg Med 2019;20(4): 681–7.

24. Singer A, Taylor M, LeBlanc D, et al. Early point-of-care testing at triage reduces care time in stable adult emergency department patients. J Emerg Med 2018; 55(2):172–8.

25. Soremekun O, Datner E, Banh S, et al. Utility of point-of-care testing in ED triage. Am J Emerg Med 2013;31(2):291–6.

26. Mathews R, Peterson E, Li S, et al. Use of emergency medical service transport among patients with ST-segment-elevation myocardial infarction. Circulation 2011;124(2):154–63.

27. Purim-Shem-Tov Y, Rumoro D, Veloso J, et al. Emergency department greeters reduce door-to-ECG time. Crit Pathw Cardiol 2007;6(4):165–8.

28. Takakuwa K, Burek G, Estepa A, et al. A method for improving arrival-to-electrocardiogram time in emergency department chest pain patients and the effect on door-to-balloon time for ST-segment elevation myocardial infarction. Acad Emerg Med 2009;16(10):921–7.

29. Coyne C, Testa N, Desai S. Improving door-to-balloon time by decreasing door-to-ECG time for walk-in STEMI patients. West J Emerg Med 2015;16(1):184–9.

30. Rivers E, Nguyen B, Havstad S, et al. Early goal-directed therapy in the treatment of severe sepsis and septic shock. N Engl J Med 2001;345(19):1368–77.

31. Mitzkewich M. Sepsis screening in triage to decrease door-to-antibiotic time. J Emerg Nurs 2019;45(3):254–6.

32. Hayden G, Tuuri R, Scott R, et al. Triage sepsis alert and sepsis protocol lower times to fluids and antibiotics in the ED. Am J Emerg Med 2016;34(1):1–9.

33. Vierheller CC. Evaluating left without being seen and against medical advice departures in a rural emergency department. J Emerg Nurs 2013;39(1):67–71.

34. Pham JC, Ho G, Hill P, et al. National study of patient, visit, and hospital characteristics associated with leaving an emergency department without being seen: predicting LWBS. Acad Emerg Med 2009;16:949–55.

35. Li D, Brennan J, Kreshak A, et al. Patients who leave the emergency department without being seen and their follow-up behavior: a retrospective descriptive analysis. J Emerg Med 2019;57(1):106–13.

36. Baker D, Stevens C, Brook R. Patients who leave a public hospital emergency department without being seen by a physician. Causes and consequences. JAMA 1991;266(8):1085–90.

37. Polevoi S, Quinn J, Kramer N. Factors associated with patients who leave without being seen. Acad Emerg Med 2005;12:232–6.

Emergency Department Operations II: Patient Flow

Evan Berg, MD*, Adam T. Weightman, MD, MBA,
David A. Druga, MD

KEYWORDS

• Crowding • Boarding • Throughput • Operations • Risk • Metrics

KEY POINTS

- Annual emergency department volume and admission rates continue to rise, leading to increased prevalence of patients boarding in emergency departments.
- Boarding has been associated with numerous risks to the quality, efficiency, and cost-effectiveness of care delivered in emergency departments.
- Administrators should benchmark their department's performance against peers using both standardized time and utilization metrics to identify and address shortcomings.
- Although no 1-size-fits-all solution exists to optimize emergency department throughput, many best practices have been identified and should be utilized where feasible to mitigate risk.

INTRODUCTION

Emergency departments (EDs) have always been busy places. According to the National Center for Health Statistics of the Centers for Disease Control and Prevention, however, ED volume across the United States grew by 6.8% between 2011 and 2016: from 136.3 million visits to 145.6 million visits annually. The number of visits by patients over 65 years of age also has grown, from 20.4 million to 23.1 million visits over the same time period, with this demographic often having more medical complexities and accounting for approximately 48% of all hospital admissions.[1] Emergency Department Benchmarking Alliance (EDBA) data have demonstrated a gradually increasing percentage of overall visits to the ED being admitted to the hospital, either as an inpatient or under observation status. In 2016%, 66% of hospitals reported that their admitted patients boarded in the ED or observation unit for 2 or more hours while awaiting an inpatient bed.[2] Recent EDBA data have demonstrated little progress in reducing median boarding minutes, defined as the interval between

Department of Emergency Medicine, Boston University Medical Center, One Boston Medical Center Place, BCD Building, 1st Floor, Room 1004, Boston, MA 02118, USA
* Corresponding author.
E-mail address: evan.berg@bmc.org

Emerg Med Clin N Am 38 (2020) 323–337
https://doi.org/10.1016/j.emc.2020.01.002
0733-8627/20/© 2020 Elsevier Inc. All rights reserved.
emed.theclinics.com

admit decision time to time of departure from the ED. EDs that serve high-volume populations and adult patients have the longest burden of boarding for admitted patients. The prolonged length of stay (LOS) for patients boarding in the ED has added risk to EDs often already dangerously over capacity.[3]

In the setting of growing ED visits, medical complexity, and boarding volume, standardized and data-driven clinical operations are essential in ensuring patient flow that is streamlined, safe, reproducible, and cost effective. Despite the existing challenges to patient flow, health systems and hospitals are expected to deliver quality, efficient, and affordable patient care. With an understanding of principles related to patient access and flow through the ED and larger health system, there are opportunities to improve on several metrics, including visit LOS, patient experience, total cost of care, and provider and staff morale. This article reviews pertinent areas of risk as well as methods to mitigate this risk as patients are evaluated and cared for throughout their ED encounters. This article reviews the basic principles of patient flow through the ED, including a focus on input, throughput, and output best practice strategies aimed at streamlining processes and mitigating risks resulting from hospital-wide overcrowding.

MODEL OF PATIENT FLOW IN THE EMERGENCY DEPARTMENT

ED patient flow encompasses the movement of patients from a point of entry to their exit from the department, including the steps involved in check-in, processing into and through a clinical area, evaluation and disposition by the treatment team, and departure from the ED to the next area of care. By standardizing and improving processes related to flow, patients are better able to navigate the system, and the treatment team is able to maximize a given space to evaluate and care for patients in a more efficient manner. In the setting of a patient volume–treatment space mismatch, improving patient flow has become a top priority for EDs and hospitals. The goal of patient flow is to minimize waste, promote continuous forward movement, and maximize parallel processes and right-sized staffing models.

ROLE OF METRICS

As ED crowding worsened over the early 2000s, the American College of Emergency Physicians (ACEP) charged hospital leadership and care providers to "quantifiably measure, analyze, and address identifiable and recurrent causes of crowding."[4] To that end, several groups of emergency medicine physicians have collaborated to craft comprehensive sets of measures and uniform definitions to facilitate understanding of the underlying factors that contributed most to crowding and to enable longitudinal research, tracking, and management of ED throughput.[5] Between 2006 and 2018, 4 Performance Measures and Benchmarking Summits were convened to define the processes by which timeliness and efficiency of ED care could be measured and performance benchmarked. Many of the resulting metrics have been adopted by the National Quality Forum and the Centers for Medicare and Medicaid Services as quality measures.[6–8]

It has been recommended that EDs benchmark themselves against peers using parameters relevant to the purpose of the comparison (eg, census, acuity, and teaching status). Using both standardized time interval (eg, arrival-to-provider time and ED LOS) and utilization metrics (eg, rate of imaging use per 100 patients and left without being seen [LWBS] rate), administrators can benchmark their performance on a granular level to identify areas for ongoing improvement.[6]

Since 2004, the EDBA has surveyed high-performing EDs in the United States to pool operational data stratified by ED volume, easing the burden of this comparative analysis. EDBA publishes an annual report detailing trends in ED performance, which can be utilized by regulatory agencies and hospital administrators alike to assess operational efficiency.[2] Once specific throughput issues have been identified, quality-improvement methodologies (eg, Six Sigma), discrete event simulation modeling, and/or the balanced scorecard can be leveraged to further evaluate and address shortcomings.[9–12]

Despite extensive research on ED operations, unfortunately, no 1-size-fits-all solution to optimizing throughput has been identified. Instead, it seems that the most common predictor of success is the presence of robust organizational support for a given intervention. Specific solutions must be nuanced and address the specific challenges faced by a particular institution.[13] This article represents a review of commonly utilized and oft-studied solutions to optimize ED operations.

INPUT AND FRONT-END STRATEGIES

Front-end patient flow concepts include steps involved with patient arrival into the ED and the triaging (ie, sorting) of patients to areas with providers and nursing staff matched to meet the acuity and needs of this patient cohort. Any effective front-end patient flow model must begin with an efficient triage process, in which a properly staffed and resourced triage team, using a triage tool (eg, Emergency Severity Index [ESI] system), can sort patients based on level of acuity and anticipated clinical resource need. ED triage should be rapid, reliable, and reproducible and should minimize bottlenecks at the patient point of entry.

SPLIT-FLOW MODEL

Once triaged, patients can be separated via a split-flow model whereby they are segmented to higher-acuity, moderate-acuity, and lower-acuity areas based on ESI score. Split-flow based on a reliable and reproducible triage tool allows for the grouping of patients requiring similar levels of care, resource requirements, and anticipated LOS into a designated geographic area with dedicated staff, space, supplies, and services designed to match the level of acuity and clinical needs. Sicker, or higher-acuity, patients (ie, ESI 1s, ESI 2s, and horizontal ESI 3s) are triaged to an area where they can be horizontal, given a longer anticipated LOS and higher likelihood of admission. So-called less sick, or lower-acuity, patients (ie, ESI 4s, ESI 5s, and vertical ESI 3s) are triaged to an area where they may be kept vertical and transitioned between evaluation and results pending or care pending spaces. Operationalization of vertical flow strategies is reviewed later. Split-flow models have been broadly adopted and are considered a best practice to shorten patients' wait time to meet a physician or other health care provider as well as their overall ED LOS.[14]

PROVIDER IN TRIAGE MODEL

Despite efforts focused on improving turnaround time within the treatment areas of the ED (including split-flow models and results pending areas), the combination of new patient arrivals and boarding patients awaiting inpatient beds results in ED overcrowding, particularly in higher-volume EDs. This volume-capacity mismatch poses a challenge to all ED patients and adds significant risk to those patients in the waiting room with undifferentiated complaints who have yet to undergo a medical screening evaluation by an ED provider. Overcrowding has been associated with higher LWBS rates, prolonged wait times, and increased medication errors.[3,15,16] In response to these challenges, the model of a provider in triage (PIT) was developed to allow for a rapid medical screening evaluation at the point of patient entry, namely triage.

The PIT provider can be a physician, physician assistant, or nurse practitioner. The PIT provider is located in the triage area and has the task of assessing and delivering care to patients queuing in the waiting room. Given that higher-acuity and more complex patients most often are directly bedded to the main ED for higher-resourced care, the PIT provider often is deployed to evaluate the lower-acuity and moderate-acuity patients, many of whom can be assessed and cared for in a vertical space. Thus, the potential advantage of a PIT provider, if fitted with the right evaluation space and resources, is to assess, treat, and place or discharge a select group of patients promptly, most often ESI 5s, ESI 4s, and vertical ESI 3s. A PIT provider tends to be most useful with lower-acuity patients and in EDs lacking an existing fast-track area to evaluate and care for this cohort. There is variability in the type of provider deployed to triage as well as whether the PIT provider is partnered with others, including a nurse, nursing assistant, or registrar. Each of these staffing resources can add significant costs, so it is important to perform a thoughtful analysis when considering the return on investment of any such model of care.

THROUGHPUT

ED throughput reflects the way in which a department handles its input and involves task, such as staffing, diagnostic testing, and treatment.[5,17–19] For the purposes of this article, throughput can be thought of as the time from physician or midlevel assessment to the time of disposition decision.[20] This section focuses on 4 specific aspects of the ED visit as they relate to enhancing throughput: optimizing staffing, reducing subcycle time intervals, utilizing results pending areas, and establishing flow coordinators.

OPTIMIZING STAFFING

Traditionally, staffing solutions have attempted to function with the fewest resources possible, which is likely why one survey revealed that respondents felt that "lack of ED staff" was one of the biggest obstacles to solving overcrowding.[17,21] As time interval metrics, such as door to electrocardiogram or door to antibiotic administration, have been increasingly scrutinized and used by regulatory bodies as markers of quality, such staffing practices must be reconsidered. At the most basic level, staffing decisions should be based on whether patients' needs can be met in a timely fashion, which suggests that the temporal distribution of staff should reflect the flow of patients in the ED.[9,22–24] Several studies using a variety of methods have found that increased staffing can have positive impacts on ED LOS, waiting times, and rates of LWBS.[25,26] Despite the inherent variability of ED arrivals, several sources suggest that ED volume now can be predicted with surprising accuracy using discrete event simulation modeling.[12,16,18,19,22–28] These data can be used reliably by administrators to guide staffing decisions.

The ACEP Emergency Medicine Practice Committee recommends specific ratios for nurses to patients (no more than 4 patients per nurse and fewer for sicker patients) and advises shifting of work to support staff when appropriate, because 1 study found that approximately 14% of nursing interventions could be performed by a non–registered nurse.[21,29,30] Thus, nurse staffing policies must take into account ED census, acuity, and nursing interventions/activities.[31–33] Resources, such as the national ED benchmark database and staffing guide, developed by the Emergency

Nurses Association (ENA), can help guide specific nurse staffing decisions, but generally the ENA recommends that staffing be "reviewed and adjusted regularly...based upon current patient acuity, length of say, patient mix and census."[29,34]

Physician scheduling must take into account utilization, or the average proportion of time in which the physicians are managing patients, which is impacted most greatly by rate of ED arrivals. The higher the physician utilization, the less ability the system has to buffer for variability. Thus, an increase in utilization typically reflects a shortage of physician workforce over a given time period.[35] Several studies have found that the use of flexible shift types with variable start times and durations (enabling overlap) allows for balanced scheduling that matches arriving patient levels to optimize physician utilization.[24,36-40] Areas for future research include optimal scheduling patterns for residents and advanced practice providers relative to attending physicians, because research in this area is limited to date.

REDUCING SUBCYCLE TIME INTERVALS

Studies have found that more than half of ED patients undergo 1 or more diagnostic screening examinations, with increased median LOS for those visits in which testing was performed.[18,19,41] It stands to reason that reduction in turnaround time for ancillary services, such as laboratory testing and radiology, would similarly reduce ED LOS. Researchers have recently embraced the designation of "time interval measurements" in lieu of the long-favored turnaround time. Ancillary service intervals are so-called subcycle intervals, in that they are but 1 facet of the overarching time interval of ED LOS.[6] Unifying mantras across testing modalities include all necessary tests should occur at the earliest possible point in a patient's stay (perhaps even in triage),[42,43] staffing of ancillary services should approximate ED volume,[20,44] and individual practitioners' utilization patterns regarding ancillary testing should be tracked.[21]

Laboratory testing can be broken down into 3 intervals: preanalytical time (order entry to arrival in laboratory), analytical time (blood arrival in laboratory to results reported), and postanalytical time (results reported to physician acknowledgment/analysis).[45,46] Several studies have analyzed interventions, such as point-of-care testing (POCT)[26,45,47-55] and satellite or stat laboratories (dedicated equipment, supplies, and personnel for prioritized ED testing),[45,56-59] with significant variability in their impact on ED LOS. One explanation is that only interventions that meaningfully decrease the time from physician order entry to physician interpretation (so-called brain-to-brain time) have an impact on ED LOS.[46,49] Bottlenecks in laboratory intervals differ among departments, although studies have revealed that delays often occur in preanalytical and postanalytical times, which are not universally impacted by implementation of POCT, satellite, or STAT laboratories.[45,46,57,60] Furthermore, improving laboratory intervals only have an impact on ED LOS when disposition decision making depends on the specific test in question, again calling into question the value of subtotal POCT.[48,54] ED administrators should evaluate their own particular laboratory processes carefully to identify bottlenecks and potential solutions, as opposed to blindly piloting laboratory alternatives.

Although less published research has focused on radiology intervals, studies have demonstrated reduced ED LOS by targeting radiology transport time[61,62] and report completion time by emergency radiologists.[63] An additional study found significant reduction in ED LOS for patients with suspected bony injuries who had imaging studies ordered from triage.[42] Radiology interval optimization is ripe for further research and quality-improvement initiatives.

UTILIZING RESULTS PENDING AREAS

In the interest of utilizing physical space as efficiently as possible to enhance functional capacity, operations experts have suggested that only patients who have a compelling clinical reason to be placed in a bed should own a bed during their visit.[21] Stated another way, patients ought to remain vertical during their stay when possible. This process can take many forms, including internal waiting rooms, results pending areas, or rapid assessment zones; but generally, vertical flow involves patients being evaluated without a stretcher or being moved from a stretcher after initial evaluation to open the space for the next patient while they await studies, treatment, and/or disposition.[64–66] Studies consistently have found significant reduction in time to physician initial assessment with variable impacts on ED LOS and LWBS rates after implementation of vertical flow.[14,64,65,67] Some researchers have suggested that selective use of vertical flow for patients with specific complaints may be the most beneficial, although exactly which conditions are best suited for this form of assessment have not been evaluated rigorously.[68] Based on the available evidence, it seems that vertical flow initiatives are likely to have the most benefit in overcrowded EDs with lower-acuity patients.[65] Although concerns regarding privacy, lower perceived acuity of vertical patients, and patient satisfaction have been raised, these have not been borne out in the published literature and may be avoided by thoughtful design of space utilized for vertical flow.[14,66,69]

FLOW COORDINATORS

A novel role within the modern ED is that of an ED flow coordinator. The ED flow coordinator is an individual (typically an experienced nurse) whose objective is to facilitate and improve movement of patients into and out of the ED, serving as a liaison between the ED and inpatient units or ancillary departments.[70,71] In departments where flow coordinators have been implemented, reductions in subcycle intervals, LWBS rates, and ED LOS have been demonstrated.[70–72] Studies evaluating the impact of physicians functioning simultaneously as clinicians and patient-flow coordinators have not demonstrated similar benefits, suggesting that this role may best be served by a nonphysician dedicated exclusively to optimizing flow.[73,74]

DISCHARGE AND ALTERNATIVE OUTPUT STRATEGIES

When working to mitigate ED overcrowding, a solution that does not inherently involve the input of other hospital departments is facilitation of expeditious discharges. Discharging patients from the ED, however, is fraught with its own risks. Ideally, the discharge process should minimize adverse outcomes to the patient as well as return visits, especially those requiring hospital admission. Special attention should be paid to higher-risk populations, such as the elderly, those with abnormal vital signs at time of discharge,[75] patients with chronic or end-stage renal disease, and those with Medicaid insurance.[76] Most return visits to the ED (even those leading to admission), however, are due to progression of illness and other factors, such as patient nonadherence, and have not been shown to reflect deficiencies in ED care during previous visit(s).[77]

A study of Medicare claims data found that 0.12% of patients died within 7 days of ED discharge. Patients discharged from EDs with admission rates in the lowest quintile had a higher 7-day mortality (0.27%) than those who were discharged from EDs with admission rates in the highest quintile (0.08%), even though the former group of patients was healthier at baseline. Several diagnoses were more common in those with early deaths after discharge: altered mental status, dyspnea, and malaise/fatigue.[78] A similar study of 7-day mortality after ED discharge found an overall death rate of 0.05% and high-risk diagnoses of noninfectious lung, renal, and ischemic heart diseases.[79]

Discharge instructions are crucial for summarizing key information from the ED visit and next steps but frequently are not understood.[80–83] Even when understood, dissatisfaction with discharge instructions is as likely to lead to medication nonadherence as lack of insurance.[84] Providing a framework for these instructions, patient interviews suggest 4 common desired outcomes after ED visits: (1) understanding the cause and expected trajectory of their symptoms, (2) reassurance, (3) symptom relief, and (4) having a plan (to manage symptoms, resolve the issue, or pursue further care).[85] In addition to verbal review of the discharge instructions, comprehension and retention can be improved with simplified written instructions[86] and using teach-back.[87]

All members of the multidisciplinary ED care team play an important part in discharges. A key role of emergency nurses is patient education and preparation for follow-up after discharge. Workload and nurse-to-patient ratios should be adequate to facilitate this discharge planning.[88] Social workers and case managers can decrease unnecessary admissions (and therefore cost), refer patients to community resources, and improve both patient and staff satisfaction. ED pharmacists can provide teaching about new medications and answer questions to improve understanding and adherence. They also can help with insurance and preauthorization issues or help prescribers to find alternatives.

Thoughtful transitions of care after ED discharge also are important. Primary care follow-up rates can be improved by discharging patients with scheduled follow-up visits, which is particularly helpful in decreasing poor outcomes and subsequent preventable admissions in patients with chronic illness.[89] Particular care should be given to geriatric patients, especially those residing in nursing homes, because they are again a high-risk population due to multiple comorbidities typically managed by multiple physicians and nonphysician providers, incomplete documentation of medical history and medication lists from facilities or patients themselves, inadequate home support, and cognitive issues affecting the ability to provide an accurate history or understand/remember discharge instructions.[90,91]

BOARDERS

Boarding admitted patients in the ED has several adverse effects on patient safety (mortality, adverse events, and so forth) and ED performance metrics (LOS and LWBS).[12,92–94] Even patients who ultimately are discharged experience longer lengths of stay because of boarding.[95] Elderly patients and those with multiple comorbidities face the greatest risk of adverse events, such as missed medication doses while boarding in the ED.[96] An Irish study found that elderly patients had the longest boarding times, the highest mortality, and the greatest chance of developing an methicillin-resistant *Staphylococcus aureus* infection during their hospital course.[97] Mental health patients have considerably longer boarding times while awaiting admission or transfer, especially when they do not have insurance.[98,99]

A contentious issue is the location of boarding patients. Many hospitals board admitted patients in the ED, which strains the staffing and resources of the department. Often, boarding patients are managed by inpatient providers, but in some cases that responsibility remains on the shoulders of the emergency physicians who also must evaluate, manage, and disposition the nonadmitted patients. Boarding patients in alternative care areas, such as inpatient hallways, post anesthesia care unit, endoscopy, and cardiac catheterization laboratories, has been shown to be as safe as patient care in inpatient beds.[100]

When asked, patients prefer to board on inpatient wards rather than in the ED, citing noise and privacy as primary concerns.[101–104] A survey of nurses revealed they generally think that unstable patients should board in the ED, but their opinions about other boarders differ. Inpatient nurses felt that boarding patients should remain in the ED whereas ED nurses (and those who have worked in EDs prior) generally felt that boarders should be moved to inpatient areas.[105] The ACEP is direct on its policy statement[106] on ED boarding: "Boarding of admitted patients in the ED represents a failure of inpatient bed management and contributes to lower quality of care, decreased patient safety, reduced timeliness of care, and reduced patient satisfaction...Because ED boarding is a hospital-wide problem, ED leadership, hospital administrators, emergency medical services directors, community leaders, state and federal officials, hospital regulators, and accrediting bodies must work together to find solutions to this problem." The policy statement calls for a variety of interventions to mitigate boarding, including having a hospital-wide contingency plan to address boarding, having additional nursing staff to manage boarders, getting patients to inpatient areas as soon as possible, and transferring patients to available inpatient beds in affiliate hospitals. Although further research on boarding solutions is needed, many proved interventions and strategies already exist and should be utilized to address hospital-specific challenges.[107]

In the future, novel strategies to address boarding doubtless will be advanced. For instance, electronic intensive care unit (ICU) telemonitoring has been shown to reduce in-hospital mortality in medical ICU boarders and facilitate their downgrade to lower levels of care.[108] Additionally, computer prediction tools may be used to reserve inpatient beds by calculating likelihood of admission and anticipated ED LOS at time of initial triage.[109]

ALTERNATIVES TO INPATIENT ADMISSION

Most patients are happier to be at home than to be admitted to the hospital.[110–112] Hospital at home programs have similar or better health outcomes as inpatient admissions[110,113,114] and, in cases of the elderly, may reduce common inpatient adverse events like delirium, nosocomial infections, and falls.[110,115–117] In the setting of ever-increasing health care costs, these programs are prudent to pursue for financial reasons as well.[110,112,113,118] A recent study of Medicare patients admitted from the ED showed an estimated difference of $4000 per patient when comparing the home health benefit and reimbursement for an inpatient admission.[119] Moreover, there are data to show that expedited discharge from the ED with home services can feasibly reduce inpatient admissions.[120] The most common reason for emergency physicians to discharge to home hospitalization is treatment of cellulitis with intravenous antibiotics,[121–123] but there is likely much benefit to be gained from expanding comfort with a range of common diagnoses and supporting robust ED case management to facilitate effective hospital at home programs.

Observation units provide another disposition option to bridge between discharge and admission. Patients presenting with conditions, such as chest pain, syncope, anaphylaxis, and transient ischemic attack, for example, commonly are kept in observation status. Observation units allow for additional monitoring, facilitation of expedited work-up, specialty consultation, procedures, and care coordination. Through these services, observation units can help mitigate risk around patients who otherwise might be discharged but for whom reliable follow-up cannot be assured.

SUMMARY

EDs across the United States continue to experience growth in visits as well as hospital admissions. In the setting of hospital-wide overcrowding, EDs face pressures related to boarding, all of which pose significant risks to patient throughput, quality of care, and patient experience. This article explores best practices related to ED input, throughput, and output processes. How these workflows can help mitigate risk related to overcrowding is reviewed and areas for ongoing operational research are identified.

DISCLOSURE

The authors have nothing to disclose.

REFERENCES

1. Centers for Disease Control and Prevention. National Center for Health Statistics (NCHS). Atlanta (GA): U.S. Department of Health and Human Services; 2016. Available at: https://www.cdc.gov/nchs/data/nhamcs/web_tables/2016_ed_web_tables.pdf. Accessed July 23, 2019.
2. Emergency Department Performance Measures. 2017 Data guide from the emergency department benchmarking alliance data. 2017. Available at: https://edba.memberclicks.net/assets/EDBA%20Final%20Report%2011.16.17.pdf. Accessed July 11, 2019.
3. Kulstad EB, Sikka R, Sweis RT, et al. Overcrowding is associated with an increased frequency of medication errors. Am J Emerg Med 2010;28(3):304–9.
4. American College of Emergency Physicians. Policy statement: crowding. Available at: https://www.acep.org/globalassets/new-pdfs/policy-statements/crowding.pdf. Accessed July 10, 2019.
5. Solberg LL, Asplin BR, Weinick RM, et al. Emergency department crowding: consensus development of potential measures. Ann Emerg Med 2003;42(6):824–34.
6. Welch SJ, Asplin BR, Stone-Griffith S, et al. Emergency department operational metrics, measures and definitions: results of the second performance measures and benchmarking summit. Ann Emerg Med 2011;58(1):33–40.
7. McHugh M, Van Dyke K, McClelland M, et al. Improving patient flow and reducing emergency department crowding: a guide for hospitals, vol. 11. Rockville, MD: Agency for Healthcare Research and Quality; 2011 (12)-0094. Available at: https://www.ahrq.gov/sites/default/files/publications/files/ptflowguide.pdf. Accessed July 10, 2019.
8. Zocchi MS, McClelland MS, Pines JM. Increasing throughput: results from a 42-hospital collaborative to improve emergency department flow. Jt Comm J Qual Patient Saf 2015;41(12):532–41.
9. Eitel DR, Rudkin SE, Malvehy A, et al. Improving service quality by understanding emergency department flow: a white paper and position statement prepared for the American Academy of Emergency Medicine. J Emerg Med 2010;38(1):70–9.
10. Holden RJ. Lean thinking in emergency departments: a critical review. Ann Emerg Med 2011;57(3):265–78.
11. Vermeulen MJ, Stuken TA, Guttmann A, et al. Evaluation of an emergency department lean process improvement program to reduce length of stay. Ann Emerg Med 2014;64(5):427–38.

12. Taylor RA, Venkatesh A, Parwani V, et al. Applying advanced analytics to guide emergency department operational decisions: a proof-of-concept study examining the effects of boarding. Am J Emerg Med 2018;36(9):1534–9.

13. Chang AM, Cohen DJ, Lin A, et al. Hospital strategies for reducing emergency department crowding: a mixed-methods study. Ann Emerg Med 2018;71(4): 497–506.

14. Garrett JS, Berry C, Wong H, et al. The effect of vertical split-flow patient management on emergency department throughput and efficiency. Am J Emerg Med 2018;36(9):1581–4.

15. Weiss SJ, Ernst AA, Derlet R, et al. Relationship between the National ED Overcrowding Scale and the number of patients who leave without being seen in an academic. Am J Emerg Med 2005;23(3):288–94.

16. Chiu I-M, Lin Y-R, Syue Y-J, et al. The influence of crowding on clinical practice in the emergency department. Am J Emerg Med 2018;36(1):56–60.

17. Bond K, Ospina M, Blitz S, et al. Interventions to reduce overcrowding in emergency departments [Technology report no 67.4]. Ottawa (Canada): Canadian Agency for Drugs and Technologies in Health; 2006.

18. Kocher KE, Meurer WJ, Desmond JS, et al. Effect of testing and treatment on emergency department length of stay using a national database. Acad Emerg Med 2012;19(5):525–34.

19. Downey LA, Zun LS. Determinates of throughput times in the emergency department. J Health Manag 2007;9(1):51–8.

20. Karpiel M. Improving emergency department flow. Healthc Exec 2004; 19(1):40–1.

21. ACEP Emergency Medicine Practice Committee. Emergency department crowding: high-impact solutions. Available at: https://www.acep.org/globalassets/sites/acep/media/crowding/empc_crowding-ip_092016.pdf. Accessed July 11, 2019.

22. Salway RJ, Valenzuela R, Shoenberger JM, et al. Emergency Department (ED) overcrowding: evidence-based answers to frequently asked questions. Rev Med Clin Condones 2017;28(2):213–9.

23. Rossetti MD, Trzcinski GF, Syverud SA. Emergency department simulation and determination of optimal attending physician staffing schedules. Proceedings of the 1999 Winter Simulation Conference: Phoenix, AZ. Available at: http://citeseerx.ist.psu.edu/viewdoc/download?doi=10.1.1.96.2019&rep=rep1&type=pdf. Accessed July 17, 2019.

24. Green LV, Soares J, Giglio JF, et al. Using queueing theory to increase the effectiveness of emergency department provider staffing. Acad Emerg Med 2006; 13(1):61–8.

25. Tabriz AA, Trogdon JG, Fried BJ. Association between adopting emergency department crowding interventions and emergency departments' core performance measures. Am J Emerg Med 2019. Available at: https://www.ajemjournal.com/article/S0735-6757(19)30273-6/pdf. Accessed July 9, 2019.

26. Hoot NR, Aronsky D. Systematic review of emergency department crowding: causes, effects, and solutions. Ann Emerg Med 2008;52(2):126–37.

27. Clark TD, Waring CW. A simulation approach to analysis of emergency services and trauma center management. Proceedings of the 1987 Winter Simulation Conference: Atlanta, GA. 1987. p. 925–34.

28. Paul JA, Lin L. Models for improving patient throughput and waiting at hospital emergency departments. J Emerg Med 2012;43(6):1119–26.

29. Ray CE, Jagim M, Agnew J, et al. ENA's new guidelines for determining emergency department nurse staffing. J Emerg Nurs 2003;29(3):245–53.

30. Svirsko AC, Norman BA, Rausch D, et al. Using mathematical modeling to improve the emergency department nurse-scheduling process. J Emerg Nurs 2019;45(4):425–32.
31. Fullam C. Acuity-based ED nurse staffing: a successful 5-year experience. J Emerg Nurs 2002;28(2):138–40.
32. Wise S, Fry M, Duffield C, et al. Ratios and nurse staffing: the vexed case of emergency departments. Australas Emerg Nurs J 2015;18(1):49–55.
33. ACEP Board of Directors. Emergency department nurse staffing. Ann Emerg Med 2017;70(1):115.
34. Velianoff GD. Benchmarking ED staffing: ENA's new database helps. J Emerg Nurs 2000;26(1):5.
35. Chaou C, Chen H, Tan P, et al. Traffic intensity of patients and physicians in the emergency department: a queueing approach for physician utilization. J Emerg Med 2018;55(5):718–25.
36. Erhard M, Schoenfelder J, Fugener A, et al. State of the art in physician scheduling. Eur J Oper Res 2018;265(1):1–18.
37. Sucov A, Sidman R, Valente J. A cost-efficiency analysis to increase clinician staffing in an academic emergency department. Acad Med 2009;84(9):1211–6.
38. Yoshida H, Rutman LE, Chen J, et al. Waterfalls and Handoffs: a novel physician staffing model to decrease handoffs in a pediatric emergency department. Ann Emerg Med 2019;73(3):248–54.
39. Coats TJ, Michalis S. Mathematical modelling of patient flow through an accident and emergency department. Emerg Med J 2001;18(3):190–2.
40. Paul SA, Reddy MC. A systematic review of simulation studies investigating emergency department Overcrowding. Simulation 2010;86(8–9):559–71.
41. Storrow AB, Zhou C, Gaddis G, et al. Decreasing lab turnaround time improves emergency department throughput and decreases emergency medical services diversion: a simulation model. Acad Emerg Med 2008;15(11):1130–5.
42. Rowe BH, Vila-Roel C, Guo X, et al. The role of triage nurse ordering on mitigating overcrowding in emergency departments: a systematic review. Acad Emerg Med 2011;18(12):1349–57.
43. Li L, Georgiou A, Vecellio E, et al. The effect of laboratory testing on emergency department length of stay: a multihospital longitudinal study applying a cross-classified random-effect modeling approach. Acad Emerg Med 2015;22(1):38–46.
44. Melton JD, Blind F, Hall AB, et al. Impact of a Hospitalwide quality improvement initiative on emergency department throughput and crowding measures. Jt Comm J Qual Patient Saf 2016;42(12):533–42.
45. Fermann GJ, Suyama J. Point of care testing in the emergency department. J Emerg Med 2002;22(4):393–404.
46. Boelstler AM, Rowland R, Theoret J, et al. Decreasing troponin turnaround time in the emergency department using the central laboratory: a process improvement study. Clin Biochem 2015;48(4–5):308–12.
47. Crocker JB, Lee-Lewandrowski E, Lewandrowski N, et al. Implementation of point-of-care testing in an ambulatory practice of an academic medical center. Am J Clin Pathol 2014;142(5):640–6.
48. Singer AJ, Ardise J, Gulla J, et al. Point-of-care testing reduces length of stay in emergency department chest pain patients. Ann Emerg Med 2005;45(6):587–91.
49. Ryan RJ, Lindsell CJ, Hollander JE, et al. A multicenter randomized controlled trial comparing central laboratory and point-of-care cardiac marker testing

strategies: the Disposition Impacted by Serial Point of Care Markers in Acute Coronary Syndromes (DISPO-ACS) trial. Ann Emerg Med 2009;53(3):321–8.

50. Murray RP, Leroux M, Sabga E, et al. Effect of point of care testing on length of stay in an adult emergency department. J Emerg Med 1999;17(5):811–4.

51. Goldstein LN, Wells M, Vincent-Lambert C. The cost of time: a randomised, controlled trial to assess the impact of upfront, point-of-care blood tests in the Emergency Centre. Afr J Emerg Med 2019;9(2):57–63.

52. Parvin CA, Lo SF, Deuser SM, et al. Impact of point-of-care testing on patients' length of stay in a large emergency department. Clin Chem 1996;42(5):711–7.

53. Kankaanpaa M, Holma-Erikkson M, Kapanen S, et al. Comparison of the use of comprehensive point-of-care test panel to conventional laboratory process in emergency department. BMC Emerg Med 2018;18(1):43.

54. Kankaanpaa M, Raitakari M, Muukkonen L, et al. Use of point-of-care testing and early assessment model reduces length of stay for ambulatory patients in an emergency department. Scand J Trauma Resusc Emerg Med 2016; 24(1):125.

55. De Freitas L, Goodacre S, O'Hara R, et al. Interventions to improve patient flow in emergency departments: an umbrella review. Emerg Med J 2018;35(10): 626–37.

56. White BA, Baron JM, Dighe AS, et al. Applying lean methodologies reduces emergency department laboratory turnaround times. Am J Emerg Med 2015; 33(11):1572–6.

57. Saxena S, Wong ET. Does the emergency department need a dedicated stat laboratory? Clin Chem 1993;100(6):606–10.

58. Yang KK, Lam SSW, Low JMW, et al. Managing emergency department crowding through improved triaging and resource allocation. Oper Res Health Care 2016;10:13–22.

59. Singer AJ, Viccellio P, Thode HC, et al. Introduction of a stat laboratory reduces emergency department length of stay. Acad Emerg Med 2008;15(4):324–8.

60. Kaushik N, Khangulov VS, O'Hara M, et al. Reduction in laboratory turnaround time decreases emergency room length of stay. Open Access Emerg Med 2018;10:37–45.

61. Hitti EA, El-Eid GR, Tamim H, et al. Improving Emergency Department radiology transportation time: a successful implementation of lean methodology. BMC Health Serv Res 2017;17(1):625.

62. White BA, Yun BJ, Lev MH, et al. Applying systems engineering reduces radiology transport cycle times in the emergency department. West J Emerg Med 2016;18(3):410–8.

63. Perotte R, Lewin GO, Tambe U, et al. Improving emergency department flow: reducing turnaround time for emergent CT scans. AMIA Annu Symp Proc 2018;2018:897–906.

64. Mandavia S, Samaniego L. Improving ED efficiency to capture additional revenue. Healthc Financ Manage 2016;70(6):66–9.

65. Bullard MJ, Villa-Roel C, Guo X, et al. The role of a rapid assessment zone/pod on reducing overcrowding in emergency departments: a systematic review. Emerg Med J 2012;29(5):372–8.

66. Fenn H, Carman M, Dermann M. Vertical patient flow: is it safe and effective? J Emerg Nurs 2015;41(3):240–1.

67. McGrath J, LeGare A, Harmanson L, et al. The impact of a flexible care area on throughput measures in an academic emergency department. J Emerg Nurs 2015;41(6):503–9.

68. McNaughton C, Self WH, Jones ID, et al. ED crowding and the use of nontraditional beds. Am J Emerg Med 2012;30(8):1474–80.
69. Liu SW, Hamedani AG, Brown DFM, et al. Established and novel initiatives to reduce crowding in emergency departments. West J Emerg Med 2012; 14(2):85–9.
70. Murphy SO, Barth BE, Carlton EF, et al. Does an ED flow coordinator improve patient throughput? J Emerg Nurs 2014;40(6):605–12.
71. Fulbrook P, Jessup M, Kinnear F. Implementation and evaluation of a 'Navigator' role to improve emergency department throughput. Australas Emerg Nurs J 2017;20(3):114–21.
72. DeAnda R. Stop the bottleneck: improving patient throughput in the emergency department. J Emerg Nurs 2018;44(6):582–5.
73. Hosking I, Boyle A, Ahmed V, et al. What do emergency physicians in charge do? A qualitative observational study. Emerg Med J 2018;35(3):186–8.
74. Oliveira MM, Marti C, Ramiawi M, et al. Impact of a patient-flow physician coordinator on waiting times and length of stay in an emergency department: a before-after cohort study. PLoS One 2018;13(12):1–8.
75. Gabayan GZ, Gould MK, Weiss RE, et al. Emergency department vital signs and outcomes after discharge. Macy ML. Acad Emerg Med 2017;24(7):846–54.
76. Gabayan GZ, Asch SM, Hsia RY, et al. Factors associated with short-term bounce-back admissions after emergency department discharge. Ann Emerg Med 2013;62(2):136–44.
77. Cheng J, Shroff A, Khan N, et al. Emergency department return visits resulting in admission: do they reflect quality of care? Am J Med Qual 2016;31(6):541–51.
78. Obermeyer Z, Cohn B, Wilson M, et al. Early death after discharge from emergency departments: analysis of national US insurance claims data. BMJ 2017; 356:j239.
79. Gabayan GZ, Derose SF, Asch SM, et al. Patterns and predictors of short-term death after emergency department discharge. Ann Emerg Med 2011;58(6): 551–8.
80. Jolly BT, Scott JL, Feied CF, et al. Functional illiteracy among emergency department patients: a preliminary study. Ann Emerg Med 1993;22(3):573–8.
81. Crane JA. Patient comprehension of doctor-patient communication on discharge from the emergency department. J Emerg Med 1997;15(1):1–7.
82. Zavala S, Shaffer C. Do patients understand discharge instructions? J Emerg Nurs 2011;37(2):138–40.
83. Engel KG, Buckley BA, Forth VE, et al. Patient understanding of emergency department discharge instructions: where are knowledge deficits greatest? Acad Emerg Med 2012;19(9):E1035–44.
84. Thomas EJ, Burstin HR, O'Neil AC, et al. Patient noncompliance with medical advice after the emergency department visit. Ann Emerg Med 1996;27(1): 49–55.
85. Vaillancourt S, Seaton MB, Schull MJ, et al. Patients' perspectives on outcomes of care after discharge from the emergency department: a qualitative study. Ann Emerg Med 2017;70(5):648–58.
86. Jolly BT, Scott JL, Sanford SM. Simplification of emergency department discharge instructions improves patient comprehension. Ann Emerg Med 1995;26(4):443–6.
87. Slater BA, Huang Y, Dalawari P. The impact of teach-back method on retention of key domains of emergency department discharge instructions. J Emerg Med 2017;53(5):e59–65.

88. Han C-Y, Barnard A, Chapman H. Discharge planning in the emergency department: a comprehensive approach. J Emerg Nurs 2009;35(6):525–7.

89. Atzema CL, Maclagan LC. The transition of care between emergency department and primary care: a scoping study. Stevenson MD. Acad Emerg Med 2017;24(2):201–15.

90. Kessler C, Williams MC, Moustoukas JN, et al. Transitions of care for the geriatric patient in the emergency department. Clin Geriatr Med 2013;29(1):49–69.

91. Cadogan MP, Phillips LR, Ziminski CE. A perfect storm: care transitions for vulnerable older adults discharged home from the emergency department without a hospital admission. Gerontologist 2016;56(2):326–34.

92. Singer AJ, Thode HC Jr, Viccellio P, et al. The Association Between Length of Emergency Department Boarding and Mortality: boarding and mortality. Acad Emerg Med 2011;18(12):1324–9.

93. Cha WC, Cho JS, Shin SD, et al. The impact of prolonged boarding of successfully resuscitated out-of-hospital cardiac arrest patients on survival-to-discharge rates. Resuscitation 2015;90:25–9.

94. Reznek MA, Upatising B, Kennedy SJ, et al. Mortality associated with emergency department boarding exposure: are there differences between patients admitted to ICU and Non-ICU settings? Med Care 2018;56(5):436–40.

95. White BA, Biddinger PD, Chang Y, et al. Boarding inpatients in the emergency department increases discharged patient length of stay. J Emerg Med 2013; 44(1):230–5.

96. Liu SW, Thomas SH, Gordon JA, et al. A pilot study examining undesirable events among emergency department–boarded patients awaiting inpatient beds. Ann Emerg Med 2009;54(3):381–5.

97. Gilligan P, Winder S, Singh I, et al. The Boarders in the Emergency Department (BED) study. Emerg Med J 2008;25(5):265–9.

98. Misek R, DeBarba A, Brill A. Predictors of psychiatric boarding in the emergency department. West J Emerg Med 2015;16(1):71–5.

99. Pearlmutter MD, Dwyer KH, Burke LG, et al. Analysis of emergency department length of stay for mental health patients at ten massachusetts emergency departments. Ann Emerg Med 2017;70(2):193–202.

100. Lee MO, Arthofer R, Callagy P, et al. Patient safety and quality outcomes for ED patients admitted to alternative care area inpatient beds. Am J Emerg Med 2019. S0735675719302943.

101. Garson C, Hollander JE, Rhodes KV, et al. Emergency department patient preferences for boarding locations when hospitals are at full capacity. Ann Emerg Med 2008;51(1):9–12.

102. Walsh P, Cortez V, Bhakta H. Patients would prefer ward to emergency department boarding while awaiting an inpatient bed. J Emerg Med 2008;34(2):221–6.

103. Richards JR, Ozery G, Notash M, et al. Patients prefer boarding in inpatient hallways: correlation with the national emergency department overcrowding score. Emerg Med Int 2011;2011:1–4.

104. Viccellio P, Zito JA, Sayage V, et al. Patients overwhelmingly prefer inpatient boarding to emergency department boarding. J Emerg Med 2013;45(6):942–6.

105. Pulliam B, Liao M, Geissler T, et al. Comparison between emergency department and inpatient nurses' perceptions of boarding of admitted patients. West J Emerg Med 2013;14(2):90–5.

106. Boarding of admitted and intensive care patients in the emergency department. Ann Emerg Med 2017;70(6):940–1.

107. Rabin E, Kocher K, McClelland M, et al. Solutions to emergency department 'boarding' and crowding are underused and may need to be legislated. Health Aff (Millwood) 2012;31(8):1757–66.
108. Kadar RB, Amici DR, Hesse K, et al. Impact of telemonitoring of critically ill emergency department patients awaiting intensive care unit transfer. Crit Care Med 2019;47(9):1201–7.
109. Qiu S, Chinnam RB, Murat A, et al. A cost sensitive inpatient bed reservation approach to reduce emergency department boarding times. Health Care Manag Sci 2015;18(1):67–85.
110. Leff B. Hospital at home: feasibility and outcomes of a program to provide hospital-level care at home for acutely ill older patients. Ann Intern Med 2005; 143(11):798.
111. Leff B, Burton L, Mader S, et al. Satisfaction with hospital at home care. J Am Geriatr Soc 2006;54(9):1355–63.
112. Edes T, Kinosian B, Vuckovic NH, et al. Better access, quality, and cost for clinically complex veterans with home-based primary care. J Am Geriatr Soc 2014; 62(10):1954–61.
113. Cryer L, Shannon SB, Van Amsterdam M, et al. Costs for 'Hospital At Home' patients were 19 percent lower, with equal or better outcomes compared to similar inpatients. Health Aff (Millwood) 2012;31(6):1237–43.
114. Leff B, Burton L, Mader SL, et al. Comparison of functional outcomes associated with hospital at home care and traditional acute hospital care. J Am Geriatr Soc 2009;57(2):273–8.
115. Creditor MC. Hazards of hospitalization of the elderly. Ann Intern Med 1993; 118(3):219.
116. Morgan VR, Mathison JH, Rice JC, et al. Hospital falls: a persistent problem. Am J Public Health 1985;75(7):775–7.
117. Saviteer SM, Samsa GP, Rutala WA. Nosocomial infections in the elderly: Increased risk per hospital day. Am J Med 1988;84(4):661–6.
118. Frick KD, Burton LC, Clark R, et al. Substitutive Hospital at Home for older persons: effects on costs. Am J Manag Care 2009;15(1):49–56.
119. Crowley C, Stuck AR, Martinez T, et al. Survey and chart review to estimate medicare cost savings for home health as an alternative to hospital admission following emergency department treatment. J Emerg Med 2016;51(6):643–7.
120. Goldsmith A, Ticona L, Thompson R, et al. Expedited discharge from an academic emergency department: a pilot program. J Emerg Med 2017;53(6): 919–23.
121. Ibrahim LF, Hopper SM, Connell TG, et al. Evaluating an admission avoidance pathway for children in the emergency department: Outpatient intravenous antibiotics for moderate/severe cellulitis. Emerg Med J 2017;34(12):780–5.
122. Stuck AR, Crowley C, Killeen J, et al. National survey of emergency physicians concerning home-based care options as alternatives to emergency department–based hospital admissions. J Emerg Med 2017;53(5):623–8.
123. Stuck AR, Crowley C, Martinez T, et al. Perspectives on home-based healthcare as an alternative to hospital admission after emergency treatment. West J Emerg Med 2017;18(4):761–9.

Supervision of Resident Physicians

Alexander Y. Sheng, MD, MHPE*, Avery Clark, MD, Cristopher Amanti, MD

KEYWORDS

- Supervision • Resident physician • Patient safety • Resident autonomy • Billing
- Entrustment

KEY POINTS

- Although studies examining the impact of supervision on patient-oriented outcomes are limited, the lack of robust objective data should not detract from the common goal of safe, high-quality patient care.
- Emergency medicine as a specialty has overall embraced the practice of 24/7 supervision for resident trainees.
- Providing appropriate level of autonomy with adequate supervision is crucial to ensuring the safe care of patients while simultaneously promoting graduated responsibility in resident trainees with the goal of independent practice upon graduation.
- Many patient, resident, and environmental factors affect entrustment in the supervisory relationship.
- Multiple strategies on the part of the supervisor, department, and institution are suggested to help physicians balance autonomy with supervision and reduce malpractice risk while providing safe, patient-centered care.

INTRODUCTION

Clinical supervision is defined as "the provision of monitoring, guidance and feedback on matters of personal, professional, and educational development in the context of the physician's care of patients."[1] There is general agreement that supervision of residents also should ensure patient safety and promote career development.[1] Nevertheless, it can be difficult to envision what appropriate resident supervision might look like in practical terms, especially in a specialty that contains such variety and complexity of knowledge, skills, attitudes, and behaviors like emergency medicine (EM). Thus, previous experts have further stipulated supervision to constitute the 3 functions/roles of oversight/management, education, and support.[1] Most of the medical literature on supervision affords little attention to discussion of theoretic models behind the concept

Department of Emergency Medicine, Boston Medical Center, Boston University School of Medicine, 800 Harrison Avenue, BCD Building, 1st Floor, Boston, MA 02118, USA
* Corresponding author.
E-mail address: alexander.sheng@bmc.org

Emerg Med Clin N Am 38 (2020) 339–351
https://doi.org/10.1016/j.emc.2020.02.004
0733-8627/20/© 2020 Elsevier Inc. All rights reserved.
emed.theclinics.com

of supervision. In essence, supervision is a complex task that encompasses multiple conceptual frameworks, including adult learning theories, experiential learning, apprenticeship, problem-based learning, social learning theories, and ideas of communities of practice.[1-4]

THE PUSH FOR INCREASED RESIDENT SUPERVISION

Since the death of Libby Zion under the care of an unsupervised resident in 1984, governing institutions and professional organizations have passed regulations and guidelines requiring resident supervision by physicians who have completed residency.[5-9]

The Institute of Medicine (IOM) report released in 2008 further intensified supervision requirements, while at the same time limiting resident duty hours and recommending fatigue-mitigation strategies, facilitation of care transitions, and increased federal oversight of the Accreditation Council for Graduate Medical Education (ACGME).[10] Furthermore, reimbursement for clinical care often is contingent on meeting specific supervision requirements laid out according to Medicare rules and health management organization guidelines.[11,12] These factors, along with increasing awareness of medical error[13,14] and public outcry calling for maximizing intensity of clinical supervision in the name of quality and safety, have led to widespread escalation of supervision of clinical trainees.[15]

EVIDENCE BASE FOR RESIDENT SUPERVISION

A review published in 1992 suggested that suboptimal supervision of junior doctors in surgery, anesthesia, EM, obstetrics, and pediatrics was associated with increased patient mortality in the United Kingdom.[16] Earlier studies in surgery and psychiatry demonstrated improved patient outcomes when residents are supervised.[17,18] More recently, a 2009 survey of residents in the United States in multiple specialties (internal medicine, obstetrics and gynecology, pediatrics, and surgery) reported few cases of inadequate supervision. In this same study, problematic supervision was positively correlated with resident perceptions of having made a significant medical error, having been belittled or humiliated, or observing others falsifying medical records. Additionally, for the small number of residents who reported inadequate supervision, there was an associated higher self-report of medical errors.[19] On the other hand, a 2018 randomized controlled trial conducted on an inpatient resident general medical service reported no significant difference in rate of medical errors between residents working under different levels of supervision. Increased supervision did result in interns speaking less and residents reporting lower autonomy. The investigators recommended increased flexibility in balancing patient safety, resident autonomy, and learner needs in graduate medical education.[20]

In the surgical literature, despite some outliers and mixed results on patient outcomes,[21-24] resident involvement in operations under direct or indirect attending supervision generally had no impact on complication rates[25-33] but may have increased operative time.[29-33] In terms of supervision of residents during surgical procedures, either directly or indirectly by the attending physician, the literature mostly reported a positive or neutral effect on patient outcomes (eg, complications, mortality, operating room time, and pain).[34]

Specific to EM, direct supervision of residents has been shown to increase compliance with guidelines, without significant impact on patients' experience of their care.[9] Other studies demonstrated significant modifications in emergency department (ED) patient management when residents were supervised.[35,36] There were significant limitations, however, in the studies' design, and the changes in treatment often were minor. Another ED study found no difference in the rate of morbidity and mortality cases between senior resident–led teams and attending-led teams, and that level of supervision appeared to have no significant impact on the standard of care provided. In this study, however, the senior resident–led team ultimately presented all cases to an attending before patient disposition.[37] Nevertheless, a 2012 systematic review across a variety of clinical settings in multiple specialties, including EM, demonstrated that increased supervision resulted in minor improvement in patient outcomes (eg, increased supervisor-initiated changes to missed or inappropriate diagnoses and increased guideline/protocol compliance) or educational outcomes (eg, improved diagnostic or procedural skills).[34]

Given the current model of medical education, it is difficult to precisely quantify the full impact of resident supervision on patient-oriented outcomes. Experts contend, however, that although further research is needed, the lack of objective data should not detract from the common goal of safe, high-quality patient care.[34] In addition, the accepted standard of care in EM is for resident-managed patients to be evaluated by an attending EM physician.

Supervision also is crucial to resident growth and development, especially when combined with focused feedback.[1] Supervision can expedite knowledge and skill acquisition. Residents who were supervised directly during continuity clinic exhibited more rapid gains in their primary care skills than those who were indirectly observed.[38] Supervision tends to be more impactful when a trainee is less experienced, and more complex cases also require closer supervision. Although behavioral changes can occur quickly from supervision, changes in attitudes take much longer. This is the case especially when there are frequent changes of the supervisor, like in EM.[1]

POLICIES AND PROCEDURES FOR SUPERVISION OF RESIDENTS

The 2009 IOM recommendations on resident physician work hours, supervision, and safety required in-house supervision for all critical care services, including EDs, intensive care units, and trauma services. In high-acuity cases, direct supervision was expected for residents by physicians who have completed residency, who should physically be available in the hospital for direct supervision.[39]

The ACGME states that supervision "provides safe and effective care to patients; ensures each resident's development of the skills, knowledge, and attitudes required to enter the unsupervised practice of medicine; and establishes a foundation for continued professional growth."[40] The ACGME common program requirements maintains that although the attending physician is ultimately responsible for patient care, other physicians share in the responsibility and accountability for their efforts. The document encourages programs and institutions to "define, communicate, and monitor" a chain of responsibility for all patient care.[40]

On a practical level, ACGME mandates that "each patient must have an identifiable and appropriately credentialed and privileged attending physician or licensed independent practitioner as specified by the applicable Residency Review Committee (RRC) who is responsible and accountable for the patient's care."[40] The respective roles for residents and faculty supervisors must be made available to providers and patients alike.[40]

In terms of specific level of supervision, flexibility exists in the ACGME common program requirements regarding the various forms supervision can take. ACGME places the burden on the program to designate "appropriate level of supervision based on resident's level of training and ability, as well as patient complexity and acuity."[40] Individual RRCs also can specify which activities require different levels of supervision.

For example, postgraduate year 1 residents should be supervised directly or indirectly with direct supervision immediately available. For many other aspects of care, supervision may be a senior resident or fellow. And for other portions of care, indirect supervision by faculty, fellow, or senior resident who is immediately available on site or by phone is acceptable. Lastly, oversight using post hoc review of resident-delivered care with feedback is adequate in some non-EM settings. ACGME requires that each resident know the limits and scope of authority. Although in certain situations, a resident is permitted to act with "conditional independence," programs must provide guidelines for cases in which residents have to communicate with supervising faculty.[40]

In the ED, EM residents must be supervised by residency-trained faculty who have been, or are in the process of getting, certified by the American Board of Emergency Medicine/American Osteopathic Board of Emergency Medicine.[41] The RRC-EM also requires specific faculty staff ratio of 4.0 patients per faculty hours or less in order to ensure "adequate clinical instruction and supervision, as well as efficient, high quality clinical operations."[41] Despite initial reluctance from certain stakeholders in the EM establishment, the culture and expectation in EM have shifted toward mandatory 24/7 attending supervision of residents. The RRC-EM, under pressure from ACEP Board of Directors and ACGME, changed their special requirements to mandate 24/7 attending supervision of EM residents.[42] The American Osteopathic Association, in their "Basic Standards for Residency Training in Emergency Medicine," also requires direct resident supervision by faculty 24 hours a day.[43]

IMPLICATION OF RESIDENT SUPERVISION ON BILLING

The 2009 IOM report encouraged the Centers for Medicare & Medicaid Services to incentivize programs and hospitals with "proven, effective levels of supervision" using graduate medical education funding.[39] In the current reimbursement model, Medicare pays for services furnished by residents within the scope of their training program through Direct Graduate Medical Education and Indirect Medical Education payments. In teaching settings, Medicare pays for services as long as they are "furnished by a resident when a teaching physician is physically present during the critical or key portions of the service" through the Medicare Physician Fee Schedule.[44]

As it relates to documentation, both residents and faculty may document physician services on a patient's chart, which must be dated and signed. Dictated/transcribed, typed, hand-written, or computer-generated method of documentation is acceptable, as long as it "sufficiently describes the specific services furnished to the specific patient on the specific date."[44] The supervising faculty must document that they "performed the service or were physically present during the critical or key portions of the service furnished by the resident" and their "participation in the management of the patient" when billing for evaluation and management services.[44] Resident documentation alone is not sufficient to establish faculty presence and participation. The combined resident and faculty entries in the chart comprise the documentation for the service, which must be supported as medically necessary.[44]

CONCERNS REGARDING LACK OF RESIDENT AUTONOMY

Over the past decade, changes in Common Program Requirements, rules on supervision and duty hours, were made with the intention of improving patient safe and quality of care. The goal was to promote a "safe and humanistic educational environment" in which residents can learn.[45] Years after the rules have been implemented, trainees still hark back to patient care experiences in which they acted relatively independently with little or no supervision and tout their perceived benefit on resident learning and development.[1] It has been stated that "excessive supervision without progressive independence may stunt residents' acquisition of knowledge and skills and ultimately hamper their progression to competency in their fields."[46] Within the ACGME 2011 Duty Hour Standards, the ACGME Task Force on Quality Care and Professionalism warns of "dire consequences if we fail to provide both supervision and independence."[47]

Therefore, ACGME requires supervising faculty delegate portion of patient care duties to residents based on trainee experience, skills, and individual patient needs. Furthermore, senior residents should supervise junior residents as they progress toward independent practice.[40] After all, the goal of graduate medical education depends on trainees receiving graduated responsibility with decreasing supervision, ending in independent practice upon graduation.[48,49] Hence, institutions should work toward systems that support residents education and independent learning while providing safe, patient-centered care.

ENTRUSTMENT IN THE SUPERVISORY RELATIONSHIP

Fortunately, resident supervision and autonomy are not mutually exclusive. Although excessive independence may have a negative impact on patient care, lack of autonomy could hinder resident learning and development.[50] It is up to attending physicians to strike a constant balance between experiential learning of the resident with patient needs for high-quality care.[51] The concept of faculty having to provide supervision while allowing suitable autonomy is termed, *entrustment*.[49,52]

Multiple factors affect entrustment of residents in the ED, including patient (eg, acuity, complexity, and family/parents), procedural (eg, complexity), environmental (eg, overcrowding, systems, and protocols), resident (eg, experience, skills, ability, and personality), and faculty (eg, confidence, risk-aversion, management style, commitment to education, and personality) (**Fig. 1**).[49,53] Regardless of patient, environment, or resident factors, however, some faculty are more likely to entrust patient care to residents than are others.[49]

Recent approaches have been developed to standardize and quantify trust in resident performance. Since ACGME announced the Milestones Project in 2008, each specialty has developed and incorporated its own competency-based assessment of residents using the milestones model.[54] The aim was to identify observable behaviors demonstrated by residents as they progress toward independent practice. By recognizing that some residents advance more rapidly in clinical competence than others, the milestones approach gives faculty permission to loosen the reins earlier, allowing more autonomy in some cases, while maintaining close supervision in others.[50] Despite the widespread incorporation of milestones in graduate medical education, however, barriers related to lack of valid assessment tools, opportunities for direct observation, proper educational infrastructure, and resources still exist in EM that hinder effective implementation of EM milestones on a program level.[55]

Entrustable professional activities (EPAs) is another approach, defined as "units of clinical practice that can be entrusted to unsupervised practice by trainees after proficiency is observed."[56] The EPAs were intended to contextualize core competencies, enabling faculty to evaluate trainees on a more holistic level as residents integrate multiple complex, interrelated behaviors during the course of patient care. EPAs can be

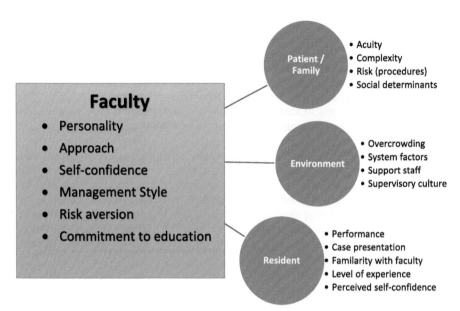

Fig. 1. Factors affecting entrustment of residents.

used to guide decisions regarding level of supervision required for each trainee and task.[53] Very recently, a consensus working group of EM educators in North America drafted 11 core EPAs for EM.[57] Both milestones and EPAs often include behaviors and skills that are applicable across a variety of situations. Although their versatility helps increase opportunities for assessment, the inter-rater reliability of milestones and EPAs suffer as a result because skills and behaviors in one setting often fail to translate to another.[55] Trainee test scores on general constructs are known to be highly case dependent.[58–60] A resident might be able to easily "manage and prioritize critically ill or injured patient" (PC1 of EM Milestones)[61] or lead a ED team (EPA 7)[57] for a presentation seen before but be less competent when managing an unfamiliar case. Nevertheless, development of specific EPAs for every condition within "The Model of the Clinical Practice of Emergency Medicine"[62] is simply unfeasible. As such, EPAs should be utilized when available but must be supplemented by other modes of supervision and entrustment for completeness.

BALANCING RESIDENT AUTONOMY WITH ADEQUATE SUPERVISION

Various strategies on an individual, departmental, and institutional level exist to assist physicians in balancing resident autonomy with appropriate supervision while reducing risk (**Fig. 2**). Previous investigators have suggested the use of a supervision contract to help balance autonomy with adequate supervision. Much like a learning contract,[63] a supervision contract can help set the structure, continuity, goals, objectives, appraisal, and assessment.[1,64] Finding time for supervision itself in the ED, however, much less developing a supervision contract, can be difficult.[1] It may be fruitful to set aside nonclinical time to review goals and expectations of supervision outside of a clinical shift.

On an individual level, effective supervisors must be knowledgeable, be clinically capable, and exhibit strong teaching and interpersonal skills. The supervisor-trainee relationship is the most important factor for effective supervision.[1] Trainees welcome

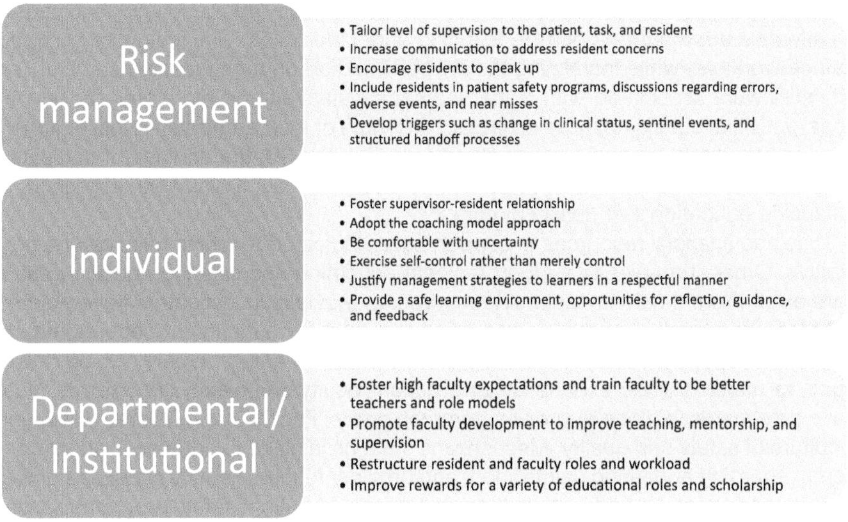

Risk management
- Tailor level of supervision to the patient, task, and resident
- Increase communication to address resident concerns
- Encourage residents to speak up
- Include residents in patient safety programs, discussions regarding errors, adverse events, and near misses
- Develop triggers such as change in clinical status, sentinel events, and structured handoff processes

Individual
- Foster supervisor-resident relationship
- Adopt the coaching model approach
- Be comfortable with uncertainty
- Exercise self-control rather than merely control
- Justify management strategies to learners in a respectful manner
- Provide a safe learning environment, opportunities for reflection, guidance, and feedback

Departmental/ Institutional
- Foster high faculty expectations and train faculty to be better teachers and role models
- Promote faculty development to improve teaching, mentorship, and supervision
- Restructure resident and faculty roles and workload
- Improve rewards for a variety of educational roles and scholarship

Fig. 2. Suggestions for optimizing resident autonomy and supervision.

behaviors such as guidance during clinical work, connecting theory to practice, shared problem solving, giving feedback, reassurance, and role modeling on the part of their supervisors. Poor empathy, rigidity, failure to offer support and address trainee concerns, lack of teaching, intolerance, not being explicit, and overemphasizing evaluations are regarded negatively.[1]

Successful faculty often adopt a coaching model[65] for supervision that involves scripted language to set trainees up for success. A simple, "This is your case, I'll be right here if you need me," can be highly effective in pushing residents to their zone of proximal development[66–68] while maintaining adequate supervision and support.[69] Faculty must be "comfortable with their own uncertainty, exercise self-control rather than merely control, and be ready to justify management strategies to learners in a respectful manner."[69] Faculty should provide a safe learning environment[70,71] and opportunities for reflection, guidance,[72–75] and feedback.[1,76]

Faculty often differ in their personalities, management styles, and tolerance for resident autonomy. Even though the need for faculty development is well recognized, most institutions lack a formal process for faculty recruitment and development that targets teaching and supervisory competencies.[1,77] Those institutions that do and are successful foster high faculty expectations and train faculty to be better teachers and role models through mentorship, learner feedback, and self-evaluation.[50] Faculty development also needs to address topics, such as teaching, assessment, counseling skills, appraisal, feedback, careers advice, interpersonal skills and the concept and purposes of supervision. Faculty development programs have been shown to be beneficial for supervisors.[1] In EM, many advanced training programs (eg, American College of Emergency Physicians/Council of Emergency Medicine Residency Directors Teaching Fellowship,[78] Academic Life in Emergency Medicine faculty and chief resident incubators,[79,80] master of health professions education, and education fellowships) already exist to augment resident and faculty skills in education. Although rewarding excellence in education has long been advocated, clinical teaching and educational scholarship still are undervalued compared with clinical service or biomedical or clinical research in medicine and academia. A more robust and holistic approach is necessary that rewards a variety of educational roles and scholarship in order to close this gap.[77]

On an operations level, restructuring resident and faculty roles and workload can be an effective approach to optimize teaching and supervision. One institution reduced trainee workload while increasing faculty participation on their teaching service. The changes were associated with higher learner satisfaction and more time for educational activities but did not have an impact on length of stay, admission rates, or adherence to standards for quality of inpatient care.[81] In the ED, the addition of dedicated teaching faculty and residents has been described as a valuable approach in balancing education and quality of care.[82,83]

Time and financial resources to support such dedicated teaching roles can be prohibitive. Other strategies to support resident education and safe high-quality patient care exist. From a risk management standpoint, previous investigators have pointed out that less experienced physicians and more complex patients/procedures require greater level of supervision.[84] Guidelines and flexible staffing models can be developed to match trainee experience and patient acuity/complexity. Physicians must have safeguards in place to prevent common errors. Faculty are crucial to cultivating a culture of safety and quality. Mechanisms must be in place to address resident concerns regarding appearing unintelligent and provider fatigue. Faculty should empower residents to speak up and include them in claims and patient safety programs as well as in discussions regarding errors, adverse events, and near misses. Triggers, such as change in clinical status and sentinel events, along with structure handoff processes can be used to mandate effective communication and decrease errors.[84]

In order to optimally balance patient safety, quality, and effective graduate medical training, all stakeholders, including physicians and patients alike, should welcome resident involvement in health care while actively encouraging appropriate level of supervision.

SUMMARY

The act of supervision entails multiple functions/roles, including oversight/management, education, and support. Despite the limited number of studies on the impact of supervision on patient outcomes, safe, high-quality patient care should be the ultimate collective aim for residents and supervising physicians alike. Residents and faculty should work together to balance autonomy with supervision in order to facilitate learning and development for resident physicians and optimize safe patient care. Although multiple patient, resident, and environmental dynamics affect entrustment in the supervisory relationship, the supervisor's personality, risk tolerance, and management styles tend to be the deciding factors. Multiple strategies can be implemented on an individual physician, departmental, or institutional level to assist supervisors in balancing autonomy with supervision while providing safe, high-quality care for patients.

DISCLOSURE

Authors have nothing to disclose.

REFERENCES

1. Kilminster SM, Jolly BC. Effective supervision in clinical practice settings: a literature review. Med Educ 2000;34(10):827–40.
2. Cruess RL, Cruess SR, Steinert Y. Medicine as a Community of Practice: Implications for Medical Education. Acad Med. 2018;93(2):185–91.

3. Boreham N, Morgan C. A sociocultural analysis of organisational learning. Oxford Rev Educ 2004;30(3):307–25.
4. Wenger E. Communities of practice: learning, meaning, and identity. Cambridge University Press; 1998.
5. Asch DA, Parker RM. The Libby Zion case. One step forward or two steps backward? N Engl J Med 1988;318(12):771–5.
6. Bell BM. Supervision, not regulation of hours, is the key to improving the quality of patient care. JAMA 1993;269(3):403–4.
7. Accreditation Council for Graduate Medical Education. *ACGME Program Requirements for Graduate Medical Education in Emergency Medicine*; 2017. Available at: https://www.acgme.org/Portals/0/PFAssets/ProgramRequirements/110_emergency_medicine_2017-07-01.pdf. Accessed May 1, 2019.
8. Working conditions and supervision for residents in internal medicine programs: recommendations. American College of Physicians. Ann Intern Med 1989;110(8):657–63.
9. Sox CM, Burstin HR, Orav EJ, et al. The effect of supervision of residents on quality of care in five university-affiliated emergency departments. Acad Med 2006;73(7):776–82.
10. Drolet BC, Spalluto LB, Fischer SA. Residents' perspectives on ACGME regulation of supervision and duty hours — a national survey. N Engl J Med 2010;363(23):e34.
11. Stern RS. Medicare reimbursement policy and teaching physicians' behavior in hospital clinics: the changes of 1996. Acad Med 2002;77(1):65–71.
12. Kuttner R. Managed care and medical education. N Engl J Med 1999;341(14):1092–6.
13. Graber M, Gordon R, Franklin N. Reducing diagnostic errors in medicine. Acad Med 2002;77(10):981–92.
14. Graber ML. The incidence of diagnostic error in medicine. BMJ Qual Saf 2013;22(suppl.2):21–8.
15. Kennedy TJT, Lingard L, Baker GR, et al. Clinical oversight: conceptualizing the relationship between supervision and safety. J Gen Intern Med 2007;22(8):1080–5.
16. McKee M, Black N. Does the current use of junior doctors in the United Kingdom affect the quality of medical care? Soc Sci Med 1992;34(5):549–58.
17. Kass F, Charles E, Eagle P, et al. Assessing the impact of supervision on outpatient evaluation in psychiatry. QRB Qual Rev Bull 1984;10(1):3–5.
18. Fallon WF, Wears RL, Tepas JJ. Resident supervision in the operating room: does this impact on outcome? J Trauma 1993;35(4):556–60 [discussion: 560–1].
19. Baldwin DC, Daugherty SR, Ryan PM, et al. Residents' ratings of their clinical supervision and their self-reported medical errors: analysis of data from 2009. J Grad Med Educ 2018;10(2):235–41.
20. Finn KM, Metlay JP, Chang Y, et al. Effect of increased inpatient attending physician supervision on medical errors, patient safety, and resident education. JAMA Intern Med 2018;178(7):952.
21. Dasani SS, Simmons KD, Wirtalla CJ, et al. Understanding the clinical implications of resident involvement in uncommon operations. J Surg Educ 2019;76(5):1319–28.
22. D'Souza N, Hashimoto DA, Gurusamy K, et al. Comparative outcomes of resident vs attending performed surgery: a systematic review and meta-analysis. J Surg Educ 2016;73(3):391–9.

23. Lee NJ, Kothari P, Kim C, et al. The impact of resident involvement in elective posterior cervical fusion. Spine (Phila Pa 1976) 2018;43(5):316–23.

24. Castleberry AW, Clary BM, Migaly J, et al. Resident education in the era of patient safety: a nationwide analysis of outcomes and complications in resident-assisted oncologic surgery. Ann Surg Oncol 2013;20(12):3715–24.

25. Wojcik BM, Lee JM, Peponis T, et al. Do not blame the resident: the impact of surgeon and surgical trainee experience on the occurrence of intraoperative adverse events (iAEs) in abdominal surgery. J Surg Educ 2018;75(6):e156–67.

26. Cvetanovich GL, Schairer WW, Haughom BD, et al. Does resident involvement have an impact on postoperative complications after total shoulder arthroplasty? An analysis of 1382 cases. J Shoulder Elbow Surg 2015;24(10):1567–73.

27. Massenburg BB, Sanati-Mehrizy P, Jablonka EM, et al. The Impact of Resident Participation in Outpatient Plastic Surgical Procedures. Aesthetic Plast Surg 2016;40(4):584–91.

28. Kshirsagar RS, Chandy Z, Mahboubi H, et al. Does resident involvement in thyroid surgery lead to increased postoperative complications? Laryngoscope 2017;127(5):1242–6.

29. Meier JC, Remenschneider AK, Gray ST, et al. The impact of surgical trainee participation on sinus surgery outcomes. Laryngoscope 2016;126(2):316–21.

30. Kim RB, Garcia RM, Smith ZA, et al. Impact of resident participation on outcomes after single-level anterior cervical diskectomy and fusion. Spine (Phila Pa 1976) 2016;41(5):E289–96.

31. Baker AB, Ong AA, O'Connell BP, et al. Impact of resident involvement in outpatient otolaryngology procedures: An analysis of 17,647 cases. Laryngoscope 2017;127(9):2026–32.

32. Vetterlein MW, Seisen T, Löppenberg B, et al. Resident involvement in radical inguinal orchiectomy for testicular cancer does not adversely impact perioperative outcomes - a retrospective study. Urol Int 2017;98(4):472–7.

33. Löppenberg B, Cheng PJ, Speed JM, et al. The effect of resident involvement on surgical outcomes for common urologic procedures: a case study of uni- and bilateral hydrocele repair. Urology 2016;94:70–6.

34. Farnan JM, Petty LA, Georgitis E, et al. A systematic review: the effect of clinical supervision on patient and residency education outcomes. Acad Med 2012; 87(4):428–42.

35. Holliman CJ, Wuerz RC, Kimak MJ, et al. Attending supervision of nonemergency medicine residents in a university hospital ED. Am J Emerg Med 1995;13(3): 259–61.

36. Sacchetti A, Carraccio C, Harris RH. Resident management of emergency department patients: is closer attending supervision needed? Ann Emerg Med 1992;21(6):749–52.

37. Van Leer PE, Lavine EK, Rabrich JS, et al. Resident supervision and patient safety: do different levels of resident supervision affect the rate of morbidity and mortality cases? J Emerg Med 2015;49(6):944–8.

38. Osborn LM, Sargent JR, Williams SD. Effects of time-in-clinic, clinic setting, and faculty supervision on the continuity clinic experience. Pediatrics 1993;91(6): 1089–93.

39. Blum AB, Shea S, Czeisler CA, et al. Implementing the 2009 Institute of Medicine recommendations on resident physician work hours, supervision, and safety. Nat Sci Sleep 2011;3:47–85.

40. Accreditation Council for Graduate Medical Education. *ACGME Common Program Requirements (Residency)*; 2018. Available at: https://www.acgme.org/Portals/0/PFAssets/ProgramRequirements/CPRResidency2019.pdf. Accessed May 5, 2019.

41. Emergency Medicine Review Committee for ACGME. *Frequently Asked Questions: Emergency Medicine*; 2017. https://www.acgme.org/Portals/0/PDFs/FAQ/110_emergency_medicine_FAQs_2017-07-01.pdf. Accessed June 28, 2019.42.

42. Zink BJ. Retrospective: When Supervision Wasn't So Super. Emerg Physicians Mon. 2016. Available at: https://epmonthly.com/article/when-supervision-wasnt-so-super/. Published 2016. Accessed June 28, 2019.

43. American Osteopathic Association, American College of Osteopathic Emergency Physicians. *Basic Standards for Residency Training in Emergency Medicine*; 2019. Available at: https://osteopathic.org/wp-content/uploads/2018/02/emergency-med-basic-standards.pdf. Accessed June 28, 2019.

44. Center for Medicare & Medicaid Services. *GUIDELINES FOR TEACHING PHYSICIANS, INTERNS, AND RESIDENTS*; 2018. Available at: https://www.cms.gov/outreach-and-education/medicare-learning-network-mln/mlnproducts/downloads/teaching-physicians-fact-sheet-icn006437.pdf. Accessed May 5, 2019.

45. Grossman RL, Heath AP, Ferretti V, et al. Residents' perspectives on ACGME regulation of supervision and duty hours — a national survey. N Engl J Med 2010;363(1):1–3.

46. Buchanan AH, Michelfelder AJ. Balancing supervision and independence in residency training. AMA J Ethics 2015;17(2):120–4.

47. ACGME Task Force on Quality Care and Professionalism. *The ACGME 2011 Duty Hour Standards: Enhancing Quality of Care, Supervision, and Resident Professional Development ACGME Task Force on Quality Care and Professionalism*. Chicago, IL; 2011. Available at: http://www.acgme.org/Portals/0/PDFs/jgme-monograph[1].pdf. Accessed May 1, 2019.

48. Saxon K, Juneja N. Establishing entrustment of residents and autonomy. Acad Emerg Med 2013;20(9):947–9.

49. Santen S, Wolff M, Saxon K, et al. Factors affecting entrustment and autonomy in emergency medicine: "how much rope do I give them? West J Emerg Med 2019;20(1):58–63.

50. Ling LJ. Teaching goldilocks to supervise: not too much, not too little, but just right. Acad Emerg Med 2013;20(9):950–1.

51. ten Cate O. Entrustability of professional activities and competency-based training. Med Educ 2005;39(12):1176–7.

52. Ten Cate O. Trust, competence, and the supervisor's role in postgraduate training. Br Med J 2006;333:748–51.

53. Tiyyagura G, Balmer D, Chaudoin L, et al. The greater good: How supervising physicians make entrustment decisions in the pediatric emergency department. Acad Pediatr 2014;14(6):597–602.

54. Beeson MS, Carter WA, Christopher TA, et al. The development of the emergency medicine milestones. Acad Emerg Med 2013;20(7):724–9.

55. Sheng A. Trials and tribulations in implementation of the emergency medicine milestones from the frontlines. West J Emerg Med 2019;20(4):647–50.

56. Ten Cate O. Nuts and bolts of entrustable professional activities. J Grad Med Educ 2013;5(1):157–8.

57. Hart D, Franzen D, Beeson M, et al. Integration of Entrustable Professional Activities with the Milestones for Emergency Medicine Residents. West J Emerg Med 2019;20(1):35–42.

58. Hodges B, Turnbull J, Cohen R, et al. Evaluating communication skills in the OSCE format: reliability and generalizability. Med Educ 1996;30(1):38–43.

59. Lurie SJ. History and practice of competency-based assessment. Med Educ 2012;46(1):49–57.

60. Miller GE. The assessment of clinical skills/competence/performance. Acad Med 1990;65(9 Suppl):S63–7.

61. Ling LJ, Beeson MS. Milestones in emergency medicine. J Acute Med 2012; 2(3):65–9.

62. EM Model Review Task Force. *2013 Model of the Clinical Practice of Emergency Medicine*; 2013. Available at: https://www.abem.org/public/docs/default-source/default-document-library/2013-em-model.pdf?sfvrsn=f498c9f4_0. Accessed May 1, 2019.

63. McGrae McDermott M, Curry RH, Stille FC, et al. Use of learning contracts in an office-based primary care clerkship. Med Educ 1999;33(5):374–81.

64. Ritter S, Norman IJ, Rentoul L, et al. A model of clinical supervision for nurses undertaking short placements in mental health care settings. J Clin Nurs 1996;5(3): 149–58.

65. LeBlanc C, Sherbino J. Coaching in emergency medicine: How is coaching different from traditional bedside teaching? CJEM 2010;12(6):520–4.

66. Vygotsky LS. Mind in society. In: Cole M, John-Steiner V, Scribner S, et al, editors. Mind in Society. Cambridge (MA): Harvard University Press; 1978. p. 19–91.

67. Yardley S, Teunissen PW, Dornan T. Experiential learning: AMEE guide no. 63. Med Teach 2012;34(2):e102–15.

68. Taylor DCM, Hamdy H. Adult learning theories: Implications for learning and teaching in medical education: AMEE Guide No. 83. Med Teach 2013;35(11): e1561–72.

69. Brunett P. Autonomy versus control: finding the sweet spot. Acad Emerg Med 2013;20(9):952–3.

70. Hutchinson L. ABC of learning and teaching: educational environment. BMJ 2003;326(7393):810–2.

71. Davies S, Lorello GR, Downey K, et al. Effective learning environments – the process of creating and maintaining an online continuing education tool. Adv Med Educ Pract 2017;8:447–52.

72. Fisher M. Using reflective practice in clinical supervision. Prof Nurse 1996;11(7): 443–4.

73. Paterson B. The view from within: perspectives of clinical teaching. Int J Nurs Stud 1994;31(4):349–60.

74. Plack MM. The reflective practitioner: reaching for excellence in practice. Pediatrics 2005;116(6):1546–52.

75. Bernard AW, Gorgas D, Greenberger S, et al. The use of reflection in emergency medicine education. Acad Emerg Med 2012;19(8):978–82.

76. Bernard A, Kman N, Khandelwal S. Feedback in the emergency medicine clerkship. West J Emerg Med 2011;12(4):537–42.

77. Irby DM, O'Sullivan PS. Developing and rewarding teachers as educators and scholars: remarkable progress and daunting challenges. Med Educ 2018; 52(1):58–67.

78. American College of Emergency Physicians. ACEP/CORD Teaching Fellowship. Available at: https://www.acep.org/education/meetings/acep—teaching-fellowship/. Accessed May 7, 2019.

79. Academic life in emergency medicine. ALiEM Chief Resident Incubator. Available at: https://www.aliem.com/aliem-chief-resident-incubator/. Accessed May 7, 2019.

80. Academic life in emergency medicine. ALiEM Faculty Incubator. Available at: https://www.aliem.com/faculty-incubator/. Accessed May 7, 2019.

81. McMahon GT, Katz JT, Thorndike ME, et al. Evaluation of a redesign initiative in an internal-medicine residency. N Engl J Med 2010;362(14):1304–11.

82. Ahn J, Golden A, Bryant A, et al. Impact of a dedicated emergency medicine teaching resident rotation at a large urban academic center. West J Emerg Med 2016;17(2):143–8.

83. Smalley C, Jacquet G, Sande M, et al. Impact of a teaching service on emergency department throughput. West J Emerg Med 2014;15(2):165–9.

84. Billingham G, Gelb A. Resident supervision and risk management. Irving, TX: ACEP Now; 2013.

Supervision of Advanced Practice Providers

Avery Clark, MD, Cristopher Amanti, MD, Alexander Y. Sheng, MD, MHPE*

KEYWORDS

- Supervision • Physician assistant • Nurse practitioner • Advanced practice provider
- Billing • Credentialing • Medicolegal

KEY POINTS

- Physician assistant (PA) and nurse practitioner (NP) training and experience are variable after completion of their respective accredited PA/NP programs.
- Supervision requirements for PAs vary state by state whereas NPs have the ability to practice independently in many jurisdictions.
- With increasing clinical experience, advanced practice providers (APPs) enjoy more autonomy and less perceived risk of malpractice from their supervisors.
- Practice models, scope of practice, credentialing, privileges, and billing for APPs vary by local and institutional policies, state laws, regulations, and insurance contracts.
- Supervision/oversight and communication issues, such as insufficient collaboration with other providers, tend to contribute to top malpractice allegation categories.

INTRODUCTION

The presence of advanced practice providers (APPs), including physician assistants (PAs) and nurse practitioners (NPs), has increased exponentially over recent years. The number of emergency department (ED) patients seen by APPs has risen from 5.5% in 1997 to 18.2% in 2011.[1] Of the 72,433 eligible practicing PAs in 2013, 6200 self-identified as practicing emergency medicine (EM).[2] In 2016, up to 62% of EDs use PAs and/or NPs,[3] up from 21.6% in 1997.[4] Of those EDs that use APPs, 72.4% have both PAs and NPs, 17.2% use only PAs, and 10.4% have only NPs.[5] The increasing demand for APP coverage in EDs is believed due to the ability of APPs to decrease wait times in ED, especially regarding lower-acuity patients, and thus increase patient satisfaction.[6]

TRAINING REQUIREMENTS FOR ADVANCED PRACTICE PROVIDERS

Training for PAs is broad and variable. They are required to have completed an approved general PA program, governed by the National Commission on Certification

Department of Emergency Medicine, Boston Medical Center, Boston University School of Medicine, 800 Harrison Avenue, BCD Building, 1st Floor, Boston, MA 02118, USA
* Corresponding author.
E-mail address: alexander.sheng@bmc.org

Emerg Med Clin N Am 38 (2020) 353–361
https://doi.org/10.1016/j.emc.2020.02.007
0733-8627/20/© 2020 Elsevier Inc. All rights reserved.
emed.theclinics.com

of Physician Assistants (NCCPA). On average, these programs last approximately 26.5 months. They usually do not have a mandatory, standardized curriculum, and there exist few postgraduate programs for PAs to obtain additional specialty training.[2,7] In 2010, the NCCPA voted to design and implement a program for certificates of added qualifications in 5 areas, 1 of which is EM. In a survey of EM attendings in 2018, however, only 40% believed that credentialing after graduation was necessary for all PAs; 36% believed it to be necessary for only new PA graduates and 23% considered additional training unnecessary for PAs at any level.[5]

Similarly, NPs enter practice with a range of prior training and experience. After completing an accredited nursing program, they then must complete either a master's degree or doctoral degree program to enter into the NP role. The Emergency Nurses Association defines the advanced practice nurse as: "a registered nurse who through advanced study at the Masters or Doctoral level has become an expert in Emergency Nursing."[8] There are some emergency NP tracks within these training programs. And various institutions offer additional credentialing courses.[9] Whether or not these advanced training options are expected/required is variable and generally differ by state.[8]

LAWS AND GUIDELINES GOVERNING SUPERVISION OF ADVANCED PRACTICE PROVIDER

Regarding regulations, individual state medical boards direct and enforce PA clinical practice in a majority of cases—43 states utilize the medical board; however, 8 states (Arizona, California, Iowa, Massachusetts, Michigan, Rhode Island, Tennessee, and Utah) also have a separate and independent regulatory board. All states require PAs to "practice within the scope of practice of the supervising physician."[2] The American Medical Association (AMA) policy states, "physician's assistants should be authorized to provide patient care services only so long as the physician assistant is functioning under the direction and supervision of a physician or group of physicians."[10] The American College of Emergency Physicians (ACEP) takes a similar regulatory stance in its policy statement.[11]

In terms of clinical supervision, Virginia is the only state to overtly require on-site physician presence in the ED. Mississippi requires temporary on-site supervision of new graduates. Although other states require physician supervision, the specifics of what supervision entails remain vague; 27% of states place restrictions on oversight of new PA graduates. Additionally, a vast majority of states regulate the number of PAs whom 1 physician can oversee, generally ranging from 2 to 6 at a given time. All states hold a physician legally responsible for the services provided by the PA. In 8 states, the hospital or physician group itself also can be held liable.[2]

This degree of oversight is in contrast to NPs who, since 2015, have the ability to practice independently in 19 jurisdictions.[12] Many still have supervisory requirements or collaboration within specific institutions that vary by state.[11]

ACEP permits the supervision of PAs and NPs to occur either directly, where a physician "personally evaluates each patient in collaboration with the midlevel," or indirectly, where "the midlevel, functioning within the constraints of the supervision agreement, evaluates and dispositions patients independently and consults with a physician as needed and as dictated by their judgment and comfort level."[11] For indirect supervision to succeed, open lines of communication must be maintained at all times without fear or reluctance from the APP to seek assistance from the supervising physician. According to ACEP, APPs may manage and disposition lower-acuity patients independently while comanaging sicker patients with their supervising physician.[11] On the other hand, the American Academy of Emergency Medicine does not support the independent practice of APPs in any capacity.[13]

FACTORS AFFECTING SUPERVISION OF ADVANCE PRACTICE PROVIDERS

Opinions regarding supervision of APPs vary greatly among practicing physicians. In a 2018 poll of ACEP council members, 51% reported that they viewed PAs and NPs as subordinate in relation to attending physicians. Of the remainder, 12% considered them to be equivalent, 0.9% similar to a medical student, and 22.9% similar to a resident. When it came to beliefs on the appropriate level of supervision, many believed NPs to have insufficient supervision compared with PAs.[5]

In a 2010 study of more than 4000 patients presenting to 63 urban EDs with acute asthma, 2% of patient were cared for by APPs without physician involvement. In such cases, the differences in patient mix (unsupervised APPs saw lower-acuity asthmatic patients) did not fully account for the decrease in guideline-concordant care (unsupervised APPs were less likely to prescribe inhaled β-agonists and systemic corticosteroids in the ED and were less likely to prescribe systemic corticosteroids at discharge) compared with physicians.[14] In contrast, a descriptive cohort study of NP patient care compared with that of residents in the Netherlands found no statistically significant difference when it came to missed injuries or inappropriate patient management. NPs demonstrated high diagnostic accuracy overall.[15]

There are a multitude of factors that appear to play into the PA-physician dynamic. One study explored the idea of "negotiated performance autonomy" as a descriptor of the progression of responsibility. The results demonstrated an inverse relationship between the time spent under direct supervision by or consulting with physicians to years of experience as a practicing PA.

This appeared consistent across specialties, including EM, primary care, and internal medicine, and surgical subspecialties. The level of autonomy allowed to APPs often correlates directly with their clinical experience. This suggests that much of autonomy is related to trust within the PA-physician relationship.[16] Similarly, a survey polling active ACEP members in 2009 found that perceived risk of PA medical malpractice decreased significantly as number of years of PA experience increased.[6] Overall, greater than 71% disagreed/strongly disagreed that PAs were more likely than physicians to commit medical malpractice in the first place. Other influential factors noted in the study were completion of a postgraduate residency program, appropriate supervision by physicians, and higher level of education.[6] Similarly, work environment plays a large role. One study found that rural PAs more often reported never having a physician in the ED and were less likely to have a physician evaluate their patients.[17]

SCOPE OF PRACTICE OF ADVANCED PRACTICE PROVIDERS

In reality, the variation of responsibilities granted to APPs is broad. Roles range from urgent care–type practice to seeing all-comers in the ED. In some instances they also are utilized as ED observation providers, or transition team members, providing ongoing care for patients awaiting admission.[8,9,18] A poll of ACEP council members reported that in 30% of EDs, PAs, and NPs saw patients who were Emergency Severity Index (ESI) level 1 whereas more than 90% of PAs and NPs overall saw patients were are ESI levels 3 to 5.[5] The main contributing factor that appears to influence such variation is the ED environment. A cross-sectional analysis of more than 200 practicing PAs in 2014 found that those in a rural practice environment were more likely to manage high acuity conditions, such as cardiac arrest, stroke, multi-system trauma, and critical illness in children. Similarly, they were more likely to have performed potentially life-saving procedures such as intubation and thoracostomy. Otherwise, there did not appear to be a significant difference in other procedures performed, such as central lines, procedural sedation, and laceration repairs.[17]

Overall, it is evident that there are many different practice models for how APPs are incorporated into the ED and which clinical and procedural privileges they are given. There is little standardization as to the scope of practice of APPs, and much is dependent on state and institutional policies. This likely will continue to evolve and broaden over the next few years as the presence of APPs within the ED continues to grow.

CREDENTIALING AND PRIVILEGES FOR ADVANCED PRACTICE PROFESSIONALS

APPs may be members of the medical staff and are subject to credentialing, privileging, and peer review processes.[19,20] The credentialing process is similar for APPs as it is for physicians; however, instead of verifying medical school and internship/residency, medical staff and credentialing services professionals (MSPs) must verify relevant graduate-level training.[20] Primary source verification needs to be obtained for all APPs. This can occur directly from the school or from a designated verification source, such as the National Student Clearinghouse. In cases of PAs, the online AMA profile service can be used. If a profile does not provide the necessary verification, the school or the National Student Clearinghouse can be contacted. In most cases, verifying undergraduate training for APPs is not required, except in rare circumstances in which an organization specifies such requirements in its credentialing policies and procedures.[19,21]

At minimum, the MSPs must verify the highest level of training that is directly related to the clinical privileges the applicant APP is requesting. Verification requirements can vary by organization. Some credentialing policies specify that all education and training must be verified. Even if it is not required by accreditation standards, an organization's policies still apply if they are stricter than the state law or accreditation requirements[19] **(Table 1)**.

In 2007 and 2008, The Joint Commission published standards regarding ongoing professional practice evaluation (OPPE) and focused professional practice evaluation (FPPE) for privileged practitioners. Although most hospitals have focused on creating such structure for medical staff members (physicians), The Joint Commission requires that the same processes be applied to NPs and PAs.[21] OPPE is the routine monitoring

Table 1		
Four basic steps in privileging advanced practice providers		
Step	**Procedure**	**Responsible Parties**
1	Establish policies and rules	MEC and governing board
2	Collect and summarize information	Management, medical staff, and MEC
3	Evaluate and recommend	Department chairs, credentialing committee, and MEC
4	Review, grant, deny, or approve	Governing board or designated agent

Abbreviation: MEC, medical executive committee.

of current competency for current medical staff members whereas FPPE is establishing current competency for new medical staff members, new privileges, and/or concerns from OPPE.

The process of credentialing and privileging NPs and PAs as well as other practitioners who provide medical care should be outlined in a hospital's staff bylaws. The credentialing process should involve verifying that individuals are properly certified, licensed, or registered with the state and that they have adequate liability insurance. As with other practitioners credentialed under the organized medical staff, hospitals should ensure that the privileges of NPs and PAs are consistent with all applicable state laws and regulations.[11,21]

BILLING ISSUES FOR ADVANCED PRACTICE PROVIDERS

Reimbursement is a challenging, ever-evolving part of medicine, particularly as it pertains to billing for services provided by APPs. The rules vary from state to state and by the various insurance carriers. Medicare requirements tend to be some of the most rigorous and well defined.[11]

In 2002, the Centers for Medicare & Medicaid Services (CMS) issued Transmittal 1776, giving APPs and their supervising physicians increased latitude for hospital and office billing of evaluation and management (E/M) services.[11,22] This allowed APPs and physicians who work for the same employer/entity to share patient visits on the same day by billing the combined work under the physician's provider number for 100% of the Medicare Physician Fee Schedule (MPFS) reimbursement.[11,23] These instructions are referred to as the Medicare split/shared visit policy and are 1 of 3 billing options for APPs, listed in **Table 2**.

The split/shared E/M visit policy applies only to selected settings: hospital inpatient, hospital outpatient, hospital observation, ED, and office and nonfacility clinics.[11,23] In order to capture 100% of the MPFS in the split/shared model, the following must be met as defined by CMS: "A split/shared E/M visit is defined by Medicare Part B payment policy as a medically necessary encounter with a patient where the physician and a qualified APP each personally perform a substantive portion of an E/M visit face-to-face with the same patient on the same date of service. A substantive portion of an E/M visit involves all or some portion of the history, exam or medical decision making key components of an E/M service. The physician and the qualified APP must be in the same group practice or be employed by the same employer."[11,22]

Specifically, documentation in the medical record must clearly identify both the APP and the emergency physician who shared in rendering the service. The emergency physician documentation should be linked to the APP documentation of the shared service and affirmatively state 1 or more elements of the encounter. This element may consist of the history, physical examination, or medical decision making.[22,23] In a shared E/M model, both parties must document the work they performed. A generic attestation of "I have seen and evaluated this patient and agree with the PA notes" or a

Table 2		
Billing options for advanced practice providers		
1		Split/shared service, receiving 100% of MPFS
2		APP's own provider number, receiving 85% of the MPFS amount
3		*Incident-to* service, receiving 100%of MPFS

notation of "seen and agreed" or "agree with above" would not qualify the service as a shared visit.[11] If this criterion for a face-to-face encounter is not met, then the claim will be filed under the APP National Provider Identifier number and reimbursed at 85% of the MPFS (option 2 above).[22,23]

The third billing option for APPs is referred to as *incident to*. This billing policy, under certain circumstances, allows a physician to bill and be paid for services that were provided by nonphysician practitioners who are employed by the physician. Services covered by Medicare *incident-to* are those furnished in a physician office. They are not applicable in a hospital setting, either inpatient or outpatient, and as such not applicable in the ED.[11,22,23]

MEDICOLEGAL CONSIDERATIONS FOR ADVANCED PRACTICE PROVIDERS

With increasing number of APPs working in EDs across the United States, there has been increasing malpractice exposure for these practitioners. Despite earlier skeptics,[24] a majority of physicians do not believe that PAs, when adequately supervised, are more likely to commit malpractice than other clinicians. As physician experience with PAs increase, their perception of malpractice risk decreases.[6] Although not the traditional focus of litigation, more and more PAs and NPs are being named as malpractice defendants. According to the National Practitioner Data Bank, there have been a rising number of claims and total indemnity paid for APPs over the past decade.[11]

A majority of claims for APPs relate to diagnosis-related (39%) and treatment-related (17%) allegations. Claims for APPs are similar to physician claims in terms of allegation categories and contributing factors (clinical judgment, communication, documentation, and technical skill). A majority of claims and amounts paid relate to diagnosis-related allegations, with cancer and infections at the top.[25]

Further analysis of APP claim reveals distinct risk factors that contribute to malpractice (**Table 3**). Scope of practice, test tracking, and informed consent are notable areas of risk.[11] The top allegation categories, however, tend to encompass supervision/oversight and communication issues, such as insufficient collaboration with other providers.[11,25]

Significant variability exists in the way APPs are supervised in EDs across the nation. Although some departments only allow APPs to independently manage lower-acuity patients (eg, ESI triage level 4 or level 5) without direct supervision or consultation, some rural EDs are staffed only with APPs.[17] In such regions, where there is severe physician shortages, autonomous practice is the norm.[26] Although no large-scale studies exist to quantify the degree of APP malpractice risk related to independent practice, anecdotal cases of poor patient outcomes and ensuing large malpractice settlements resulting from haphazard supervision abound.[27] The authors strongly recommend airing on the side of caution by normalizing healthy supervisory practices and creating an atmosphere of collaboration between APPs and physicians.

Other contributing factors for malpractice involving APPs include poor documentation, improper credentialing, failure to comply with regulatory and billing standards, medical board licensing issues, and failure to follow policies and procedures.[11] One of the largest malpractice awards paid in US history, with a settlement sum of more than $200 million, pertains to a careless credentialing error made in the case of an unlicensed PA.[20] Therefore, administrators and physicians must be proactive in defining policies for APP oversight that comply with state regulations and organization standards.[25]

Table 3
Major areas of malpractice risk for advanced practice providers and potential ways to address them

Area of Risk for Advance Practice Providers	Potential Ways to Avoid Allegations
Delay referral to supervising physician	Maintain positive professional relationship and open lines of communication. Provide time for consultation. Exercise good judgment. Outline specific situations that require consultation with the supervising physician.
Practicing beyond scope of care	Develop clear understanding of state-specific regulations on scope of practice, requirements for supervision, and collaboration. Develop guidelines/practice agreements to define APP roles and responsibilities
Failure to address all test results	Establish test tracking processes to ensure clinician review, patient notification, and decision-making documentation related to the result. Develop protocol to follow-up pending results that require clinician response and patient notification.
Lack of informed consent related to the care that APPs provide	Ensure patients' awareness of provider options and understanding of APP role in their care. Accommodate patient requests for evaluation by physician instead of APP.

SUMMARY

The integration of APPs in the form of PAs and NPs has been extensive and rapid in EDs across the nation over recent years. APP training and experience are variable after completion of their respective accredited PA/NP programs. A key difference between PAs and NPs is that supervision requirements for PAs vary state by state whereas NPs have the ability to practice independently in many jurisdictions. It is understandable that, with more clinical experience, APPs enjoy increasing autonomy and decreasing perceived risk of malpractice. Departments and hospitals must maintain their practice models, scope of practice, credentialing, privileges, and billing processes for APPs that are compliant with local and institutional policies, state laws, and regulations and by insurance contract. Although malpractice claims for APPs are similar to physician claims in terms of allegation, administrators and individual clinicians must remain vigilant regarding APP-specific malpractice risks, which include supervision/oversight and communication issues, such as insufficient collaboration with other providers.

REFERENCES

1. Reiter M, Wen LS, Allen BW. The emergency medicine workforce: profile and projections. J Emerg Med 2016;50(4):690–3.
2. Wiler JL, Ginde AA. State laws governing physician assistant practice in the united states and the impact on emergency medicine. J Emerg Med 2015;48(2):e49–58.
3. Augustine J. More advanced practice providers working in emergency departments. *ACEP Now.* 2017. Available at: https://www.acepnow.com/article/advanced-practice-providers-working-emergency-departments/2/. Accessed May 1, 2019.

4. Ellis GL, Brandt TE. Use of physician extenders and fast tracks in United States emergency departments. Am J Emerg Med 1997;15(3):229–32.
5. Phillips AW, Klauer KM, Kessler CS. Emergency physician evaluation of PA and NP practice patterns. J Am Acad Physician Assist 2018;31(5):38–43.
6. Gifford A, Hyde M, Stoehr JD. JAAPA PAs in the ED: do physicians think they increase the malpractice risk. JAAPA 2011;24(6):34–8.
7. Cooper RA, Henderson T, Dietrich CL. Roles of nonphysician clinicians as autonomous providers of patient care. J Am Med Assoc 1998;280(9):795–802.
8. Chang E, Daly J, Hawkins A, et al. An evaluation of the nurse practitioner role in a major rural emergency department. J Adv Nurs 1999;30(1):260–8.
9. Cole FL, Kleinpell R. Expanding acute care nurse practitioner practice: focus on emergency department practice. J Am Acad Nurse Pract 2006;18(5):187–9.
10. American Medical Association. State law chart - physician assistants' scope of practice 2018.
11. ACEP Board of Directors. Advanced practice providers (physician assistant and nurse practitioner) medical-legal issues 2016.
12. Hooker RS. Is physician assistant autonomy inevitable? J Am Acad Physician Assist 2015;28(1):18–20.
13. American Academy of Emergency Medicine. Updated position statement on advanced practice providers 2019.
14. Tsai CL, Sullivan AF, Ginde AA, et al. Quality of emergency care provided by physician assistants and nurse practitioners in acute asthma. Am J Emerg Med 2010;28(4):485–91.
15. van der Linden C, Reijnen R, de Vos R. Diagnostic accuracy of emergency nurse practitioners versus physicians related to minor illnesses and injuries. J Emerg Nurs 2010;36(4):311–6.
16. Cawley JF, Bush E. Levels of supervision among practicing physician assistants. J Am Acad Physician Assist 2015;28(1):61–2.
17. Sawyer BT, Ginde AA. Scope of practice and autonomy of physician assistants in rural versus urban emergency departments. Acad Emerg Med 2014;21(5):520–5.
18. Ganapathy S, Zwemer FL. Coping with a crowded ED: an expanded unique role for midlevel providers. Am J Emerg Med 2003;21(2):125–8.
19. Credentialing Resource Center. Credentialing advance practice professionals. Credentialing Resour Cent Dig 2018. Available at: https://credentialingresource center.com/articles/credentialing-advanced-practice-professionals. Published 2018. Accessed May 1, 2019.
20. Cascella LM. Credentialing and privileging advanced practice providers: reducing risk through due diligence. Fort Wayne,IN: MedPro Group Inc; 2017.
21. The Joint Commission. Credentialing and privileging - requirements for physician assistants and advanced practice registered nurses. Jt Comm 2019. Available at: https://www.jointcommission.org/standards_information/jcfaqdetails.aspx?Standards FaqId=1880&ProgramId=46. Published 2019. Accessed May 1, 2019.
22. Centers for Medicare & Medicaid Services. Medicare claims processing manual chapter 12 - physicians/nonphysician practitioners 2018.
23. Baklid-Kunz E. Rules for Medicare's split/shared visit policy can be a lot to choke down. Here's our simplified interpretation to make it easier to digest. AAPC. Available at: https://www.aapc.com/blog/23741-medicares-splitshared-visit-policy/. Published 2008. Accessed May 1, 2019.
24. Hall GJ. Physician assistants in control: ED mayhem. Am J Emerg Med 1996;14(3):338–9.

25. Cascella LM. Supervision of advanced practice providers foreseeing the risks and considering ways to reduce liability; MedPro Group Inc: Fort Wayne,IN.
26. Klauer K. Issues concerning the PA & NP in the ED. Medium. 2016..Accessed May 1, 2019. Available at: https://medium.com/@emabstracts/issues-concerning-the-pa-np-in-the-ed-2dd133daea5f.
27. Crane M. NPs and PAs: what's the malpractice risk? Med Econ 2000;6:205–8.

Practice Makes Perfect

Simulation in Emergency Medicine Risk Management

Barbara M. Walsh, MD[a], Ambrose H. Wong, MD, MSEd[b],
Jessica M. Ray, PhD[b], Alise Frallicciardi, MD, MBA, MS[c],
Thomas Nowicki, MD[d], Ron Medzon, MD[e],
Suzanne Bentley, MD, MPH[f,g], Stephanie Stapleton, MD[e,*]

KEYWORDS

- Simulation • Risk mitigation • Teams training • In situ simulation • Patient safety
- Medical procedure

KEY POINTS

- Simulation has been steadily changing the safety culture in the health care industry.
- Simulation allows individual clinicians and interdisciplinary teams to be proactive in the culture of risk reduction and improves patient safety.
- Literature has demonstrated improved patient outcomes, improved team-based skills, systems testing, and mitigation of latent safety threats.
- Simulation may be incorporated into practice via different modalities; the simulation laboratory is helpful for individual procedures, in situ simulation (ISS) for system testing and teamwork, community outreach ISS for sharing of best practices, content resource experts and systems testing, and finally, serious medical gaming is becoming a good adjunct in medical education.

[a] Division of Pediatric Emergency Medicine, Boston University School of Medicine, Boston Medical Center, 801 Albany St, 4th floor, Boston, MA 02118, USA; [b] Department of Emergency Medicine, Yale School of Medicine, 464 Congress Avenue, Suite 260, New Haven, CT 06519, USA; [c] Department of Emergency Department, University of Connecticut School of Medicine, University of Connecticut Emergency Department, c/o Lynda Burns, 263 Farmington Avenue, Farmington, CT 06030, USA; [d] Department of Emergency Medicine, University of Connecticut School of Medicine, Hartford Hospital, 22 Jefferson Street, Hartford, CT 06106, USA; [e] Department of Emergency Medicine, Boston University School of Medicine, Boston Medical Center, One Boston Medical Center Place, BCD Building, 1st Floor, Boston, MA 02118, USA; [f] Department of Emergency Medicine, Icahn School of Medicine at Mount Sinai, NYC Health + Hospitals/Elmhurst, 79 01 Broadway, Elmhurst, NY 11375, USA; [g] Department of Medical Education, Icahn School of Medicine at Mount Sinai, NYC Health + Hospitals/Elmhurst, 79 01 Broadway, Elmhurst, NY 11375, USA
* Corresponding author.
E-mail address: snstaple@bu.edu

Emerg Med Clin N Am 38 (2020) 363–382
https://doi.org/10.1016/j.emc.2020.02.003
0733-8627/20/© 2020 Elsevier Inc. All rights reserved.

INTRODUCTION

Simulation-based medical education (SBME) has steadily grown to become a standard in medical training. From simple task trainers to high-cost and technologically advanced human patient simulators, these can all be used to address risk. The true benefit of simulation is in its ability to teach the clinician safer patient care, how to provide this care with fewer errors, and how to communicate better with patients and their families to promote these goals. Whether the simulation will require a simple task trainer for psychomotor repetition (such as an intravenous task trainer arm), an airway model for higher level motor tasks, or a simulated patient manikin in a dedicated space run by trained simulation educators, will depend on the learners and the patient safety objective.

HISTORY

The aviation industry was the forerunner to the use of occupational simulation, and the medical field followed the direction. Both aviation and medical fields placed incredible importance on safety and quality. In 1999, the National Institute of Medicine's publication of *To Err Is Human*[1] highlighted the magnitude and impact of medical errors. This publication, along with a growing focus on patient safety and quality, helped drive the desire to change medical education and helped pave the way for the adoption of SBME. Every pilot is mandated to spend hundreds of hours in a flight simulator, being confronted by rare, high-risk scenarios. Now, with the advent of hospital-based simulation centers, a parallel process is becoming true for medical training. It requires highly trained educators, and it is costly. It is early in its adoption, and research is ongoing to determine how effective various simulation modalities are on patient safety outcomes and risk.

REDUCING RISK USING SIMULATION

The use of simulation in risk management can be approached from 2 sides: the reactive versus the proactive. An emergency department (ED) group can use frequent occurrences as the trigger for a department-wide program. If there are errors related to handoffs for example, then scenarios can be designed to create a focused debrief discussion on a standardized hand-off procedure. This is important and useful, although it is training reacting to an error. There are disadvantages to this approach. Although the programs generally are extremely good at resolving the issue in a time-sensitive manner, the lack of ongoing training means that there is a decay in the knowledge as staff turns over and time passes. In addition, staff can be missed if a concentrated but short-term program is designed.

The second approach is to be proactive. Programs in the ED are designed to standardize behavioral best practices within the group. For example, to introduce a new device into the clinical space, using the safety of the simulation, staff are permitted to make errors, have a constructive dialogue around these errors, repeat the scenario and fix the errors, and thereby prevent an occurrence from ever happening.

Finally, there are other intangible risk reduction benefits to having teams use simulation. Closed-loop communication can be practiced during any scenario. Having the ability to step back during the debrief, look at the situation without the time pressure of an actual patient present, is invaluable for the team's cohesiveness and can prevent errors in areas such as medication dosing, handoffs, correct procedure–correct patient, and crisis resource management. Some centers are using simulations for interprofessional high-risk scenarios, such as the interface between trauma surgery and emergency medicine (EM) and patient care, or high-risk airway emergencies.[2]

GUIDE TO ARTICLE

This article serves as a brief guide to the risk management specific applications of simulation in EM. If you are wondering how this applies to you and your practice, ask yourself how you and your hospital practice skills without harming patients? The answer is the same way airline pilots practice landing without crashing a plane full of passengers: simulation. You may practice via computer models, airway sessions, and "dry runs" in the trauma bay; these are all methods that fall under the broad umbrella of simulation. For this article, the definition of simulation includes use of task trainers, animal models, manikins, standardized patients, or computer-assisted scenarios.

The article begins with a brief overview of the simulation process and terms defined (**Table 1**). The 4 fundamental simulation modalities (ie, procedural, individual, team, and multiteam) are described in detail regarding their use in risk management with discussion on core design (summarized in **Table 2**). Last lies a reference list of free practical simulation resources (**Table 3**). Given the degree of potential complexity, we recommend discussing any simulation program with an expert who will help guide the program's and professionals' success.

SIMULATION PROCESS OVERVIEW

Simulation has been shown to provide many advantages, such as improvement in patient safety and reduction in health costs through the improvement of provider and staff competencies.[3–5] Simulation uses are broad and ever expanding across educational, evaluative, and systems testing scopes. This may present in a wide range of manners, such as individual skills practice, team communication evaluation, or in situ testing a new trauma room with multiple teams.

All simulation programs should be designed to closely serve predefined objectives. Design may be approached via an educational paradigm such as Kern's 6 steps of curricula[6] or the quality improvement tools such as plan do study act (PDSA) model of quality improvement. **Table 4** compares the steps for each. Given our focus on risk management, the PDSA model was selected to exhibit core elements of simulation.

Plan

Planning must begin with a needs assessment or gap analysis to delineate and define the problem or task at hand. This assessment should then inform the creation of specific objectives, selection of personnel, equipment, and location, and a program evaluation plan to guide ongoing iterative improvement. The needs may be identified by malpractice claims, expert consensus, event root cause analyses, challenging clinical cases, or in response to a specific patient outcome.[7] Every ED is different and will have different gaps to fill, as well as different priorities for what to simulate.

Select appropriate combinations of personnel, equipment, and location to align with program goals. Personnel may be an individual clinician who wishes to practice a new central venous catheter (CVC) technique or interprofessional education systems testing of the new cardiac catheterization laboratory activation system, requiring both EM and cardiac catheterization laboratory teams. Equipment is the type of material used during the simulation. From the prior example, this may be a CVC task trainer or a manikin that allows catheterization. Location depends heavily on goals, balanced also with resources. The CVC trainer could be used in a sim center or peri-clinical suite. However, the catheterization laboratory activation testing has to be done "in situ" in the ED and conclude in the catheterization laboratory to test all systems and teams, if systems testing is the objective.

Table 1
Common simulation terms and meaning

Term	Definition
Debrief	Period of facilitated reflective learning within or after a simulation.
In situ simulation	Simulation occurring in the clinical setting. Ex: EM and trauma surgery teams respond to a pedestrian struck simulated patient in the trauma bay.
Just-in-time simulation	Simulation occurring in the peri-clinical setting immediately before clinical performance. Ex: An EM physician practices with a pacer kit immediately before placing it in a patient.
Manikins	Computer-controlled life-size "patients" that exhibit a broad range of acute medical conditions and responses to interventions. Common features include changeable airways, physical examination sounds, intravenous and intraoral sites, and cardiac arrhythmias. All features are adaptable in real time to show the intervention effect or lack thereof. Ex: Laerdal Simman, Gaumard HAL
Procedural model/ Task trainer	Model designed to practice the key elements of a procedure. Ex: Homemade abscess model, CVC Trainer
Procedural simulation	Practicing procedures on models designed for key procedure elements. Ex: Practicing CVC placement on a CVC Trainer
Safe learning environment	Environment in which learners are comfortable to explore their weaknesses and trust educators to help them improve without fear of negative impact on patient care or personal embarrassment.
Scenario	The clinical vignette with anticipated flow, branch points and debriefing points.
Scenario-based simulation	Simulation centers around a clinical vignette that the learner must go through as if it is really occurring. Based on given information, the learners make diagnostic and therapeutic decisions that have real-time consequences for their "patient." After a scenario is completed, the facilitator leads a debrief that provides a safe reflective learning space. Ex: A confused "patient" needs to be diagnosed with a blast crisis requiring the learner to organize an exchange transfusion.
Shared mental model	Team members have a shared understanding of their task and work required.
Simulation center	Separate dedicated simulation space that is not a part of the clinical space.
Standardized patients	Actors who are trained to play patients exhibiting and providing formative feedback on the clinician's performance. Ex: Actor plays the role of a bereaved mother who killed her child.

Abbreviations: CVC, central venous catheter; EM, emergency medicine; Ex, example.

Adapted from Lioce L. (Ed.), Downing D., Chang T.P., Robertson J.M., Anderson M., Diaz D.A., and Spain A.E. (Assoc. Eds.) and the Terminology and Concepts Working Group (2020), Healthcare Simulation Dictionary –Second Edition. Rockville, MD: Agency for Healthcare Research and Quality; January 2020. AHRQ Publication No. 20-0019. DOI: https://doi.org/10.23970/simulationv2.

Do

Carry out your simulation with a postsimulation debriefing facilitated by a simulation expert. The facilitator will determine which debriefing techniques are most suited to the topic and event. Ensure a safe reflective learning environment to maximize effectiveness.

Table 4
Simulation design methods

Process Section	PDSA	Kerns
Development	Plan	Problem identification and general needs assessment
		Targeted needs assessment
		Goals and objectives
		Educational strategies
Implementation	Do	Implementation and
Evaluation	Study	Evaluation and feedback
	Act	

Study

Clearly evaluate the program's effectiveness and room for improvement immediately after the program if possible. Both quantitative and qualitative methods are recommended, as they allow for a synergistic comprehensive assessment. Data should measure impact and provide evidence of efficacy. If personnel evaluations are part of the program, they should be kept separately from program evaluations. Evaluative methods are numerous and include direct observation, self-efficacy surveys, checklist use, and clinical/process outcomes.

Act

Continue to improve the program through an iterative process. Apply feedback and observations to the program and assess for changing needs. This process aligns with evidence-based strategies to improve quality of care through iterative testing and change management using simulation technology.[8]

ROLE OF PROCEDURAL SIMULATION TRAINING IN EMERGENCY MEDICINE RISK MANAGEMENT

Procedural training is one of the many domains of simulation that can be used to address risk management in EM. Simulation-based (SB) procedural training enables health care professionals to learn and master complex technical skills with no risk to patients. In this section, we review the important facets of procedural training in EM, how SB procedural training can impact risk management, and the key factors in implementing an SB procedural training program for risk management.

EM is a field that requires a broad span of expertise. Emergency physicians are required to master and perform numerous procedures competently and successfully, even when the opportunity for practice may not present itself on a regular basis.[9] The 2016 Council of Residency Directors in EM Model of Clinical Practice delineates 70 procedures that span from the routine to the rare.[10] Each of these procedures, when performed in the ever-varying environment of the ED, present numerous opportunities for patient safety risks.[9]

SB education provides a solution to training on procedural skills in EM. Deliberate practice is used in SB procedural training, where a procedure may be practiced repetitively to achieve proficiency. In the SB environment, errors demonstrate a performance gap that provides an opportunity for improvement, rather than cause a patient safety risk.[11,12] Simulation can be used in EM for training learners or ensuring provider competency in new areas. There is a great variety of physical task training models to practice technical skills for EM procedures, including simple models, cadaveric models, complex procedure–specific models, realistic high-tech procedural simulators, and ever-advancing virtual reality simulators.[13]

The use of simulation training for procedural skills has been linked to better patient care and improved patient safety with ever-expanding research showing the positive impact of SB procedural training on EM risk management initiatives.[4,14–17]

Several procedural areas have significant evidence to support the utilization of simulation procedural training to improve patient safety, most notably airway training and CVC insertion. SB airway training is used extensively and effectively in EM training programs. A meta-analysis looking at health care professionals at all levels showed increased knowledge and technical skills with simulation training.[18] Because high-risk airway experiences are often infrequent, SB airway training is also useful for the experienced professional to maintain management skills between clinical experiences.[19] Significant evidence exists to support the utilization of simulation for CVC insertion training to decrease medical errors and improve patient safety. Barsuk and colleagues[20] showed that SB training programs outperformed traditional training on improvement of performance and decreased errors among resident physicians. This same team also showed that this training subsequently led to fewer catheter-related bloodstream infections in their intensive care unit.[21–24]

Many other procedures beyond airway training and CVC placement lend themselves to SB training to improve patient safety and outcomes, including lumbar puncture, peripherally inserted central catheter line placement, and obstetric deliveries.[3] Excellent procedural skills are paramount to all emergency physicians. Evidence shows SB practice decreases risk by improving patient outcomes across numerous procedures.

INDIVIDUAL SIMULATION IN RISK MANAGEMENT

Individual-based simulation is a simulation designed and executed for the development of the single health care professional. This often takes the form of scenario-based learning designed to develop diagnostic, critical thinking, and interpersonal skills.

This modality works best for independent practice and evaluation or individual remedial work as a safe space to dissect out an individual's thought process without distraction and judgment. This modality may overlap with others, but the focus will be on the individual clinician and is adaptable to his or her needs. This section discusses the core uses of individual simulation in risk management regarding error identification, correction, and prevention.

Using Simulation to Identify Error

The ED is one of the highest-risk areas of the hospital due to high patient and staff turnover, limited information, constant interruption, and time constraints. With all systems and persons in flux, errors and near misses are not infrequent. We must learn from error to improve patient safety[1] and thus manage the risk otherwise inherent in EM. To learn from error, we must first identify and categorize it as diagnostic, therapeutic, anticipatory, medication, or systems.[1] The error source must be clearly and systematically identified to mitigate it. This aligns with American College of Emergency Physicians 2013 risk management guidelines[25] to perform chart review and quality improvement.

There are many nonsimulation methods to identify error (eg, root cause analysis, 6 whys). Simulation is an additional tool that may be used to identify errors. This may even begin as a tabletop exercise to practice and do a root cause analysis using simulated charts. There is a growing call to use simulation to recreate immersive patient safety events so the clinician (and others) can identify error source. Using simulation to recreate the events encourages people to act out what could or did happen rather than what they think occurred.

Simulation Practice Reduces Patient Harm

The core of simulation usefulness and success is allowing clinicians to learn from their mistakes without the risk of patient harm or medicolegal culpability.[13,26] When compared with routine practice, those with simulation practice exhibit increased knowledge and skills with a small to moderate benefit for patient-related outcomes.[5] Numerous studies illustrate improved clinical behavior and problem solving with simulation. This is best illustrated in the pediatric EM literature, where multiple studies show increased adherence to neonatal and pediatric code algorithms,[27] significantly improved trauma care, and improved patient care handoffs/transitions of care.[3]

Crisis resource management (CRM) simulation decreases nontechnical errors. Seventy percent of clinical errors are the result of nontechnical skills, such as communication, situational awareness, resource utilization, or leadership.[28] CRM is a tool adapted from aviation that helps clinicians develop these nontechnical skills.[29] It was largely credited to decrease airplane crashes[28,30] and has been widely adapted in anesthesia practice with good effect.[31–34] Multiple CRM simulation trials show significant increase in these nonclinical skills after 1 session.[29,30,35]

Simulation practice prevents clinical skills degradation without patient risk. There is significant evidence that skills degrade when unused for 6 months.[36,37] Physicians, like all adult humans, are limited in their global self-assessment over time, and skills can quietly rust until a rare case arrives and the practice gap becomes apparent. As no ED physician sees everything in his or her clinical practice, simulation allows physicians to practice and reflect on their performance on rare cases and preemptively change before patient error.

Individual simulation fosters clinical resilience as measured by unanticipated complex problem solving.[38] This expert-level skill is developed by deliberate practice, which is a technique of focused reiterative learning. Motivated learners practice a well-defined task with specific goals, after which they are given feedback and opportunity to gradually refine their performance.[39] This practice reduces the risk of errors in complex situations and theoretically decreases frustration, regret, and burnout. Obstetrics has used this type of simulation to decrease malpractice rates; there is great opportunity to adapt this model to EM to increase patient safety and decrease provider risk.

In summary, individual-based simulation is a simulation designed and executed for the development of the single health care professional to identify errors and reduce patient harm. This modality serves as a framework for other types of simulation, such as team-based, multiteam, and in situ.

TEAM-BASED SIMULATION

Teamwork is a critical component in error reduction and increased quality of care for EM.[40] Teamwork requires both the social and cognitive nontechnical skills referenced earlier.[41,42] Simulation provides a proven and powerful tool in the development of these skills.[43,44] Care of critically ill patients often requires the coordination of interprofessional teams within the ED as well as multidisciplinary consultant teams that are brought into the care of the patient. By creating a safe environment in which to practice both routine and low-frequency clinical scenarios, simulation provides the opportunity to develop and practice team-based skills, including roles and responsibilities, closed-loop communication, situational awareness, and shared mental models.[45,46]

Team-based simulations are generally created to understand and develop nontechnical skills used by medical care teams.[47] A needs assessment should focus on team organization, group challenges, and the unit environment. Learning objectives need to be shared among team members. This might include communication skills, such as check backs or summaries for the development of a shared mental model. Team science experts point to both task structure and context as key contributors for the quality of teamwork.[42] When considering teamwork skills within the clinical environment, it is also crucial to consider the technological interfaces used (eg, Electronic Medical Record, intubation materials, Pyxis).[48] Tracking development of teamwork skills during simulation is a key component of risk management, and multiple surveys and direct observation guides exist to assess health care teamwork.[49] These assessment tools ultimately guide improvement of teamwork and safety culture, thus reducing risk.

Team-based scenarios can be created for multiple simulation training settings and purposes; different modalities are used for each, such as tabletop, simulation laboratory based, or in situ simulation (ISS). The optimal simulation modality and fidelity is determined via the learning objectives needed to illicit the social and cognitive features required to meet the objectives. For example, a session focused on the initial development of a new team's structure and process coordination might best be suited for tabletop simulation. Communication patterns, necessary to support this new team, could then be further developed in laboratory-based simulations. Finally, this new team should be integrated into the larger clinical care system via ISSs. This progression provides the opportunity to further test and refine the team-based skills and processes generated in earlier simulations.

Key Elements of Team-Based Simulations in EM Risk Management

Interprofessional team-based simulations use the same planning paradigm but require significantly greater resources, coordination, and planning than simulations for individuals or participants from a single profession. **Table 5** describes the potential challenges, major strategies, and key examples involved in the development, implementation, and evaluation phases for successful use of team-based simulation sessions in EM risk management.[50]

The development phase needs to ensure that learning objectives and simulation design align with the desired effective team-based processes to improve safety in emergency care. Some of these are related to communication emphasized in Team-STEPPS,[51] like programming. All interprofessional participants need to have a significant and balanced role in demonstrating those skills during the case. Barriers in planning include scheduling learners from different professions/disciplines, finances, and facilitators to debrief the sessions.[52] Other barriers to effective interprofessional communication often stem from hierarchical division of labor and differences in professional identity.[53] These social contexts need to be re-created in the scenario to uncover potential issues and address them during the debriefing.

To ensure success in the implementation phase, recruitment of "champions" or early adopters from each profession/discipline is critical.[54] These champions help overcome potential resistance, as team-based simulations can involve a range of difficult interactions linked to inequalities of authority and political tensions between professional groups. A prebriefing sets up clear expectations of participants who may have variable simulation experiences. This allows the debriefer to set the stage for constructive, open dialogue, focusing the discussion on shared consensus toward

Table 5
Key challenges and strategies for team-based simulations to address risk management in EM

Challenge	Strategy	Example
Development phase		
Maximizing participant engagement	Focus on team-based objectives such as communication and leadership skills. Design scenarios relevant to all professions and disciplines.	An interdisciplinary EM/OBGYN simulation was created using an obstetric simulator. Emergency physicians manage the airway of a pregnant patient while obstetricians emergently deliver the fetus.
Complex logistics	Leverage existing opportunities and mandatory training as team-based simulation time.	Incorporation of a team-based simulation into annual in-service of ED nurses in conjunction with intern orientation.
Unaddressed interprofessional tension	Recreate the power, hierarchical, and cultural complexities in the scenario that exists in the clinical environment.	Team-based scenario was designed with both surgery and EM residents participating jointly to unmask potential safety issues that arise when patient comanagement results in conflicting orders to nurses.
Implementation phase		
Participant or group reluctance	Recruit interprofessional champions or change agents from each group as collaborators.	A well-respected senior nurse helps recruit nursing colleagues to join sessions and allay feelings of intimidation and fear of judgment.
Denial of simulation to life error translation	Prebrief the participants to clarify expectations of cooperation, shared learning, and expected actions or mechanics of the simulation.	Facilitators ask all participants to introduce their first names and clinical professions and orients them to the high-fidelity manikin by pointing out locations where pulses can be palpated and defibrillator leads attach.
Domineering participants	Encourage all participants to freely express views that reflect different professional identities or levels of experience but focus on safety rather than individual behaviors and work toward consensus-based solutions.	A nurse educator and physician administrator co-debrief together and support contrasting views on communication challenges between nursing and provider participants.
Evaluation phase		
Difficulty evaluating program impact	Measure both quantitative (eg, surveys, process/patient outcomes) and qualitative (eg, interviews, focus groups) metrics and focus on team assessment.	An observer uses a structured instrument during each simulation and debriefing to record and track performance and suggested solutions.
Disappointment in limited changes and results	Embed team-based simulation into a broader mandate for interprofessional practice and quality assurance efforts to show value. Circulate results of simulation with stakeholders and front-line staff.	Identified latent safety threats and potential solutions from the simulations are regularly presented at the administrative leadership meeting and posted on staff notice board.

Abbreviations: ED, emergency department; EM, emergency medicine; OBGYN, obstetrics gynecology.

generalizable solutions for improving safety rather than on individual behaviors or personal disagreements.[55]

The evaluation phase is crucial for program adaptation, efficacy, and impact. These results also provide concrete evidence for return on investment and meaningful change with stakeholders and front-line staff, emphasizing alignment of risk management goals for the larger organization and health system.

Teams of Teams Simulation

Teams of teams simulation is a step further than team-based simulation. It involves orchestration of multiple interdisciplinary teams that coordinate care in the ED. For example, management of complex cases, such as trauma or postpartum hemorrhage, often require the ED and subspecialty consult teams to work smoothly together. Interpersonal dynamics and clinical care priorities are often disparate across departments and significant benefits from simulation training were demonstrated in a recent review of teamwork for interdisciplinary trauma resuscitation simulations in 12 studies.[44]

Team of teams simulation is often helpful in disaster preparedness, such as a mass casualty incident (MCI). This event overwhelms the local health care system, where casualty numbers vastly exceed local resources and capabilities in a short time.[56] MCIs are low frequency but very high stakes and require rapid decision making with limited information. A variety of simulations have been implemented to address MCI preparedness, such as a "SimWars" format (eg, triage during an MCI gas line explosion).[57] Many SB initiatives have been conducted surrounding disaster and MCI preparedness and management, ranging from tailored, narrow-scope drills (eg, initial triage), through large-scale, MCI drills conducted from a prehospital setting through operative procedures. These include a multiagency, multijurisdictional, multidisciplinary exercise conducted by 17 hospitals simulating a train derailment and chemical spill. The objective of the massive scale drill was to assess each hospital in 5 areas: communications, command structure, decontamination, staffing, and patient tracking. It revealed many deficiencies yet opportunities for improvement. The authors concluded that tabletop exercises are inadequate to expose operational and logistic gaps in disaster response, compared with those elicited through systematic simulation of an MCI.[58]

IN SITU SIMULATION

In situ or unit-based simulation (ISS) takes simulation out of the simulation center and into the workplace. ISS offers opportunity for interdisciplinary teams to practice together in their actual work setting using unit equipment and resources.[59] Deliberate practice and integration of teamwork skills in the time-pressured clinical environment provides great realism and a rich resource to identify latent threats and system issues that can compromise patient safety, and aligns more closely with the actual "work as done" by the health care team.[46] This "crash testing the dummy"[46] provides a method to improve reliability, resilience, and safety in high-risk areas, such as the ED. Potential applications include its use to examine workflow, improve culture, practice teamwork and communication, orient staff, identify systems issues, uncover latent safety threats (LSTs), and practice rare events.[46,60,61] It allows teams to test their effectiveness in a controlled manner and to interrogate departmental and hospital processes in real time and in real locations.[60] The rationale for ISS is "to introduce anomalies, errors and system failures for human operators to experience, mitigate, control, and learn from in a safe environment without human lives at stake."[62]

ISS can be used to proactively evaluate system competence and areas of weakness predisposing to medical error after near-miss or critical event. It offers opportunities to identify LSTs in the clinical system that may not be discoverable in the simulation center.[46] Studies demonstrate that ISS leads to a higher rate of detection of LST than that seen in the simulation center. This technique has helped EDs beta test newly constructed areas before opening for patient care. One ED found missing laryngoscope blades, thoracostomy tubes, and defibrillator connector cables, among other LSTs. Because of the ISS, they were able to mitigate risks to the patients.[46]

Most ISS studies focus on nontechnical skills and interprofessional teamwork, both paramount for patient safety, and have demonstrated effectiveness in improving patient outcomes.[63] ED providers often care for critically ill and rapidly deteriorating patients. Studies suggest that many providers feel inadequately prepared and report high anxiety when managing cardiopulmonary arrests, and interprofessional training using ISS for these cases offers an example of optimal management of these events while simultaneously teaching and reinforcing knowledge, technical skills, and teamwork.[63]

Other notable uses and outcomes using ISS include contribution to changing the safety culture of the system[46] and ISS as a catalyst for change in clinical care systems, leading to improved clinical outcomes.[46] In addition, ISS allows routine opportunity to formally debrief participants, something that rarely occurs after actual patient encounters. This debriefing encourages sharing of information and perceptions between multidisciplinary team members[63] and encourages post-critical incident debriefing.

In conclusion, ISS is an emerging and expanding strategy with increasing studies and data to support its efficacy. A programmatic approach to training and assessment based on system thinking is required for a sustained improvement of team-based performance and patient safety.[46,60,63]

SIMULATION-BASED RISK MITIGATION IN COMMUNITY EMERGENCY MEDICINE

As discussed in prior sections, simulation has been used for at least a decade in most academic centers for education, training, and to assist in maintaining critical skills for physicians and nurses in patient care.[64–70] Community sites may have access to local simulation centers or have purchased simulation equipment; however, they may not have the expertise of simulation-trained facilitators or content experts in disciplines outside EM (eg, obstetrics, pediatric EM [PEM], anesthesia) to maximize the value of simulation training.[71] Patient populations, pathology ,and service availability differ widely among EDs, which can lead to differences in team comfort with patient management.[72,73] This is where sharing of best practices through collaboration between academic and community/rural ED sites using simulation training has become an innovative approach for decreasing patient risk and improving the quality of care in the ED setting.[74–79]

EXISTING ACADEMIC COMMUNITY PARTNERSHIPS

There are different programs that have been launched throughout the United States and abroad where an academic specialty performs in situ training at community sites, right in the environment of that particular unit's care (eg, trauma bay, operating room unit, delivery room).[76,80,81] Both academic and community teams benefit from this exchange. The academic teams use their expertise in simulation and content to help bridge gaps in care (eg, improving sepsis care by following critical care guidelines), whereas the community teams present reminders of variable practice environments (eg, limited specialists and pediatric equipment). For the purpose of this article, we discuss 2 well-established programs and share the process of program development to create a sustainable community-based program. While PEM based, they are unique and illustrate the power of academic partnerships with community ED sites.

Community Outreach Mobile Education Training (COMET)[82] is a New England regional program where PEM interprofessional subspecialists partner with community sites to perform in situ training sessions geared toward each site's unique practice. This type of program enables (1) sharing of best pediatric acute care practices, (2) education and training of site teams regarding common but life-threatening pediatric presentations, (3) focus on improving teamwork and communication, and finally, (4) evaluation of system issues and LSTs.

Improving Pediatric Acute Care Through Simulation (ImPACTS) is a larger, national collaborative that uses simulation as a research tool to study gaps in emergency care provided to pediatric patients across a spectrum of EDs. The mission of the collaborative is to improve health outcomes and survival for acutely ill and injured infants and children through these SB interventions and quality improvement processes.

KEY ELEMENTS OF COMMUNITY-BASED SIMULATIONS IN EMERGENCY MEDICINE RISK MANAGEMENT

Community-based simulation follows the previously mentioned design and implementation process with some potential adaptations. The needs assessment might be based on referral patterns, consensus meetings of transfer data, focus groups, or an onsite needs assessment using initial simulations. Goals and objectives are site specific and should reflect the needs across disciplines and professions. The simulation scenarios need to be developed, tested, and refined for case flow and subject matter. **Table 3** lists numerous freely accessible materials on simulation design and implementation.

Implementation can be a more involved process. Buy-in needs to occur across professions, levels, and sites if partnering with an academic group. This includes physicians, nurses, support staff, and their leaders. Day-of criteria need to be established, for instance, a "no-go" agreement if the department clinical needs are at a critical high. The day-of involves bringing equipment to the sites: simulators, cables, mock medication trays, and supplementary material, such as radiographs or electrocardiograms pertinent to the cases. If these are inaugural simulations, participants may need encouragement to care for the simulated patient as they would a human one.

Following each simulation case, a debrief is done in the room in real time. It is crucial to maintain the safe learning and reflecting environment, so participants are comfortable verbalizing their observations, questions, and exploring solutions. At the conclusion of the session, a formal evaluation should be distributed to participants. This is essential to the program growth and development, especially in reaction to revealed LSTs and systems issues. This then allows a collaboration to help implement change in the deficits uncovered through the simulations.

FUTURE DIRECTIONS IN SIMULATION: AUGMENTED REALITY/VIRTUAL REALITY/ SERIOUS GAMES

As the simulation field has evolved, simulation experts have turned to other innovative approaches to enhance and augment training. Younger generations of trainees are more tech savvy and request more engaging learning methods, and medical education is changing to meet these learner needs. As such, serious medical games are gaining momentum in medical education.

Serious medical games encompass screen-based simulation (SBS), virtual reality (VR) and virtual trainers (VT). The SBS has the advantage for brief asynchronous learning on a

Table 2
Alignment of personnel, equipment, and environment to training needs

		Procedural	Individual	Teams	Teams of Teams	Systems Testing
Simulation needs						
Example		Clinician wishes to practice their CVC skills on a task trainer	Clinician wishes to practice a case with an atypical arrhythmia	An ED care team of clinicians, RNs, CNAs are running a GI bleed case	The ED and trauma surgery teams are running a blunt trauma case requiring massive transfusion	The ED is opening new trauma bays and needs to "dry run" patient care to ensure flow and equipment function
Equipment						
Task trainer	$	Simulation equipment and consumables	Simulation equipment and consumables	Simulation equipment pay RN/support staff	Simulation equipment pay RN/support staff	Simulation equipment pay RN/support staff
	T	Clinician	1 clinician:1 facilitator	Staff, clinician, 1 facilitator	Staff, clinician, ≥1 facilitator per team	Staff, clinician, ≥1 facilitator per team
Manikin	$	Simulation equipment and consumables	Simulation equipment and consumables	Simulation equipment pay RN/support staff	Simulation equipment pay RN/support staff	Simulation equipment pay RN/support staff
	T	Clinician	1 clinician:1 facilitator	Staff, clinician, 1 facilitator	Staff, clinician, ≥1 facilitator per team	Staff, clinician, ≥1 facilitator per team
Standardized patient	$	Actor and consumables	Actor and consumables	Actor, consumables, RN/support staff	Actor, consumables, RN/support staff	Actor, consumables, RN/support staff
	T	Clinician	1 clinician:1 facilitator	Staff, clinician, 1 facilitator	Staff, clinician, ≥1 facilitator per team	Staff, clinician, ≥1 facilitator per team
Virtual	$	Game hardware and software	Game hardware and software	Game hardware and software	Game hardware and software	Game hardware and software, would need to be site specific design
	T	Clinician	Clinician	Staff, clinician	Staff, clinician	Staff, clinician

(continued on next page)

Table 2
(continued)

Environment		Procedural	Individual	Teams	Teams of Teams	Systems Testing
Simulation center	$	Simulation center, sim staff, equipment and consumables	Simulation center, sim staff, equipment and consumables	Simulation center, sim staff, equipment and consumables pay RN/support staff	Simulation center, sim staff, equipment and consumables pay RN/support staff	Simulation center, sim staff, equipment and consumables pay RN/support staff
	T	Clinician	1 clinician:1 facilitator	Staff, clinician, 1 facilitator	Staff, clinician, $\geq$1 facilitator per team	Staff, clinician, $\geq$1 facilitator per team
In situ	$	Simulation equipment and consumables	Simulation equipment and consumables	Simulation equipment pay RN/support staff	Simulation equipment pay RN/support staff	Simulation equipment pay RN/support staff
	T	Clinician	1 clinician:1 facilitator	Staff, clinician, 1 facilitator	Staff, clinician, $\geq$1 facilitator per team	Staff, clinician, $\geq$1 facilitator per team
Virtual	$	Game hardware and software	Game hardware and software	Game hardware and software	Game hardware and software	Game hardware and software, would need to be site specific design
	T	Clinician	Clinician	Staff, clinician	Staff, clinician	Staff, clinician

Abbreviations: $, denotes cost; CNA, certified nursing assistant; ED, emergency department; GI, gastrointestinal; RN, registered nurse; sim staff, simulation staff; T, denotes time.

Table 3
Simulation resources

Type	Organization	Web Site
Professional societies	International Pediatric Simulation Society	https://www.ipssglobal.org/ipssw-2019/
	Society for Academic Emergency Medicine	https://www.saem.org/simulation
	Society for Simulation in Healthcare	https://www.ssih.org/
Simulation scenarios	EM SIM cases	https://emsimcases.com/
	Med- Ed Portal	https://www.mededportal.org/
	The Sim Book	https://thesimbook.com/
University-associated organizations	Center for Medical Simulation	https://harvardmedsim.org/
	COMET: Community Outreach Mobile Education Training	https://www.bmc.org/medical-professionals/solomont-sim-center/community-outreach-mobile-education-training-comet
	ImPACTS: Improving Pediatric Acute Care Through Simulation	https://medicine.yale.edu/lab/impacts/

computer, tablet, or smartphone. Its portability and potential for lower cost overall can be attractive to hospitals and training centers. VR is a high-fidelity virtual world in which one navigates their avatar between environments and interactions with other potential avatars to coordinate patient care.[83] VT involves technical learning using a screen-based component with a haptic simulator that approximates the actual device used in a particular procedure. For example, with intubation you would practice the mechanics on a physical simulator while looking at a screen that simulates the anatomic airway.

SBS is a relatively young but rapidly growing field. Research teams are evaluating its utility for education, its role compared with manikin-based simulation, and its long-term engagement of learners. This developing field has great potential and exciting avenues to explore.

SUMMARY

Simulation has been part of evolving medical education, postgraduate-level training, and all health care disciplines (eg, emergency medical services, registered nurses) for more than a decade. It has been steadily changing the safety culture and team dynamics in the health care industry and allowing individual clinicians and interdisciplinary teams to be proactive in the culture of risk reduction and improved patient safety. Simulation literature has demonstrated improved patient outcomes, improved team-based skills, systems testing, and mitigation of LSTs. There are many options in using simulation methodology and incorporating it into one's hospital system. All modalities serve a purpose: the simulation laboratory is helpful for individual procedures; ISS for system testing and teamwork; community outreach ISS for sharing of best practices, content resource experts, and systems testing; and finally, serious medical gaming is becoming a good adjunct in medical education. All types of simulation are demonstrating efficacy in making significant strides in patient safety.

DISCLOSURE

Dr. Wong is supported by the Robert E. Leet and Clara Guthrie Patterson Trust Mentored Research Award and the National Institutes of Health (NIH) National Center for Advancing Translational Sciences (grant KL2TR001862). The funders had no role in the design and conduct of the study; collection, management, analysis, and interpretation of the data; preparation, review, or approval of the manuscript; and decision to submit the manuscript for publication. The other authors have no disclosures.

REFERENCES

1. Institute of Medicine (US), Committee on Quality of Health Care in America. To err is human: building a safer health system. In: Kohn LT, Corrigan JM, Donaldson MS, editors. Washington, DC: National Academies Press (US); 2000. Available at: http://www.ncbi.nlm.nih.gov/books/NBK225182/. Accessed January 28, 2020.
2. Crimlisk JT, Krisciunas GP, Grillone GA, et al. Emergency airway response team simulation training: a nursing perspective. Dimens Crit Care Nurs 2017;36(5): 290–7.
3. Griswold S, Fralliccardi A, Boulet J, et al. Simulation-based education to ensure provider competency within the health care system. Acad Emerg Med 2018; 25(2):168–76.
4. Zendejas B, Brydges R, Wang AT, et al. Patient outcomes in simulation-based medical education: a systematic review. J Gen Intern Med 2013;28(8):1078–89.
5. Cook DA, Brydges R, Hamstra SJ, et al. Comparative effectiveness of technology-enhanced simulation versus other instructional methods: a systematic review and meta-analysis. Simul Healthc 2012;7(5):308–20.
6. Thomas PA, Kern DE, Hughes MT, et al, editors. Curriculum development for medical education: a six-step approach. 3rd edition. Baltimore (MD): Johns Hopkins University Press; 2016.
7. Macrae C. Imitating incidents: how simulation can improve safety investigation and learning from adverse events. Simul Healthc 2018;13(4):227–32.
8. Geis GL, Pio B, Pendergrass TL, et al. Simulation to assess the safety of new healthcare teams and new facilities. Simul Healthc 2011;6(3):125–33.
9. McLaughlin S, Fitch MT, Goyal DG, et al. Simulation in graduate medical education 2008: a review for emergency medicine. Acad Emerg Med 2008;15(11): 1117–29.
10. Chapman DM, Hayden S, Sanders AB, et al. Integrating the Accreditation Council for Graduate Medical Education Core competencies into the model of the clinical practice of emergency medicine. Ann Emerg Med 2004;43(6):756–69.
11. Aggarwal R, Grantcharov T, Moorthy K, et al. A competency-based virtual reality training curriculum for the acquisition of laparoscopic psychomotor skill. Am J Surg 2006;191(1):128–33.
12. Aggarwal R, Mytton OT, Derbrew M, et al. Training and simulation for patient safety. Qual Saf Health Care 2010;19(Suppl 2):i34–43.
13. Ziv Stephen D Small Paul Root Wolpe A. Patient safety and simulation-based medical education. Med Teach 2000;22(5):489–95.
14. McGaghie WC, Issenberg SB, Cohen ER, et al. Does simulation-based medical education with deliberate practice yield better results than traditional clinical education? A meta-analytic comparative review of the evidence. Acad Med 2011; 86(6):706–11.
15. Ross JG. Simulation and psychomotor skill acquisition: a review of the literature. Clin Simul Nurs 2012;8(9):e429–35.
16. Sawyer T, White M, Zaveri P, et al. Learn, see, practice, prove, do, maintain: an evidence-based pedagogical framework for procedural skill training in medicine. Acad Med 2015;90(8):1025–33.

17. McGaghie WC, Siddall VJ, Mazmanian PE, et al. Lessons for continuing medical education from simulation research in undergraduate and graduate medical education: effectiveness of continuing medical education: American College of Chest Physicians Evidence-Based Educational Guidelines. Chest 2009;135(3 Suppl):62S–8S.

18. Kennedy CC, Cannon EK, Warner DO, et al. Advanced airway management simulation training in medical education: a systematic review and meta-analysis. Crit Care Med 2014;42(1):169–78.

19. Boet S, Borges BCR, Naik VN, et al. Complex procedural skills are retained for a minimum of 1 yr after a single high-fidelity simulation training session. Br J Anaesth 2011;107(4):533–9.

20. Barsuk JH, Cohen ER, McGaghie WC, et al. Long-term retention of central venous catheter insertion skills after simulation-based mastery learning. Acad Med 2010; 85(10 Suppl):S9–12.

21. Barsuk JH, McGaghie WC, Cohen ER, et al. Simulation-based mastery learning reduces complications during central venous catheter insertion in a medical intensive care unit. Crit Care Med 2009;37(10):2697–701.

22. Barsuk JH, Cohen ER, Feinglass J, et al. Use of simulation-based education to reduce catheter-related bloodstream infections. Arch Intern Med 2009;169(15): 1420–3.

23. Barsuk JH, Cohen ER, Potts S, et al. Dissemination of a simulation-based mastery learning intervention reduces central line-associated bloodstream infections. BMJ Qual Saf 2014;23(9):749–56.

24. Barsuk JH, McGaghie WC, Cohen ER, et al. Use of simulation-based mastery learning to improve the quality of central venous catheter placement in a medical intensive care unit. J Hosp Med 2009;4(7):397–403.

25. A risk management program for emergency medicine; basic components and considerations. Available at: https://www.acep.org/globalassets/uploads/uploaded-files/acep/clinical-and-practice-management/resources/medical-legal/risk-mgmt-infopaper_jan2013.pdf. Accessed January 27, 2020.

26. Kobayashi L, Patterson MD, Overly FL, et al. Educational and research implications of portable human patient simulation in acute care medicine. Acad Emerg Med 2008;15(11):1166–74.

27. Lee MO, Brown LL, Bender J, et al. A medical simulation-based educational intervention for emergency medicine residents in neonatal resuscitation. Acad Emerg Med 2012;19(5):577–85.

28. Bleetman A, Sanusi S, Dale T, et al. Human factors and error prevention in emergency medicine. Emerg Med J 2012;29(5):389–93.

29. Truta TS, Boeriu CM, Copotoiu SM, et al. Improving nontechnical skills of an interprofessional emergency medical team through a one day crisis resource management training. Medicine (Baltimore) 2018;97(32):e11828.

30. Hicks CM, Kiss A, Bandiera GW, et al. Crisis Resources for Emergency Workers (CREW II): results of a pilot study and simulation-based crisis resource management course for emergency medicine residents. CJEM 2012;14(6):354–62.

31. Holzman RS, Cooper JB, Gaba DM, et al. Anesthesia crisis resource management: real-life simulation training in operating room crises. J Clin Anesth 1995; 7(8):675–87.

32. Weinger MB, Banerjee A, Burden AR, et al. Simulation-based assessment of the management of critical events by board-certified anesthesiologists. Anesthesiology 2017;127(3):475–89.

33. Howard SK, Gaba DM, Fish KJ, et al. Anesthesia crisis resource management training: teaching anesthesiologists to handle critical incidents. Aviat Space Environ Med 1992;63(9):763–70.

34. Gaba DM. Crisis resource management and teamwork training in anaesthesia. Br J Anaesth 2010;105(1):3–6.

35. Kim J, Neilipovitz D, Cardinal P, et al. A pilot study using high-fidelity simulation to formally evaluate performance in the resuscitation of critically ill patients: The University of Ottawa Critical Care Medicine, High-Fidelity Simulation, and Crisis Resource Management I Study. Crit Care Med 2006;34(8):2167–74.

36. Yang C-W, Yen Z-S, McGowan JE, et al. A systematic review of retention of adult advanced life support knowledge and skills in healthcare providers. Resuscitation 2012;83(9):1055–60.

37. Nestel D, Groom J, Eikeland-Husebø S, et al. Simulation for learning and teaching procedural skills: the state of the science. Simul Healthc 2011;6(Suppl):S10–3.

38. Paige JT, Kozmenko V, Yang T, et al. Attitudinal changes resulting from repetitive training of operating room personnel using of high-fidelity simulation at the point of care. Am Surg 2009;75(7):584–90 [discussion: 590–1].

39. Ericsson KA. Deliberate practice and acquisition of expert performance: a general overview. Acad Emerg Med 2008;15(11):988–94.

40. Risser DT, Rice MM, Salisbury ML, et al. The potential for improved teamwork to reduce medical errors in the emergency department. The MedTeams Research Consortium. Ann Emerg Med 1999;34(3):373–83.

41. Gordon M, Baker P, Catchpole K, et al. Devising a consensus definition and framework for non-technical skills in healthcare to support educational design: a modified Delphi study. Med Teach 2015;37(6):572–7.

42. Rosen MA, DiazGranados D, Dietz AS, et al. Teamwork in healthcare: key discoveries enabling safer, high-quality care. Am Psychol 2018;73(4):433–50.

43. Murphy M, McCloughen A, Curtis K. The impact of simulated multidisciplinary Trauma Team Training on team performance: a qualitative study. Australas Emerg Care 2019;22(1):1–7.

44. McLaughlin C, Barry W, Barin E, et al. Multidisciplinary simulation-based team training for trauma resuscitation: a scoping review. J Surg Educ 2019;76(6):1669–80.

45. Shapiro MJ, Gardner R, Godwin SA, et al. Defining team performance for simulation-based training: methodology, metrics, and opportunities for emergency medicine. Acad Emerg Med 2008;15(11):1088–97.

46. Patterson MD, Blike GT, Nadkarni VM. In situ simulation: challenges and results. In: Henriksen K, Battles JB, Keyes MA, et al, editors. Advances in patient safety: new directions and alternative approaches (vol. 3: performance and tools). Advances in patient safety. Rockville (MD): Agency for Healthcare Research and Quality (US); 2008. Available at: http://www.ncbi.nlm.nih.gov/books/NBK43682/. Accessed January 27, 2020.

47. Rosen MA, Hunt EA, Pronovost PJ, et al. In situ simulation in continuing education for the health care professions: a systematic review. J Contin Educ Health Prof 2012;32(4):243–54.

48. Carayon P, Wetterneck TB, Rivera-Rodriguez AJ, et al. Human factors systems approach to healthcare quality and patient safety. Appl Ergon 2014;45(1):14–25.

49. Havyer RDA, Wingo MT, Comfere NI, et al. Teamwork assessment in internal medicine: a systematic review of validity evidence and outcomes. J Gen Intern Med 2014;29(6):894–910.

50. Boet S, Bould MD, Layat Burn C, et al. Twelve tips for a successful interprofessional team-based high-fidelity simulation education session. Med Teach 2014; 36(10):853–7.
51. TeamStepps | Agency for Health Research and Quality. Available at: https://www.ahrq.gov/teamstepps/index.html. Accessed January 28, 2020.
52. Reeves S, van Schaik S. Simulation: a panacea for interprofessional learning? J Interprof Care 2012;26(3):167–9.
53. Sharma S, Boet S, Kitto S, et al. Interprofessional simulated learning: the need for "sociological fidelity. J Interprof Care 2011;25(2):81–3.
54. D'Amour D, Oandasan I. Interprofessionality as the field of interprofessional practice and interprofessional education: an emerging concept. J Interprof Care 2005;19(Suppl 1):8–20.
55. Lindqvist SM, Reeves S. Facilitators' perceptions of delivering interprofessional education: a qualitative study. Med Teach 2007;29(4):403–5.
56. Ben-Ishay O, Mitaritonno M, Catena F, et al. Mass casualty incidents - time to engage. World J Emerg Surg 2016;11:8.
57. Bentley S, Iavicoli L, Boehm L, et al. A simulated mass casualty incident triage exercise: SimWars. MedEdPORTAL 2019;15:10823.
58. Klima DA, Seiler SH, Peterson JB, et al. Full-scale regional exercises: closing the gaps in disaster preparedness. J Trauma Acute Care Surg 2012;73(3):592–7 [discussion: 597–8].
59. Wheeler DS, Geis G, Mack EH, et al. High-reliability emergency response teams in the hospital: improving quality and safety using in situ simulation training. BMJ Qual Saf 2013;22(6):507–14.
60. Spurr J, Gatward J, Joshi N, et al. Top 10 (+1) tips to get started with in situ simulation in emergency and critical care departments. Emerg Med J 2016;33(7): 514–6.
61. Petrosoniak A, Auerbach M, Wong AH, et al. In situ simulation in emergency medicine: moving beyond the simulation lab. Emerg Med Australas 2017;29(1):83–8.
62. Shabot MM. New tools for high reliability healthcare. BMJ Qual Saf 2015;24(7): 423–4.
63. Zimmermann K, Holzinger IB, Ganassi L, et al. Inter-professional in-situ simulated team and resuscitation training for patient safety: description and impact of a programmatic approach. BMC Med Educ 2015;15:189.
64. Pucher PH, Darzi A, Aggarwal R. Development of an evidence-based curriculum for training of ward-based surgical care. Am J Surg 2014;207(2):213–7.
65. Casey MM, Wholey D, Moscovice IS. Rural emergency department staffing and participation in emergency certification and training programs. J Rural Health 2008;24(3):253–62.
66. Tamariz VP, Fuchs S, Baren JM, et al. Pediatric emergency medicine education in emergency medicine training programs. SAEM Pediatric Education Training Task Force. Society for Academic Emergency Medicine. Acad Emerg Med 2000;7(7): 774–8.
67. Christopher N. Pediatric emergency medicine education in emergency medicine training programs. Acad Emerg Med 2000;7(7):797–9.
68. Wayne DB, Barsuk JH, O'Leary KJ, et al. Mastery learning of thoracentesis skills by internal medicine residents using simulation technology and deliberate practice. J Hosp Med 2008;3(1):48–54.
69. Wayne DB, Butter J, Siddall VJ, et al. Mastery learning of advanced cardiac life support skills by internal medicine residents using simulation technology and deliberate practice. J Gen Intern Med 2006;21(3):251–6.

70. Allan CK, Thiagarajan RR, Beke D, et al. Simulation-based training delivered directly to the pediatric cardiac intensive care unit engenders preparedness, comfort, and decreased anxiety among multidisciplinary resuscitation teams. J Thorac Cardiovasc Surg 2010;140(3):646–52.

71. McGaghie WC. Medical education research as translational science. Sci Transl Med 2010;2(19):19cm8.

72. Simon HK, Sullivan F. Confidence in performance of pediatric emergency medicine procedures by community emergency practitioners. Pediatr Emerg Care 1996;12(5):336–9.

73. Katznelson JH, Mills WA, Forsythe CS, et al. Project CAPE: a high-fidelity, in situ simulation program to increase critical access hospital emergency department provider comfort with seriously ill pediatric patients. Pediatr Emerg Care 2014; 30(6):397–402.

74. Hunt EA, Duval-Arnould JM, Nelson-McMillan KL, et al. Pediatric resident resuscitation skills improve after "rapid cycle deliberate practice" training. Resuscitation 2014;85(7):945–51.

75. Abulebda K, Lutfi R, Whitfill T, et al. A collaborative in situ simulation-based pediatric readiness improvement program for community emergency departments. Acad Emerg Med 2018;25(2):177–85.

76. Ullman E, Kennedy M, Di Delupis FD, et al. The Tuscan Mobile Simulation Program: a description of a program for the delivery of in situ simulation training. Intern Emerg Med 2016;11(6):837–41.

77. Auerbach M, Whitfill T, Gawel M, et al. Differences in the quality of pediatric resuscitative care across a spectrum of emergency departments. JAMA Pediatr 2016; 170(10):987–94.

78. Kessler DO, Walsh B, Whitfill T, et al. Disparities in adherence to pediatric sepsis guidelines across a spectrum of emergency departments: a multicenter, cross-sectional observational in situ simulation study. J Emerg Med 2016;50(3): 403–15.e1-3.

79. Walsh BM, Gangadharan S, Whitfill T, et al. Safety threats during the care of infants with hypoglycemic seizures in the emergency department: a multicenter, simulation-based prospective cohort study. J Emerg Med 2017;53(4):467–74.e7.

80. Bayouth L, Ashley S, Brady J, et al. An in-situ simulation-based educational outreach project for pediatric trauma care in a rural trauma system. J Pediatr Surg 2018;53(2):367–71.

81. Amiel I, Arad J, Gutman M, et al. Mobile trauma simulation in an emergency department of a rural hospital in a conflict area in Israel. Harefuah 2015;154(5): 303–7, 339 [in Hebrew].

82. COMET Program Inquiry | Boston Medical Center. Available at: https://www.bmc. org/comet-inquiry. Accessed January 28, 2020.

83. Youngblood P, Harter PM, Srivastava S, et al. Design, development, and evaluation of an online virtual emergency department for training trauma teams. Simul Healthc 2008;3(3):146–53.

High-risk Pediatric Emergencies

B. Lorrie Edwards, MD*, David Dorfman, MD

KEYWORDS

- Pediatric emergency medicine • Pediatric emergency malpractice • Medicolegal
- Risk management • Medical error

KEY POINTS

- Pediatric medical malpractice cases occur less commonly than adult cases but with potentially higher indemnity payments.
- The most common diagnoses associated with pediatric malpractice cases in the emergency department are cardiac/cardiopulmonary arrest, meningitis, pneumonia, appendicitis, testicular torsion, and fracture.
- The most common causes of pediatric malpractice litigation are missed diagnosis and delayed diagnosis.
- In cases of suspected child abuse, physicians have immunity against liability when reporting suspected abuse if reports are made in good faith, although details of that immunity vary by state.

Medical malpractice is a serious challenge for physicians who take care of children in the emergency department (ED). Although the frequency of medical malpractice claims against pediatricians is one of the lowest of all specialties, the payments made when awarded are among the highest,[1,2] perhaps due to the lifelong consequences that may result from an injury sustained at an early age. For emergency physicians who take care of children, the medicolegal risk is higher; more than half of pediatric malpractice suits arise from the ED.[3,4] The diagnoses associated with malpractice claims vary by age and have evolved over time, currently focused on the significant morbidity and mortality of cardiac and cardiorespiratory arrest.[5] Other diagnoses commonly associated with pediatric ED malpractice claims include meningitis, respiratory illness in infants, appendicitis, testicular torsion, and fracture.[3,5] **Table 1** lists these diagnoses according to the age of the patient and demonstrates the change in epidemiology over the past few decades. This review focuses on the management of these high-risk diagnoses, with emphasis on specific pitfalls that

Department of Pediatrics, Division of Pediatric Emergency Medicine, Boston University School of Medicine, 4th floor, 801 Albany Street, Boston, MA, 02119, USA
* Corresponding author.
E-mail address: lorrie.edwards@bmc.org

Emerg Med Clin N Am 38 (2020) 383–400
https://doi.org/10.1016/j.emc.2020.01.004
0733-8627/20/© 2020 Elsevier Inc. All rights reserved.

may contribute to increased medicolegal liability. Discussion of cardiac and cardiopulmonary arrest in children is deferred, because there are few data exploring the underlying cause of malpractice in these cases, and a full review of pediatric cardiopulmonary resuscitation is beyond the scope of this article.

MENINGITIS

Key Points

- Meningitis in children can progress rapidly and can lead to serious morbidity and mortality.
- Any child with suspected meningitis should have an urgent lumbar puncture, unless contraindicated by the severity of illness.
- Antibiotics should be administered as soon as is feasible after necessary testing but should not be delayed should complications with testing (such as difficulty with lumbar puncture) arise.
- Children, in particular infants, may present with nonspecific signs of infection prior to development of more classic signs of meningitis.
- Seizure outside the classic age for febrile seizure, irritability, bulging fontanelle, and neck stiffness are red flag symptoms and should raise concern for meningitis.
- Published low-risk decision rules can be a valuable evidence-based tool for the evaluation of fever in very young infants. Care should be taken to use them only in patients for whom they are designed.

Meningitis has been one of the most common diagnoses associated with pediatric malpractice cases over the past few decades.[3,5] In patients under the age of 2, it now falls behind only pulmonary illness and cardiac arrest.[5] Nonetheless, a majority of meningitis claims are in pediatric patients, with 60% of those cases involving patients under the age of 2 years.[2] This is likely because the incidence of meningitis is dramatically higher in this age group, with a peak incidence of 80.69 cases per 100,000 infants less than 2 months of age and 6.91 per 100,000 children 2 months to 23 months, compared with 0.56 cases per 100,000 children and 0.43 cases per 100,000 children in ages 2 years to 10 years and 11 years to 17 years, respectively.[6] Although it is rare, the high morbidity and mortality of meningitis in the youngest of children make it a diagnosis that cannot be missed.

Delayed and missed diagnosis of meningitis remain the most commonly cited causes of malpractice. In a review of pediatric meningitis malpractice, only 12.3% of suits had an initial diagnosis of meningitis.[2] The most common alternative diagnoses were viral infection or influenza, other, or otitis media. Correctly identifying patients at risk for meningitis, therefore, is critical on the initial presentation. It has been demonstrated that delay to antibiotics of greater than 24 hours from symptom onset in cases of bacterial meningitis is independently associated with adverse neurologic outcomes,[7] and death from meningococcal infection can occur within a few hours of symptom onset.[8]

Identifying patients at risk, especially in the very young, can be quite challenging. Patients with meningitis can present with nonspecific symptoms.[2] Among meningitis malpractice cases, 74% of children presented with fever, whereas 49% presented with nausea and vomiting.[2] In older children, the classic presentation of fever, photophobia, headache, and mental status change is seen more often, but these symptoms are by no means present in all patients with meningitis.[8,9] Infants often present with

Table 1
Most common diagnoses involved in pediatric emergency department malpractice claims

Patient Age: Years Studied	First	Second	Third
0-2 y: 1985–2000	Meningitis	Impaired neonate	Pneumonia
0-2 y: 2001–2015	Cardiac or cardiorespiratory arrest	Diseases of lung	Meningitis
3-5 y: 1985–2000	Fracture	Meningitis	Appendicitis
3-5 y: 2001–2015	Cardiac or cardiorespiratory arrest	Appendicitis	Fracture of the radius or ulna
6–11 y: 1985–2000	Fracture	Appendicitis	Meningitis
6–11 y: 2001–2015	Cardiac or cardiorespiratory arrest	Appendicitis	Malunion of fracture, meningitis, disorder of male genital organs, aseptic necrosis of bone
12–17 y: 1985–2000	Disorder of male genitalia	Cardiac or cardiorespiratory arrest	Encephalopathy (not further defined), appendicitis
12–17 y: 2001–2015	Fracture	Appendicitis	Testicular torsion

Data from Selbst SM, Friedman MJ, Singh SB. Epidemiology and etiology of malpractice lawsuits involving children in US emergency departments and urgent care centers. *Pediatric emergency care.* 2005;21(3):165-169. and Glerum KM, Selbst SM, Parikh PD, Zonfrillo MR. Pediatric Malpractice Claims in the Emergency Department and Urgent Care Settings From 2001 to 2015. *Pediatric emergency care.* 2018;00.

fever but also may present with hypothermia.[9] Nonspecific symptoms, such as jaundice, poor feeding, vomiting, and irritability, also are common in infants.[9] Certain red flag features can be identified, including a bulging fontanelle or neck stiffness in an infant, seizure outside the typical age range for febrile seizure, irritability or toxic appearance, and any mental status change or sign of meningeal irritation.[8,9] For meningococcal infection in particular, symptoms of sepsis, such as fever, change in skin color, coolness in the hands and feet, leg pain, and irritability, have been noted as earlier signs of the disease than the more classic signs of neck stiffness or petechial rash.[8]

In the very youngest patients, in particular those under 2 months of age, in whom the risk of meningitis is highest, fever may be the only presenting sign within the first 24 hours of illness. Any febrile infant in this age group who is not well appearing to the examiner should have a full sepsis evaluation, including complete blood cell count, blood culture, urinalysis, urine culture, and lumbar puncture. In well-appearing young infants, the rate of serious bacterial infection is 8% to 13%,[10] and many studies have attempted to determine which of these infants may need invasive testing and antibiotic treatment. Several low-risk criteria have been developed, including the Rochester, Philadelphia, and Pediatric Emergency Care Applied Research Network (PECARN) low-risk rule, and the step-by-step rule,[10–12] which aim to identify febrile infants who can be discharged without lumbar puncture or antibiotic therapy. Proper use of low risk criteria can allow approximately 30% of febrile infants to avoid lumbar puncture and be treated with observation alone.[13] A comparison of these rules can be seen in **Table 2**. All of these low-risk rules have exclusion criteria, including infants with prematurity, recent antibiotic use, infants with chronic underlying illness, and infants who are ill appearing on examination.[10,12,14] The step-by-step rule is designed to assess risk for patients with invasive bacterial infections, which includes bacteremia and meningitis but not urinary tract infections.[12] The PECARN low-risk rule was published in 2018 and has yet to be externally validated by additional studies.[10] It should be used with particular caution in infants less than 29 days old in whom the risk of meningitis is highest.

Low-risk decision rules for evaluation of febrile infants also have been cited in several published clinical practice guidelines (CPGs), which use the data to systematically evaluate young febrile infants.[15,16] CPGs have been shown to improve flow and reduce unnecessary testing[17] and may be useful references for emergency providers faced with these challenging patients. Citation of nationally published CPGs, such as those published by the American Heart Association, have been used successfully to defend against malpractice litigation,[18] although it has not yet been demonstrated that institutional CPGs carry similar legal protection. These clinical decisions should be discussed with families, who also may be able to share in decision making around comfort with testing versus risk.

Because no clinical rule or clinical evaluation can be perfect, it is essential that any patient presenting with signs or symptoms of infection, regardless of severity at the time of initial diagnosis, have a solid plan for follow-up. Signs and symptoms of worsening illness should be discussed in detail with the parent or guardian prior to discharge, and strict return precaution for worsening symptoms always should be clear.

PNEUMONIA

Key Points

Cough and fever are common in pediatric pneumonia, but chest pain, hypoxia, and increased work of breathing are more specific clinical signs of concern. Absence of tachypnea is associated with lower risk of pneumonia compared with other respiratory illness.

Identification of children with respiratory distress is critical. Symptoms include tachypnea, grunting, nasal flaring, apnea, cyanosis, altered mental status, and hypoxemia.

Any child with respiratory distress or severe disease should undergo chest radiograph (CXR) and be admitted to the hospital for close respiratory monitoring and therapy.

CXR is not required in children with suspected pneumonia who have mild disease and are deemed well enough for outpatient therapy.

Anticipatory guidance regarding the possibility progression of illness is important for any child who is discharged home with a diagnosis of pneumonia. Families should be given a clear and specific follow-up plan.

In infants presenting to the ED, pneumonia and lung disease remain among the top diagnoses involved in medical malpractice cases, likely because they can be associated with significant patient morbidity or mortality.[2,3,5] It is a common diagnosis, with an annual incidence of 3 to 4 cases per 100 children in the developed world.[19] Although pediatric pneumonia often can be managed in the outpatient setting, failure to identify severe disease can lead not only to respiratory failure but also to severe sequelae, including septic shock and even death. Although there have been no formal studies evaluating the specifics of pediatric pneumonia malpractice cases, selected

Table 2
Comparison of low-risk decision rules for febrile young infants

Rule	Modified Philadelphia Criteria	PECARN Low-risk Rule	Step-by-Step Rule
Age range (d)	29–56	≤60	22–90
Urinalysis	<10 WBC/HPF, -LE, -nitrite	≤5WBC/HPF, - LE, -nitrite	≤5WBC/ HPF, -LE, -nitrite
Blood testing	WBC ≥5 and ≤15 I:T ratio of <0.2	ANC ≤4090/μL Procalcitonin ≤1.71 ng/mL	ANC ≤10,000 Procalcitonin <0.5 CRP ≤20
Sensitivity	98.5%	97.7%	92.0%
NPV	97.1%	99.6%	99.3%

Abbreviations: ANC, absolute neutrophil count; CRP, C-reactive protein; HPF, high-power field; I:T,immature neutrophils:total neutrophils; LE, leukocyte esterase; NPV, negative predictive value; WBC, white blood cell count.

Data from Garra G, Cunningham SJ, Crain EF. Reappraisal of Criteria Used to Predict Serious Bacterial Illness in Febrile Infants Less than 8 Weeks of Age. *Acad Emerg Med.* 2005;12(10):921-925; Kuppermann N, Holmes JF, Dayan PS, et al. Identification of children at very low risk of clinically-important brain injuries after head trauma: a prospective cohort study. *Lancet.* 2009;374:1160-1170; and Gomez B, Mintegi S, Bressan S, et al. Validation of the "Step-by-Step" Approach in the Management of Young Febrile Infants. *Pediatrics.* 2016;138(2).

case reviews note suits related primarily to missed diagnosis or failure to recognize severity of illness, including failure to hospitalize.[20–22]

Although cough and fever are seen in up to 80% of children with pneumonia, a systematic review of signs and symptoms of pneumonia in children found that chest pain, hypoxia, and increased work of breathing were the clinical observations which most successfully identified children with pneumonia compared with other respiratory illnesses.[23] The presence of tachypnea was not found to increase the likelihood of pneumonia, although the absence of tachypnea was found to be associated with a lower likelihood of pneumonia.[23] It is critical to remember that respiratory rate varies significantly by age, and recognition of respiratory distress is dependent on knowing these values. World Health Organization criteria for tachypnea are noted in **Table 3**. Other signs of respiratory distress at any age include dyspnea, retractions, grunting, nasal flaring, apnea, altered mental status, and hypoxemia (pulse oximetry <90% on room air).[19] Such patients should be admitted to the hospital for close monitoring and treatment.

When clinical concern is high enough, the diagnosis can be confirmed with CXR. Routine CXR is not required, however, for children suspected of mild disease who

Table 3
World Health Organization criteria for tachypnea

Age	Respiratory Rate (Breaths/min)
0–2 mo	>60
2–12 mo	>50
1–5 y	>40
>5 y	>20

Adapted from Bradley JS, Byington CL, Shah SS, et al. The management of community-acquired pneumonia in infants and children older than 3 months of age: clinical practice guidelines by the Pediatric Infectious Diseases Society and the Infectious Diseases Society of America. *Clinical Infectious Diseases.* 2011;53(7):e25-e76.

are well enough to be treated as outpatients. Children with severe disease, however, defined as fever greater than or equal to 38.5°C, moderate to severe respiratory distress, cyanosis, altered mental status, dehydration or poor feeding, or other signs of sepsis,[19] should have a CXR performed to evaluate for complications of pneumonia, such as pleural effusion, empyema, pneumothorax, and abscess. Children with diagnosed community-acquired pneumonia should be admitted to the hospital for any of the following criteria: respiratory distress, hypoxemia, age less than 6 months, suspected pathogen with increased virulence such as methicillin-resistant *Staphylococcus aureus* (MRSA), and concern about adequate follow-up and home observation.[19] Anticipatory guidance regarding the potential for worsening of respiratory symptoms is critical in patients who are deemed well enough to be discharged home.

First-line treatment of pediatric pneumonia suspected to be of bacterial origin is with oral amoxicillin, 90 mg/kg/day, divided twice a day in infants, preschool-aged children, and school-aged children. Consideration also can be given to macrolide therapy for school-aged patients with a more indolent clinical course suspected of atypical infection, such as *Mycoplasma pneumoniae*. The child in need of hospitalization should be treated with intravenous ampicillin or penicillin G, if immunized against *Streptococcus pneumoniae*, or with a third-generation cephalosporin, such as ceftriaxone, if not fully immunized against pneumococcal strains (usually completed at approximately age 6 months).

Coinfection with influenza should prompt additional scrutiny; 30% to 40% of patients hospitalized with influenza are found to have pneumonia,[24] and although any child with influenza may develop bacterial pneumonia, the highest risk of coinfection is found in children under age 5.[24] Children with pneumonia who are coinfected with influenza have an increased risk of requiring intensive care admissions and have longer hospital lengths of stay.[25] Whereas children without influenza coinfection are most likely to have *S pneumoniae,* children with influenza coinfection are more likely to be infected with *S aureus,* with a high prevalence of MRSA.[25] Therefore, in children with pneumonia and influenza, empirical therapy should always include coverage for MRSA, with a low threshold for hospitalization in any child who is not well appearing. Additional antimicrobial therapy should be directed at specific pathogens based on local susceptibility data.

APPENDICITIS

Key Points

Children with appendicitis commonly present with atypical features, particularly in younger ages. Consider the diagnosis in children with nonspecific complaints, such as generalized abdominal pain, fever, or vomiting, and, if unsure, consider supplementing the clinical history and examination with additional laboratory or imaging studies.

Pediatric appendicitis is most likely to be missed in the first 24 hours of presentation, and extra attention should be paid to this patient population.

Clinical prediction rules can aid in diagnosis but lack the sensitivity to make a definitive diagnosis of appendicitis. They may be used in the context of a broader clinical care pathway.

Ultrasound is the imaging modality of choice for pediatric appendicitis. If ultrasound is not available, other alternatives include magnetic resonance imaging (MRI) or surgical consultation. Computed tomography (CT) should be avoided if possible, to reduce exposure to ionizing radiation.

Acute appendicitis occurs in approximately 70,000 pediatric patients every year.[26] For several reasons, including its high incidence, the potential for significant morbidity and mortality, and multiple clinical factors relating to its presentation, acute appendicitis is the second most common diagnosis associated with malpractice suits in school-aged children.[3,5,26]

A review of pediatric appendicitis malpractice claims from 1984 to 2013 notes that more than 75% of claims cite delay to diagnosis or misdiagnosis as the breach of care, with the remainder of claims citing operative/perioperative issues.[26] Emergency physicians were named in 20.2% of cases, hospital groups in 38.3%, and pediatricians in 29%.[26] Consequences of missed appendicitis can include perforation, abscess formation, obstruction, sepsis, and death.[27] Importantly, the cases of delayed or missed diagnosis in this case series had a 19.9% mortality rate,[26] and although selection bias certainly plays a role in which cases proceed to lawsuits, this fact highlights the importance of making this diagnosis at the first presentation.

Unfortunately, children with acute appendicitis present unique clinical challenges, increasing the risk of missed diagnosis. Although practitioners may be on the lookout for the textbook signs and symptoms of periumbilical pain followed by development of nausea, right lower quadrant pain, fever, and finally peritoneal signs, this classic progression is seen only in up to 50% of adults and even less often in children.[28] Fever is absent in up to 83% of patients, Rovsing sign is absent in 68%, 52% have absence of rebound pain, and 32% have absence of pain in the right lower quadrant.[28]

Not surprisingly, patients who present with nonspecific chief complaints less suggestive of appendicitis, such as fever, vomiting, and dehydration, have an increased rate of missed diagnosis compared with children presenting with a chief complaint of generalized abdominal pain or right lower quadrant pain,[29] leading to a delayed/missed diagnosis rate of 7.5% to 37% in pediatric patients.[30] The most common incorrect diagnosis in these cases is acute gastroenteritis.[26,30]

Overall, the perforation rate in cases of missed pediatric appendicitis is more than 70%.[30] Younger patients are especially vulnerable. Patients ages 5 years to 12 years have a perforation rate of 7% at less than 24 hours after symptom onset and 38% at 24 hours to 48 hours, and at greater than 48 hours the rate climbs to greater than 98%.[31] Patients under 3 years of age have a 70% rate of perforation at less than 48 hours.[31]

The fact that children frequently have atypical presentations of appendicitis makes it difficult for the emergency practitioner to recognize and diagnose. The extensive literature on diagnosis of pediatric appendicitis is constantly evolving, but consensus often relies on the use of clinical prediction rules, such as the Pediatric Appendicitis Score (PAS) or the refined Low-Risk Appendicitis Rule, to assess patients with symptoms concerning for appendicitis. Pertinent positive and negative findings on these scoring systems should be documented thoroughly if utilized.

The PAS is a scoring system that assigns points to historical, examination, and laboratory variables (**Table 4**).[32] A score of less than or equal to 3 suggests a low risk of appendicitis, whereas a score of greater than or equal to 7 indicates a 78% to 96% risk of appendicitis. This suggests that patients with a score of 7 or higher on the PAS warrant additional work-up with either imaging or surgical consultation. Patients with PAS scores of 4 to 6, however, are of indeterminate risk, and further evaluation with imaging is indicated. Although a high score is not sufficient to rule in appendicitis completely, clinical pathways that make use of the PAS have been reported to have sensitivity and specificity of 92.3% and 94.7%, respectively.[33]

The refined Low-Risk Appendicitis Rule defines patients as low risk for appendicitis if they meet 1 of 2 criteria: (1) absolute neutrophil count of $6.75 \times 10^3/\mu L$ or less without maximal tenderness in the right lower quadrant or (2) absolute neutrophil count of

6.75 × 10³/μL or less with maximal tenderness in the right lower quadrant and without abdominal pain with walking/jumping or coughing.[34] This score has been validated with a sensitivity of 98.1% and specificity of 23.7%, with a negative predictive value of 95.3% in identifying children without appendicitis.[34] This rule is not designed to identify children who do have appendicitis.

Neither of these clinical prediction rules makes use of imaging studies. Although CT is both sensitive and specific for pediatric appendicitis, exposure to ionizing radiation makes its use less desirable than other modalities. Sensitivity of ultrasound for pediatric appendicitis is as high as 92% to 94%, with sensitivity of 93.76% to 91.2%,[35] making it the first choice for evaluation of pediatric appendicitis. Availability of ultrasound, however, may be limited at certain institutions, and the study has been shown to be highly operator dependent.[35] MRI also has been demonstrated to have a 96% sensitivity and 96% specificity for pediatric appendicitis, but, again, MRI availability may be limited. When optimal imaging is unavailable and patients are clinically equivocal for appendicitis, surgical consultation or transfer to a facility with pediatric radiology and pediatric surgical availability may be warranted.

Despite use of clinical decision rules and imaging, missing a diagnosis of appendicitis in a child remains a risk, especially at the early stages of presentation, when historical and examination findings can be nonspecific. It is, therefore, critical for a provider to establish a clear plan for follow-up to ensure that the examination findings have not substantially worsened or changed. There is no evidence-based timeline for when follow-up should occur for discharged patients, but, given the high morbidity and mortality of perforated appendicitis, follow-up within 24 hours is appropriate. Proper anticipatory guidance also should include detailed instructions for ED reevaluation for all red flag symptoms that were not present on initial evaluation, including fever, vomiting, migration of pain to the right lower quadrant, or significant worsening of pain. These conversations should be thorough and well-documented in a patient's medical record.

TESTICULAR TORSION

Key Points

Boys and men of any age presenting to the ED with a chief complaint of genital and/or abdominal pain always should have a full testicular examination performed.

A combination approach using history, physical examination findings, and ultrasound should be used when determining risk for testicular torsion.

Scrotal ultrasound with doppler has a sensitivity of up to 96% for testicular torsion, but this test is not perfect, and results should not be used as the sole factor in diagnosis.

When high clinical suspicion for testicular torsion exists based on any of these criteria, urologic consultation is warranted, regardless of specific examination findings or ultrasound results.

Testicular torsion has been cited as the third most common diagnosis involved in cases of medical malpractice in adolescent patients.[5] Although relatively rare, occurring in 4.5 per every 100,000 male patients under age 25,[36] the frequency of its appearance in medical malpractice suits underscores the significant morbidity of infarction of the testicle and emphasizes the need for specific attention to this diagnosis.

Table 4	
Pediatric appendicitis score	
Variable	**Points**
Nausea/vomiting	1
Anorexia	1
Migration of pain to the right lower quadrant	1
Fever $\geq$38°C	1
Right lower quadrant tenderness	2
Tenderness with cough/percussion/hopping	2
Leukocytosis (>10,000)	1
Left shift (>75% neutrophilia)	1
Total possible score	10

Adapted from Samuel, M. Pediatric appendicitis score. *J Pediatr Surg* 2002; 37:877.

Testicular torsion in male adolescents most often is due to twisting of the spermatic cord within the tunica vaginalis, leading to increased venous pressure and decreased arterial flow, ultimately resulting in testicular ischemia if not corrected. The classic patient with testicular torsion is a male adolescent with acute onset of severe, unilateral testicular pain of less than 6 hours duration prior to presentation, often with associated nausea and vomiting. His testicular examination reveals a tender and edematous testicle, which may be high-riding with horizontal orientation within the scrotum and absence of a cremasteric reflex.[37]

Unfortunately, although this classic presentation remains the most common, atypical presentations can lead to missed or delayed diagnosis, with significant risk of morbidity. Case series reviews have found that 5% to 12.5% of patients who ultimately were diagnosed with testicular torsion by surgical exploration did not present with a chief complaint of testicular pain.[38] In a review of medical malpractice appellant cases for testicular torsion, 31% of cases listed a chief complaint of abdominal pain alone.[39] Importantly, the lack of testicular examination in such cases commonly is cited as the breach of standard of care.[39,40] Other classic historical features, such as the acute onset of pain for a short period of time, also have been refuted. Testicular torsion has been shown to present with gradual onset of pain in multiple cases, whereas alternative diagnoses for acute scrotum, such as epididymitis, which classically has a more insidious onset, can present relatively acutely.[38]

On examination, patients may present with a vertical lie to the affected testicle, even in cases of torsion, as often as 17% to 54% of the time.[38] Scrotal edema and testicular swelling are not unique to torsion and may be confused with other causes of acute scrotum, such as epididymo-orchitis or torsion of the appendix testis.[38] Even the absence of the cremasteric reflex, long touted as the pathognomonic sign of testicular torsion,[41] has been found to be both absent in cases of normal testes, and present in cases of confirmed testicular torsion.[38] In short, reliance on the clinical history or the physical examination alone may result in missed or delayed diagnosis.

It also is critical to remember that testicular torsion also can present in younger children, with 10% of cases occurring in the neonatal period.[42] In neonates, patients initially may present with painless scrotal swelling or with nonspecific signs of discomfort, such as irritability or poor feeding. Findings on testicular examination in neonates may include scrotal swelling with or without signs of inflammation.[37] Keeping testicular torsion on the differential diagnosis of the fussy neonate and performing a thorough testicular examination for any infant boy with nonspecific symptoms may help catch these especially challenging cases.

Supplementing the history and the physical examination with high-resolution ultrasonography with color Doppler, therefore, often is recommended to evaluate both for sonographic features of testicular torsion–such as the spermatic whirlpool sign and redundant spermatic cord—and, particularly, for evidence of asymmetric perfusion to the affected testicle.[37,43] Doppler ultrasonography has an 88.9% to 96% sensitivity, with greater than 98% specificity.[40,44] False-negative ultrasound reports have been cited in multiple malpractice cases[39,40] as the proximal cause of morbidity. It, therefore, should be emphasized that when clinical suspicion is high enough, a urologist should be consulted. This is supported by review of litigated cases, noting that although ordering an ultrasound is not correlated with successful defense, consultation with urology has been shown to lead to more successful legal outcomes.[40]

Awaiting the ultrasound should never delay urologic consultation in cases of sufficiently high clinical suspicion of torsion, because delay in making this diagnosis can lead to significant morbidity for affected patients. Although missed diagnosis is the most common cause of malpractice litigation, delay to hospital admission and delay to urology consultation account for up to 35% of appellate cases.[39] Nor should providers slow their approach for patients complaining of prolonged testicular pain—the classic teaching that testicular ischemia is irreversible after 6 hours to 8 hours of torsion has been demonstrated to be quite untrue.[45] A systematic review by Mellick and colleagues[45] noted that although testicular survival does diminish significantly with increasing duration of pain, there is an up to 18.1% chance of testicular recovery even after 24 hours of torsion. The adage, "time is testicle," is a valid one, and a decision to act on the diagnosis, therefore, should be made as expeditiously as possible.

FRACTURES AND ORTHOPEDIC INJURIES

Key Points

Elbow fractures are common, but the findings can be subtle on radiography (look for posterior fat pad in lateral view)—have high suspicion for supracondylar, lateral condyle, and medial condyle fractures in patients presenting with focal elbow pain or tenderness.

Injury patterns differ depending on the age of the child, due to changes in activity with development as well as anatomic changes due to growth.

Children with growth plates can sustain Salter-Harris fractures. Management depends on grade and location. Salter-Harris types III and IV fractures should have orthopedic consultation.

Legg-Calvé-Perthes disease (LCP) and slipped capital femoral epiphysis (SCFE) are seen best in the anteroposterior (AP) and frog leg views of the pelvis. Early presentations may not be apparent on plain films.

Approximately half of all children will suffer at least 1 fracture during their childhood, with an annual incidence as high as 400 cases per 100,000 children per year.[46,47] Malpractice litigation for fracture is common, and a majority of cases are due to redisplacement of a previously reduced fracture, dissatisfaction in healing, and missed fracture diagnosis.[48] In 1 case series, the sites most commonly involved in litigation were the elbow, the forearm, the humerus (transcondylar), the femur, and the hand.[49] With any fracture, neurovascular compromise is a potential complication, and a complete and thorough neurovascular examination always should be performed and well documented.

Elbow Fractures

The most difficult joint in which to diagnose a fracture in children is the elbow. It is a common site for fracture and when fractured can lead to long-term morbidity. The most common elbow fracture in the pediatric patient is the supracondylar fracture.[50] These can be subtle and often can only be seen in a lateral x-ray view—the sail sign, an overly large anterior fat pad, or the presence of the posterior fat pad, which is not normally seen. It is, therefore, essential to make sure the lateral view is taken correctly, determined by the presence of a figure 8 or teardrop shape,[51] with the upper extremity directed anteriorly rather than externally rotated.

Type I supracondylar fracture describes a nondisplaced fracture with radiographic evidence of elbow effusion (anterior sail and/or posterior fat pad signs). Type II supracondylar fracture refers to a displaced fracture with an intact posterior periosteum. Type III supracondylar fracture is a displaced fracture with disrupted anterior and posterior periosteum. Recognizing the degree of displacement is critical for the emergency physician, because a type I supracondylar fracture can be splinted and referred to orthopedics. Orthopedics should be consulted, however, immediately for type II and type III supracondylar fractures, because nerve and vascular damage is of concern with these fractures.

Lateral condyle fractures are the second most common elbow fracture in children[52] and have a worrisome risk of nonunion, malunion, and avascular necrosis.[53,54] Even nondisplaced lateral condyle fractures may be unstable despite casting or splinting. All children with this fracture should be seen within a few days by an orthopedist. Medial humeral condyle fractures also are of concern, because they require casting in flexion and the forearm in neutral position, even with no displacement. Slight displacement (>2 mm) is generally treated operatively.[55] Unfortunately, both lateral and medial condyle fractures can be missed on initial radiographs. Children with elbow swelling, limited range of motion, or point tenderness should be followed closely and referred to orthopedics if symptoms do not resolve in a timely fashion.

Forearm Fractures

The distal radius and ulnar frequently are broken. Some of these fractures are obvious, with marked angulation. Children, however, are prone to buckle fractures (torus fractures), which may have more subtle presentations. Such buckle fractures of the distal radius or ulna routinely heal well. A removable splint that a family can remove for bathing is the preferred treatment.[56]

Midshaft fractures of the radius and ulna, on the other hand, are more commonly involved in litigation, with most cases citing redisplacement of the fracture after reduction as the cause of complaint.[48] Although this can be a known complication of fracture reduction, anticipatory guidance for families regarding timely follow-up with orthopedics is key as are signs and symptoms of worsening pain, swelling, or deformity, which should prompt more urgent return to care.

Foot Fractures

The most commonly missed pediatric fractures involve the phalanges and metatarsals. The most commonly missed metatarsal fracture is at the base of the fifth metatarsal, often caused by ankle inversion.[57] Children have an apophysis at the base of the fifth metatarsal, which lies along the long axis of the metatarsal. In some instances, it is mistaken for a fracture. In other instances, fractures of the fifth metatarsal are mistaken for the apophysis. Knowing the developmental anatomy of the metatarsal, and correlating radiographic findings with tenderness on examination protect against this error.

Salter-Harris Fractures

No review of pediatric fractures would be complete without a discussion of Salter-Harris fractures. In growing children, the physeal plates often are the weakest part of the bone and many pediatric fractures go completely or partially through the growth plate. Salter-Harris type I fractures involve only the physis. They may be radiologically obscure. A subtle sign may be widening of the affected growth plate. Salter-Harris type II fractures go through the physis and into the metaphysis. Salter-Harris type III fractures involve the physis and the epiphysis. Salter-Harris type IV fractures include the physis and both the epiphysis and metaphysis. Finally, Salter-Harris type V fractures are a crush injury with compression of the physis and involving both the epiphysis and metaphysis.

Some Salter-Harris fractures are relatively trivial and heal well. Salter-Harris type I and small nondisplaced Salter-Harris type II fractures of the distal fibula are treated in the same manner as ankle sprains and are shown to heal without complication.[58] Salter-Harris type III fractures of the anterolateral distal tibia with avulsion of the lateral tibial epiphysis (Tillaux fracture) are the most common Salter-Harris type III fracture in children and typically occur in young teenagers but can be difficult fractures to recognize. The patient often has anterior ankle swelling. It is best seen in the AP view of the ankle and appears as a vertical line through the epiphysis. If there is displacement of the epiphyseal fragment, determined by CT, surgery may be needed. Close follow-up with orthopedics is required for patients with this injury.

Another, rather complicated fracture of the distal tibia seen in young adolescents prior to fusion is the triplane fracture or Salter-Harris type IV fracture. It involves 3 planes (hence its name) and incorporates Salter-Harris types I, II, and III that are joined together. This fracture generally is seen most clearly in the lateral view. CT and urgent orthopedic referral are required.

Hip Pathology

Limp is a common cause for ED visits by young children. The differential includes malignancy, Lyme disease, osteomyelitis, fracture, and abuse but also muscle strain and hand foot and mouth disease. Two entities deserve special mention from a medicolegal standpoint. Idiopathic avascular necrosis of the femoral head (LCP) generally presents with a subacute course, most frequently in school-aged children (range 3–12 years; peak 6 years).[59] The diagnosis may be made on plain radiographs (AP and frog leg radiographs of the pelvis, including both hips for comparison are the standard views) but early on in its course these films may be normal. If a child has persistent pain and LCP is suspected, bone scan or MRI can detect early changes that are not seen on radiographs. The treatment of LCP is controversial but this diagnosis may lead to legal risk if missed.

The other entity that is often missed, sometimes leading to increased morbidity, is SCFE. SCFE, separation of the capital femoral epiphysis from the femoral neck through the physis, most often presents in children in early adolescence, prior to closure of the femoral physis. It is one on the most common hip disorders among adolescents. It may present as an acute, acute on chronic, or chronic phase. Diagnosis is suggested by limp, hip pain, or even medial thigh or knee pain in a child 10 years to 15 years of age and typically is associated with obesity. It may occur earlier in girls. A diagnosis generally is made by plain film, AP, and frog leg views of the pelvis and hips. Comparison of the 2 hips is helpful to detect subtle slippage. SCFE may occur in both hips. In very early cases, it even may present in a preslip phase, in which the only radiologic evidence of SCFE is relative physeal widening. Slippage also may worsen over time.[60] Thus, the treatment involves non–weight bearing and immediate orthopedic referral for surgical pinning.

CHILD ABUSE

Key Points

Physicians have a duty to report suspected cases of child abuse and should be aware of the specifics of reporting laws in the state in which they practice.

Physicians may be criminally or civilly liable for failure to report child mistreatment but have immunity, which limits liability for reporting in most states.

Patients presenting with frequent injuries or red flag historical or examination features should be evaluated for child abuse, and a report should be made to the appropriate child protective service.

Child abuse is a diagnosis that no physician wishes to make. More than 2 million reports of suspected child maltreatment are made each year, 650,000 of which ultimately are substantiated, leading to an estimated 1500 annual fatalities annually.[61] Adult reports of childhood abuse suggest that these data consistently underreport the problem.[61] Although child abuse cases are not among the more common diagnoses associated with medical malpractice cases, the anxiety associated with the potential legal ramifications of child abuse reporting merits inclusion of child abuse in this review. To prevent significant and potentially long-term morbidity or mortality, physicians are required by state and national laws to report suspected child abuse to the appropriate protective authorities. Nationally, the Federal Child Abuse Prevention and Treatment Act requires reporting of abuse by certain parties responsible for child welfare, including physicians.[62] All 50 states impose criminal penalties on physicians who fail to report child abuse, with some states providing additional civil liability in such cases,[62] although states differ in the exact definition of findings that require reporting.[63]

Although private malpractice suits regarding missed diagnoses of child abuse are not especially common, they do exist.[64,65] Cases generally stem from a failure to report suspected abuse in patients whose injuries might have otherwise raised red flags, as seen in the landmark case of *Landeros v Flood*, the case of an 11 month old whose initial ED visit for bruising and multiple fractures was not recognized as inflicted until she re-presented suffering from severe abusive head trauma at a later date.[63]

On the other end of the spectrum, physicians are relatively protected against liability in cases in which a report is made but ultimately unsubstantiated. Although every state is different, and physicians should be aware of the statutes of the states in which they practice, every state provides some degree of immunity to physician reporters. A few states provide absolute immunity for all reporters.[62] Others provide an immunity defense only for reports made in good faith, sometimes including a presumption that physician reports are in good faith unless affirmatively proved otherwise.[62,63] In practice, it is rare that physicians are found liable for reporting suspected child abuse. In a survey of child abuse physicians, 16% reported having been sued for malpractice but none successfully.[66]

Injuries are one of the most commonly presenting pediatric complaints to EDs, and determining which injuries might be nonaccidental can be challenging. **Table 5** lists historical and examination features that may raise suspicions for child abuse in the pediatric patient. In particular, physicians should be wary of injuries in children with explanations that do not seem to be consistent with the injury or with the appropriate developmental stage of the child. A nonambulatory infant is unlikely to suffer fractures accidently, unless the history specifically addresses the injuries present. Once ambulatory, bruises in children are common but should be located on areas typical for simple falls and contusions. Bruising rarely includes the torso, neck, or abdomen, and those locations should prompt further evaluation. Red flags for pediatric fractures include multiple fractures, fractures in different stages of healing, rib fractures, infants or toddlers with midshaft humeral or femoral fractures, high-impact fractures such as the scapula or sternum, and classic metaphyseal lesions of the long bones.

Once child abuse is suspected, evaluation should include consultation with a child abuse specialist as early as possible to guide further management. In children under age 2 years, a skeletal survey should be obtained to evaluate for occult fracture, which is seen in up to 11% of studies.[61] Screening liver and pancreatic enzymes should be sent to evaluate for occult abdominal trauma. If severe trauma is suspected in an infant, head imaging also is recommended to evaluate for abusive head trauma.[61] Documentation should be clear and thorough and should include documentation of all findings as well as the likelihood of accidental versus nonaccidental injury. Disposition may be dependent on the response of local child protective services, but admission to the hospital may be warranted if there are safety concerns.

Table 5 Historical and examination features suggestive of child abuse	
Historical Features	**Physical Examination Findings**
Significant injury with vague or no explanation	Any injury to a preambulatory infant
Denial of trauma in a child with obvious injury	Injuries to multiple organ systems
Details of explanation change in a substantial way	Multiple injuries in different stages of healing
Explanation of events is inconsistent with injury	Patterned injuries (eg, object-shaped bruises, object-shaped or immersion burns, bite marks)
Explanation of events is inconsistent with developmental capabilities of the child	Injuries to nonbony or unusual locations (eg, torso, ears, face, neck, upper arms)
Unexplained notable delay in seeking medical care	Significant unexplained injuries
Different witnesses provide substantially different explanations	Additional evidence of child neglect

Adapted from Christian CW, Committee on Child Abuse and Neglect, American Academy of Pediatrics. The evaluation of suspected child physical abuse. *Pediatrics.* 2015;135(5):e1337-1354.

SUMMARY

Children are not small adults. The diagnoses associated with malpractice are unique to the pediatric population and vary by age. All providers who take care of children in the emergency setting should be cognizant of the medicolegal risk associated with this population, not only to protect against liability but also to increase awareness of the pitfalls of these critical but complex diagnoses in order to improve outcomes for all pediatric patients.

DISCLOSURE

The authors have nothing to disclose.

REFERENCES

1. Jena AB, Chandra A, Seabury SA. Malpractice risk among US pediatricians. Pediatrics 2013;131(6):1148–54.
2. McAbee GN, Donn SM, Mendelson RA, et al. Medical diagnoses commonly associated with pediatric malpractice lawsuits in the United States. Pediatrics 2008; 122(6):e1282–6.
3. Selbst SM, Friedman MJ, Singh SB. Epidemiology and etiology of malpractice lawsuits involving children in US emergency departments and urgent care centers. Pediatr Emerg Care 2005;21(3):165–9.
4. Najaf-Zadeh A, Dubos F, Aurel M, et al. Epidemiology of malpractice lawsuits in paediatrics. Acta Paediatr 2008;97(11):1486–91.
5. Glerum KM, Selbst SM, Parikh PD, et al. Pediatric malpractice claims in the emergency department and urgent care settings from 2001 to 2015. Pediatr Emerg Care 2018. [Epub ahead of print].
6. Thigpen MC, Whitney CG, Messonnier NE, et al. Bacterial meningitis in the United States, 1998-2007. N Engl J Med 2011;364(21):2016–25.
7. Bargui F, D'Agostino I, Mariani-Kurkdjian P, et al. Factors influencing neurological outcome of children with bacterial meningitis at the emergency department. Eur J Pediatr 2012;171:1365–71.
8. Thompson MJ, Ninis N, Perera R, et al. Clinical recognition of meningococcal disease in children and adolescents. Lancet 2006;367(9508):397–403.
9. Curtis S, Stobart K, Vandermeer B, et al. Clinical features suggestive of meningitis in children: a systematic review of prospective data. Pediatrics 2010;126(5): 952–60.
10. Kuppermann N, Dayan PS, Levine DA, et al. A clinical prediction rule to identify febrile infants 60 days and younger at low risk for serious bacterial infections. JAMA Pediatr 2019;173(4):342–51.
11. Anbar RD, Richardson de Corral V, O'Malley PJ. Difficulties in universal application of criteria identifying infants at low risk for serious bacterial infection. J Pediatr 1986;109:483–5.
12. Gomez B, Mintegi S, Bressan S, et al. Validation of the "step-by-step" approach in the management of young febrile infants. Pediatrics 2016;138(2) [pii: e20154381].
13. Huppler AR, Eickhoff JC, Wald ER. Performance of low-risk criteria in the evaluation of young infants with fever: review of the literature. Pediatrics 2010;125(2): 228–33.

14. Garra G, Cunningham SJ, Crain EF. Reappraisal of criteria used to predict serious bacterial illness in febrile infants less than 8 weeks of age. Acad Emerg Med 2005;12(10):921–5.

15. Scarfone R, Gala R, Murray A, et al. ED pathway for evaluation/treatment of febrile young infants (0-56 days old). 2010. Available at: https://www.chop.edu/clinical-pathway/febrile-infant-emergent-evaluation-clinical-pathway. Accessed July 1, 2019.

16. Bishop J, Ackley H, Fenstermacher S, et al. Seattle children's hospital neonatal fever pathway. Available at: http://www.seattlechildrens.org/pdf/neonatal-fever-pathway.pdf. Accessed July 1, 2019.

17. Kuppermann N, Holmes JF, Dayan PS, et al. Identification of children at very low risk of clinically-important brain injuries after head trauma: a prospective cohort study. Lancet 2009;374:1160–70.

18. Mackey TK, Liang BA. The role of practice guidelines in medical malpractice litigation. Virtual Mentor 2011;13(1):36–41.

19. Bradley JS, Byington CL, Shah SS, et al. The management of community-acquired pneumonia in infants and children older than 3 months of age: clinical practice guidelines by the Pediatric Infectious Diseases Society and the Infectious Diseases Society of America. Clin Infect Dis 2011;53(7):e25–76.

20. Selbst SM. Legal briefs. Pediatr Emerg Care 2010;26(4):316–9.

21. Selbst SM. Legal briefs. Pediatr Emerg Care 2014;30(8):583–5.

22. Selbst SM. Legal briefs. Pediatr Emerg Care 2013;29(6):770–2.

23. Shah SS, Bachur RG, Simel DL, et al. Does this child have pneumonia? The rational clinical examination systematic review. JAMA 2017;318(5):462–71.

24. Kalil AC, Thomas PG. Influenza virus-related critical illness: pathophysiology and epidemiology. Crit Care 2019;23(1):258.

25. Williams DJ, Hall M, Brogan TV, et al. Influenza coinfection and outcomes in children with complicated pneumonia. Arch Pediatr Adolesc Med 2011;165(6):506–12.

26. Sullins VF, Rouch JD, Lee SL. Malpractice in cases of pediatric appendicitis. Clin Pediatr (Phila) 2017;56(3):226–30.

27. Hamid KA, Mohamed MA, Salih A. Acute appendicitis in young children: a persistent diagnostic challenge for clinicians. Cureus 2018;10(3):e2347.

28. Becker T, Kharbanda A, Bachur R. Atypical clinical features of pediatric appendicitis. Acad Emerg Med 2007;14(2):124–9.

29. Drapkin Z, Dunnick J, Madsen TE, et al. Pediatric appendicitis: association of chief complaint with missed appendicitis. Pediatr Emerg Care 2018. [Epub ahead of print].

30. Chang YJ, Chao HC, Kong MS, et al. Misdiagnosed acute appendicitis in children in the emergency department. Chang Gung Med J 2010;33(5):551–7.

31. Marzuillo P, Germani C, Krauss BS, et al. Appendicitis in children less than five years old: a challenge for the general practitioner. World J Clin Pediatr 2015;4(2):19–24.

32. Samuel M. Pediatric appendicitis score. J Pediatr Surg 2002;37(6):877–81.

33. Saucier A, Huang EY, Emeremni CA, et al. Prospective evaluation of a clinical pathway for suspected appendicitis. Pediatrics 2014;133(1):e88–95.

34. Kharbanda AB, Dudley NC, Bajaj L, et al. Validation and refinement of a prediction rule to identify children at low risk for acute appendicitis. Arch Pediatr Adolesc Med 2012;166(8):738–44.

35. Mangona KLM, Guillerman RP, Mangona VS, et al. Diagnostic performance of ultrasonography for pediatric appendicitis: a night and day difference? Acad Radiol 2017;24(12):1616–20.
36. Bass JB, Couperus KS, Pfaff JL, et al. A pair of testicular torsion medicolegal cases with caveats: the Ball's in your court. Clin Pract Cases Emerg Med 2018; 2(4):283–5.
37. Sharp VJ, Kieran K, Arlen AM. Testicular torsion: diagnosis, evaluation, and management. Am Fam Physician 2013;88(12):835–40.
38. Mellick LB. Torsion of the Testicle: It is time to stop tossing the dice. Pediatr Emerg Care 2012;28:80–6.
39. Gaither TW, Copp HL. State appellant cases for testicular torsion: Case review from 1985 to 2015. J Pediatr Urol 2016;12(5):291.e1-5.
40. Colaco M, Heavner M, Sunaryo P, et al. malpractice litigation and testicular torsion: a legal database review. J Emerg Med 2015;49(6):849–54.
41. Kadish HA, Bolte RG. A retrospective review of pediatric patients with epididymitis, testicular torsion, and torsion of testicular appendages. Pediatrics 1998; 102(1 Pt 1):73–6.
42. Kaye JD, Levitt SB, Friedman SC, et al. Neonatal torsion: a 14-year experience and proposed algorithm for management. J Urol 2008;179(6):2377–83.
43. Bandarkar AN, Blask AR. Testicular torsion with preserved flow: key sonographic features and value-added approach to diagnosis. Pediatr Radiol 2018;48(5): 735–44.
44. Baker LA, Sigman D, Mathews RI, et al. An analysis of clinical outcomes using color doppler testicular ultrasound for testicular torsion. Pediatrics 2000;105: 604–7.
45. Mellick LB, Sinex JE, Gibson RW, et al. A systematic review of testicle survival time after a torsion event. Pediatr Emerg Care 2019;35(12):821–5.
46. Jones IE, Williams SM, Dow N, et al. How many children remain fracture-free during growth? A longitudinal study of children and adolescents participating in the Dunedin Multidisciplinary Health and Development Study. Osteoporos Int 2002; 13(12):990–5.
47. Khosla S, Melton LJ 3rd, Dekutoski MB, et al. Incidence of childhood distal forearm fractures over 30 years: a population-based study. JAMA 2003;290(11): 1479–85.
48. Wong C, Bodtker S, Buxbom P, et al. A closed-claim analysis of complaints after paediatric antebrachial fractures. Dan Med J 2017;64(12) [pii:A5430].
49. Vinz H, Neu J. Out of court settlement of malpractice claims relating to the treatment of fractures in children: experience of the arbitration board of the North German Medical Associations. Dtsch Arztebl Int 2009;106(30):491–8.
50. Lins RE, Simovitch RW, Waters PM. Pediatric elbow trauma. Orthop Clin North Am 1999;30(1):119–32.
51. Grayson DE. The elbow: radiologic imaging pearls and pitfalls. Semin Roentgenol 2005;40(3):223–47.
52. Della-Giustina K, Della-Giustina DA. Emergency department evaluation and treatment of pediatric orthopedic injuries. Emerg Med Clin North Am 1999;17(4): 895–922, vii.
53. Gogola GR. Pediatric humeral condyle fractures. Hand Clin 2006;22(1):77–85.
54. Flynn JC. Nonunion of slightly displaced fractures of the lateral humeral condyle in children: an update. J Pediatr Orthop 1989;9(6):691–6.
55. Goodwin RC, Kuivila TE. Pediatric elbow and forearm fractures requiring surgical treatment. Hand Clin 2002;18(1):135–48.

56. Plint AC, Perry JJ, Correll R, et al. A randomized, controlled trial of removable splinting versus casting for wrist buckle fractures in children. Pediatrics 2006; 117(3):691–7.

57. Singer G, Cichocki M, Schalamon J, et al. A study of metatarsal fractures in children. J Bone Joint Surg Am 2008;90(4):772–6.

58. Boutis K, Willan AR, Babyn P, et al. A randomized, controlled trial of a removable brace versus casting in children with low-risk ankle fractures. Pediatrics 2007; 119(6):e1256–63.

59. Perry DC, Skellorn PJ, Bruce CE. The lognormal age of onset distribution in Perthes' disease: an analysis from a large well-defined cohort. Bone Joint J 2016;98-B(5):710–4.

60. Kocher MS, Bishop JA, Weed B, et al. Delay in diagnosis of slipped capital femoral epiphysis. Pediatrics 2004;113(4):e322–5.

61. Christian CW, Committee on Child Abuse and Neglect, American Academy of Pediatrics. The evaluation of suspected child physical abuse. Pediatrics 2015; 135(5):e1337-54.

62. Richardson C. Physician/hospital liability for negligently reporting child abuse. J Leg Med 2002;23:131–50.

63. Clayton EW. Potential liability in cases of child abuse and neglect. Pediatr Ann 1997;26(3):173–7.

64. Selbst SM. Legal briefs. Pediatr Emerg Care 2006;22(7):533–6.

65. Selbst SM. Legal briefs. Pediatr Emerg Care 2011;27(8):784–6.

66. Flaherty EG, Schwartz K, Jones RD, et al. Child abuse physicians: coping with challenges. Eval Health Prof 2013;36(2):163–73.

The High-Risk Airway

Jorge L. Cabrera, DO[a],*, Jonathan S. Auerbach, MD[a],
Andrew H. Merelman, BS[b], Richard M. Levitan, MD[c]

KEYWORDS

• Airway • RSI • Intubation • Awake intubation • Difficult airway • High-risk airway

KEY POINTS

- Emergency airways are, by definition, higher risk because of the underlying life-threatening processes requiring airway management.
- High-risk airways can be broadly divided into those that are anatomically challenging and those that are physiologically challenging.
- Widespread adoption of video laryngoscopes (both conventional and hyperangulated blades) have made anatomically challenging airways more manageable, but there remain situations involving upper airway pathology in which indirect elevation of the epiglottis may not work (even with video assistance).
- On rare occasions, emergency physicians need to avoid rapid-sequence intubation and use alternative techniques, such as delayed sequence intubation, ketamine-only breathing intubation, and awake intubation.
- Cricothyrotomy may be required in dynamically deteriorating patients with altered upper airway anatomy, and situations of overwhelming fluids in the airway.

 Video content accompanies this article at http://www.emed.theclinics.com.

INTRODUCTION

Airway management is one of the highest risk procedures performed in the emergency department. Providers must be confident and competent during airway-related emergencies and have a thorough understanding of the anatomic and physiologic factors involved. This review addresses some important considerations in the management of high-risk airways. For the emergency provider, composure under stress, having the right tools for the job, and prior deliberate practice with those tools will mitigate the risk of the challenging airway.

[a] University of Miami Miller School of Medicine, 1600 NW 10th Ave, Miami, FL 33136, USA;
[b] Rocky Vista University College of Osteopathic Medicine, 8401 S. Chambers Rd, Parker, CO 80134, USA; [c] Department of Medicine, Dartmouth Geisel School of Medicine, Dartmouth-Hitchcock Medical Center, 853 Rt 25a, Orford, NH 03777, USA
* Corresponding author.
E-mail address: jcabrera@med.miami.edu
Twitter: @In10sivist (J.L.C.); @amerelman (A.H.M.); @airwaycam (R.M.L.)

Emerg Med Clin N Am 38 (2020) 401–417
https://doi.org/10.1016/j.emc.2020.01.008
0733-8627/20/© 2020 Elsevier Inc. All rights reserved.

GENERAL PHYSIOLOGIC CONSIDERATIONS

Emergent airway management has traditionally focused on airway procedural aspects and neglected to address physiologic parameters that can lead to significant morbidity and mortality. Recently, practice has shifted toward addressing essential peri-intubation factors, including oxygenation, hemodynamics, and acid-base disorders, which contribute to poor outcomes.[1-3] Because there is minimal evidence supporting specific methods to address some of these factors, the authors of this paper encourage the reader to prepare for every airway as though it were a high-risk airway, for this is impossible to predict. We recommend an essential set of tools be available for the management of every airway, as listed in **Table 1**.

Oxygenation

Oxygenation must be maintained through all phases of intubation. Preoxygenation is the most important intervention to prevent desaturation peri-intubation.[4] The best method of preoxygenation is dependent on the patient condition, environment, and available resources. A general approach to preoxygenation is as follows:

- Use basic airway maneuvers, such as jaw thrust, to maintain a patent airway
- Apply a nasal cannula (NC) at $\geq$15 L/min during preoxygenation
- In addition to NC, consider the following methods to maximize preoxygenation:
  o Non-rebreather (NRB) mask at flush rate (ie, turn the flow meter counterclockwise until it cannot be rotated farther) for patients with no significant respiratory disease
  o Continuous or bilevel positive airway pressure for patients with hypoxemia (oxygen saturation <96% on NRB) or respiratory disease
  o Bag-valve-mask (BVM) ventilation with positive end-expiratory pressure (PEEP) for patients with diminished respiratory effort

During the intubation attempt, NO DESAT (nasal oxygenation during efforts to secure a tube) using an NC at $\geq$15 L/min should be performed.[5] During the time after sedative administration but before the onset of paralysis (apneic period), airway patency must be maintained with a jaw thrust or oropharyngeal airway for apneic oxygenation to be effective. In patients who have a high likelihood of desaturation

Table 1 Recommended intubation tool kit	
Primary airway equipment	
Bag-valve-mask with oxygen source	Positive end-expiratory pressure valve
Suction set up	End-tidal CO_2
Nasal cannula	Bougie
Direct laryngoscope (low profile Mac 4)	Video laryngoscope
Backup equipment	
Supraglottic airway device (SGA)	Flexible endoscope
Magill forceps	
Surgical airway	
Scalpel (#10)	Bougie
Medications	
Push-dose vasopressors	Crystalloids with pressure bag
Ketamine	Rocuronium

(eg, pulmonary shunt), BVM ventilation may be appropriate during the apneic period. It is essential that ventilation is performed diligently and with the head of the patient raised above the level of the stomach to reduce the risk of gastric insufflation. This includes a 2-person technique, low tidal volume, and slow rate with a PEEP valve in place,[6] or can also be performed by one provider with relative ease using a supraglottic airway device.

If an intubation attempt is unsuccessful, ventilation must be performed to restore oxygen saturation. The trigger to abandon an intubation attempt and provide BVM ventilation is typically a decrease in oxygen saturation below a limit that is established by the team before intubation attempt. In a patient with normal oxygenation to start, this limit is usually 92% to 94%; however, in patients with lower preintubation oxygen saturation, the limit should be adjusted. A team member must be assigned to monitor the oxygen saturation and inform the intubating provider if it reaches the preestablished threshold. When this happens, BVM ventilation is performed using a 2-person, low-pressure, slow-rate technique to avoid stomach insufflation, ideally with ongoing use of continuous capnography. Once the oxygen saturation is restored, further airway procedures may be undertaken.

Hemodynamics

Patients intubated emergently often have a high risk of hemodynamic compromise. The rapid-sequence intubation (RSI) procedure causes decreases in blood pressure due to the effects of sedative and neuromuscular blocking agents as well as the abrupt transition from negative-pressure to positive-pressure ventilation.[7] These cardiovascular effects can be mitigated by managing hemodynamic concerns before intubation is undertaken by using the following principles:

- Patients who are hypotensive before intubation must be resuscitated before undertaking RSI. This may include blood or fluid administration and/or initiation of vasoactive support.
- Medications should be chosen and dosed to minimize cardiovascular effects (**Table 2**).
- Given the significant risk of hemodynamic deterioration during airway management, push-dose vasopressors should be available.[9] Epinephrine is typically used, with a dose of 5 to 20 µg at a time after diluting to 10 µg/mL.

METABOLIC ACIDOSIS

The most common acid-base disorder causing deteriorating during intubation is metabolic acidosis (MA). MA is seen frequently in diabetic ketoacidosis and salicylate toxicity and also can be present in many other conditions. Apnea, intentionally caused by sedation and paralysis, can lead to acute drops in pH and potentially worsen outcomes. To minimize clinical deterioration in patients with MA who potentially require intubation,

- Avoid intubation of patients with severe MA when possible
- If intubation must be undertaken, ensure that the patient has been resuscitated before the procedure, including correction of acidosis as much as feasible
- For patients with severe MA, consider awake intubation or ketamine-only breathing intubation[10] to maintain respiratory compensation
- After intubation, the ventilator settings should attempt to match the patient's prior minute ventilation

Table 2
Induction and paralytic dosing

	Dosing-Low Shock Index	Dosing- High Shock Index[18]	Dissociative Dosing in Shock	Contraindications
Induction				
Ketamine[10,19,20]	1–2 mg/kg IBW	0.5 mg/kg IBW	20 mg every 30 s as needed	1. ACS 2. Acute aortic dissection
Etomidate[21–23]	0.3 mg/kg LBW	0.1 mg/kg LBW		Adrenal insufficiency[21]
Paralytic				
Rocuronium[24]	1.2 mg/kg IBW	2.4 mg/kg IBW		
Succinylcholine[25–27]	1.5 mg/kg TBW (1 mg/kg TBW in obese)	2 mg/kg TBW		1. Hyperkalemia 2. Crush, burns, strokes with residual sx >72 h 3. Neurologic disorders 4. Malignant hyperthermia 5. Renal failure and rhabdomyolysis

Abbreviations: ACS, acute coronary syndrome; IBW, ideal body weight; Sx, symptoms; TBW, total body weight.
  Data from Refs.[10,18–27]

ANATOMIC CONSIDERATIONS
Positioning

Proper positioning is crucial for successful intubation. Ear to sternal notch positioning (**Fig. 1**) optimizes airway visualization, and elevating the head above the level of the stomach optimizes preoxygenation and reduces the risk of aspiration.[11–13] In patients

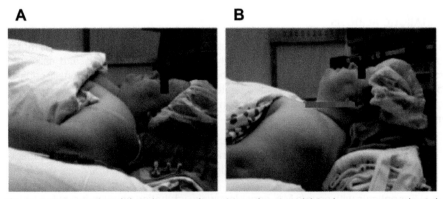

A   **B**

Fig. 1. A supine patient (*A*) and a properly positioned patient (*B*) in the ear to sternal notch position. (*From* Collins J, Lemmens H, Brodsky J, et al. Laryngoscopy and Morbid Obesity: a Comparison of the "Sniff" and "Ramped" Positions. *Obesity Surgery.* 2004;14(9):1171-1175; with permission.)

who cannot be bent because of spinal precautions, position in a reverse Trendelenburg position at 30° to optimize preoxygenation and laryngoscopy.

During the apneic period, various maneuvers should be performed to optimize apneic oxygenation.[4] Head elevation and jaw thrust should be performed in all patients if safe and feasible. Some patients (obese and/or obstructive sleep apnea) may require nasal or oral airways. Use a nasal trumpet as first line in all of these patients, provided there is no facial trauma or coagulopathy, as it can be placed in the awake patient because it is more tolerable and does not induce the gag reflex.

Obesity

Obese patients have decreased lung volumes and lung capacities, leading to less physiologic reserve.[14] Therefore, obese patients should be intubated in a sitting or ramped position (**Fig. 2**).[15]

THE BOUGIE

The endotracheal tube (ETT) introducer is an essential item to have in any high-risk airway toolbox. A recent single-center randomized controlled trial showed that routine bougie use in emergency intubation performed by emergency physicians had higher first-attempt success than endotracheal tube with stylet.[16] One benefit of the bougie is its smaller outer diameter than most adult ETTs, which allows more space for the operator to maintain visualization with the glottic inlet when inserted in the mouth. To use the bougie, the operator places the coudé tip above the interarytenoid notch, pointing the tip anteriorly at 12 o'clock (**Fig. 3**) to guide the device into the trachea and not the esophagus.

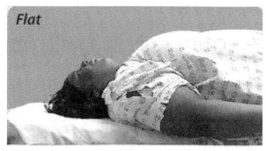

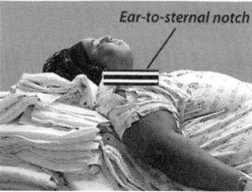

Fig. 2. An example of an obese patient being ramped. (*Courtesy of* Richard Levitan, Franklin, NH; with permission.)

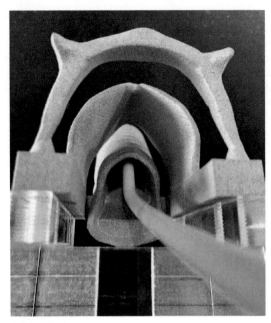

Fig. 3. Bougie tip at 12 o'clock

Tracheal placement is quickly confirmed with the palpation of tracheal clicks, which are vibrations produced when the bougie slides over the anterior tracheal rings. Tracheal clicks are a reliable method of confirming tracheal placement.[16,17] This is improved if the operator deliberately trains to recognize this vibratory feedback. In the minority of the cases in which the coudé tip does not reach the anterior trachea (ie, saber sheath trachea depicted in **Fig. 4**), careful rotation of the tip toward the 10 o'clock position (**Fig. 5**) or 2 o'clock position (**Fig. 6**) will elicit tracheal clicks in most cases.

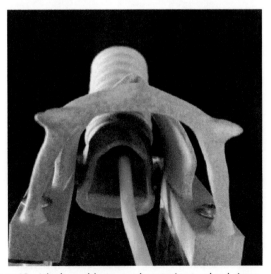

Fig. 4. Bougie tip at 12 o'clock unable to reach anterior tracheal rings

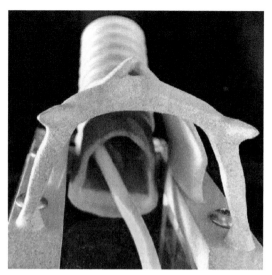

Fig. 5. Bougie tip rotated towards 10 o'clock contacts anterior tracheal rings

The ETT is then advanced over the bougie and the bougie is removed. This can be accomplished by having an assistant remove the bougie or a single operator can use the "hand-off" method. This is when the bougie is moved to the operator's left hand against the laryngoscope while the right hand loads the ETT onto the bougie (Video 1).

INTUBATION MEDICATIONS

In the high-risk airway, preparation is essential. The clinician must have an easily accessible list of medications and dosing to manage patients safely (**Table 2**). In general, we prefer the use of rocuronium over succinylcholine. There is only one

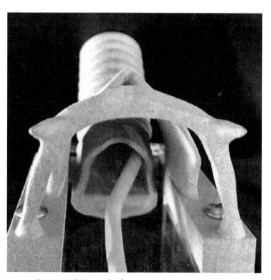

Fig. 6. Bougie tip rotated towards 2 o'clock contacts anterior tracheal rings

contraindication to its use (prior allergic reaction) and it provides prolonged paralysis, obviating the need for redosing of medications in difficult airway attempts. We also prefer ketamine to etomidate for induction because of its safety profile and hemodynamic benefit. However, not all locations have rocuronium and ketamine, therefore knowledge of dosing of other agents is important. For patient safety during intubation, all medications given must be clearly labeled and confirmation of correct dosing must be performed.

AWAKE INTUBATION

A provider may choose to perform an awake endoscopic intubation for several reasons, including the following:

- Anticipated anatomically difficult airway, for example, limited mouth opening, fused cervical spines
- Suspected upper airway obstruction, for example, angioedema, obstruction causing stridor
- Patients who are physiologically difficult, for example, right heart failure or severe MA, in whom induction agents, apnea, and conversion to positive-pressure ventilation pose a significant risk of precipitating further clinical deterioration

There are a few contraindications to performing an awake intubation. The only absolute contraindication is an allergy to lidocaine. The following are relative contraindications to awake intubation:

- Soiled airways in which blood or vomit can obscure the endoscopic view
- Rapidly deteriorating or uncooperative patient in whom there is insufficient time to topicalize the upper airway

When performing awake intubation, it is necessary to understand the basic anatomy. It is important to consider that sensation from the posterior one-third of the tongue to the epiglottis (afferent limb of the gag reflex) is provided by the glossopharyngeal nerve, whereas the vagus nerve covers sensation from the underside of the epiglottis to the vocal cords through the internal branch of the superior laryngeal nerve (**Fig. 7**).

1. Ensure all RSI medications and equipment are readily available, including the necessary tools to perform a surgical airway.
2. As you are gathering the necessary equipment and logistical support, give an antisialagogue, such as glycopyrrolate, 0.2 mg to 0.4 mg intravenously (IV) to dry the mucosa.
3. Use atomized lidocaine to topicalize from the oral/nasal mucosa all the way down to the vocal cords using the EZ-Spray atomizer or the Mucosal Atomization Device; 4% to 5% lidocaine paste applied to the posterior tongue using a tongue depressor works well for the oral route.
4. Spray oxymetazoline into each nostril if using the nasal route.
5. If using the oral approach, have an assistant pull on the patient's tongue with a gauze or use an intubating oral airway and stay midline as you enter the mouth with the ETT preloaded on the flexible endoscope.
6. Identify the larynx.
7. Enter the trachea and advance until you reach the carina with the scope.
8. Railroad the ETT while applying a counterclockwise rotation.
9. Withdraw the scope slowly while visually confirming ETT placement in the trachea.
10. Secure the tube and ventilate the patient.
11. Ensure adequate sedation to prevent self-extubation.

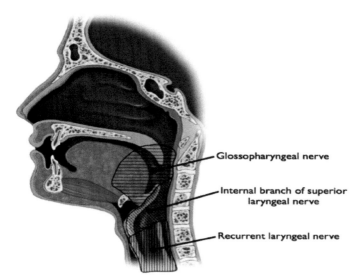

Fig. 7. Innervation of the upper airway. (*From* Kovacs G and Law A. Airway Management in Emergencies: The Infinity Edition.; 2018; with permission.)

12. If choosing the nasal route, lubricate and insert a size 6.5 to 7.5 ETT to a depth of approximately 12 to 14 cm, then insert the flexible endoscope and visualize the larynx.
13. Repeat steps 7 to 11 described above (Video 2).

Note: although lidocaine toxicity may occur at IV doses greater than 4 to 5 mg/kg,[28,29] atomized particles have much lower systemic absorption.

BOUGIE-ASSISTED SURGICAL CRICOTHYROTOMY

A cricothyrotomy is one of the most feared procedures of airway providers. Those managing airways must be trained to perform a surgical airway and recognize that it is an essential, and sometimes expected, step in any airway algorithm. The "failed airway" is better thought of as the "surgically inevitable airway." Indeed, all that is required is a 1-inch incision to save the patient's life. The recommended technique for emergency surgical airway in the adult patient is the bougie-assisted surgical cricothyrotomy, which has been shown to be more effective than other techniques.[30–32]

The following are indications for a surgical airway:

- Inability to ventilate or oxygenate
- Patients with significant upper airway deformity in whom oral or nasal airway attempts are unlikely to be successful (eg, facial trauma, large amount of airway soiling, or certain anatomic variants)

The basic procedure for bougie-assisted surgical cricothyrotomy is a stepwise process:

1. Preoxygenate the patient.
2. Stand on the same side of the patient as your dominant hand.
3. Lay the patient flat with the neck extended.
4. Use a laryngeal handshake (**Fig. 8**) to identify and stabilize the thyroid cartilage with your nondominant hand and palpate the thyroid prominence, the cricothyroid membrane (CTM), and the cricoid cartilage with your index finger.

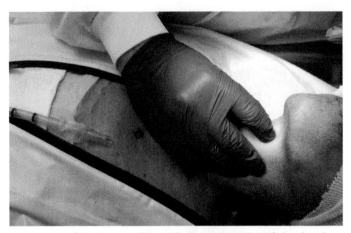

Fig. 8. Demonstration of the laryngeal handshake used to identify landmarks.

5. Make a vertical incision from the thyroid prominence to the cricoid cartilage and place the index finger of your nondominant hand inside the incision to feel for the CTM. NOTE: you do not need to know the exact location of the CTM when you start the procedure. Once the vertical incision is made, your index finger will identify the location of the CTM.
6. Pierce the CTM and make a horizontal incision, bringing the scalpel toward you. Extend the incision by rotating the blade and cutting away from you. Remove the scalpel.
7. Place the index finger of the nondominant hand in the airway and slide a bougie next to it, pointing caudad toward the carina. Insert the bougie into the trachea 8 to 12 cm.
8. Advance the tracheostomy tube or a size 6.0 ETT over the bougie until the proximal cuff enters the airway. Inflate the cuff and remove the bougie.
9. Confirm placement with waveform capnography.
10. Ventilate the patient and secure airway (Video 3).

SPECIFIC AIRWAY SCENARIOS
Traumatic Brain Injury and Cervical Spine Injury

Often in severe head injury there is a pathologic respiratory disturbance that can worsen patient outcomes due to derangements in CO_2 levels. In addition, patients with severe head injury and altered mental status often cannot maintain their own airway.

Intubation of a head-injured patient should be done slowly and cautiously, as laryngoscopy can increase intracranial pressure (ICP). The provider may consider using a bougie to limit manipulation of the patient.

After intubation, patients with head injury must have their ventilation strictly controlled and should not be hyperventilated or hypoventilated. End-tidal CO_2 ($ETCO_2$) should be used to guide ventilation, with a goal of 35 to 40 mm Hg.[33,34] Hyperventilation should be performed only if the patient has evidence of acute brainstem herniation, evidenced by seizure activity, dramatic increase in blood pressure, decrease in heart rate, or dilation of 1 pupil. Hyperventilation to an $ETCO_2$ of 30 mm Hg can be used in cases of impending herniation for a maximum of 10 minutes as a rescue treatment.[35]

As for medication choice, ketamine is safe in patients with increased ICP,[36,37] and is the preferred induction agent in most intubations, including trauma patients, for its hemodynamic benefit (see **Box 1**).

In addition, after intubation, patients with head injury should be kept upright or in the reverse Trendelenburg position, as this will help reduce ICP by facilitating blood and cerebrospinal fluid drainage.

Airway management in known or suspected cervical spine injury is difficult because of the need for manual inline stabilization during laryngoscopy.[38] We advocate the use of a video laryngoscopy (VL)/direct laryngoscopy (DL) device in these patients, as VL can provide a better view with less cervical manipulation whereas DL can be deployed if blood or vomit obscure the camera lens. If using DL, a bougie should be used, as it can typically be placed in the airway with less glottic exposure.

Inline stabilization is performed by removing the anterior portion of the cervical collar and having an assistant stand at either the head or side of the bed and use his or her fingers and palms to stabilize the patient's mastoid process and occiput. The patient's collar should be replaced postintubation.[38]

Asthma and Chronic Obstructive Pulmonary Disease

Patients with reactive airway disease can present in severe respiratory distress and require intubation. These patients can be difficult to intubate, as induction agents and positive-pressure ventilation have the potential to worsen the patient's condition.

Before intubation, these patients must be maximally preoxygenated. A fluid bolus should be considered, as increased intrathoracic pressure may result in hypotension due to impaired venous return. Point-of-care ultrasound using the parasternal short-axis view of the heart, focusing on the shape and motion of the septum can identify those patients with septal flattening in which further fluid boluses may restrict left ventricular filling due to ventricular interdependence. Providers should have a low threshold to initiate vasopressors before intubation in these patients.

After intubation, these patients must have their ventilation managed properly to prevent worsening of their condition. Usually, there is a need for a prolonged expiratory phase, which may be obtained via BVM or with mechanical ventilation by lowering respiratory rate as low as necessary to allow the capnography waveform to return to zero after exhalation (typically 8–10 breaths/min). In addition, the clinician must monitor for auto-PEEP postintubation. Achieving ideal ventilation may require ongoing neuromuscular blockade. If exhalation is not allowed or the patient has severe

---

Box 1
Necessary equipment for awake intubation

- Atomizer device (because of the larger droplets produced, atomizers are more effective than nebulizers at anesthetizing the upper airway)[8]

- 5 to 10 mL of a 4% lidocaine solution

- 4% to 5% lidocaine paste or ointment

- Tongue depressor if using the oral approach

- If choosing a nasal route, a vasoconstrictor such as oxymetazoline can facilitate passage of the endotracheal tube while minimizing trauma

From Kovacs G, Law A. Airway Management in Emergencies: The Infinity Edition. http://aimeairway.ca/book#. Published 2018; with permission and *Data from* Walls R, Murphy M. *Manual of Emergency Airway Management.* Lippincott Williams & Wilkins; 2012.

bronchoconstriction, air trapping can occur within the alveoli. This causes an increasing intrathoracic pressure that can result in decreased venous return or pneumothorax with clinical signs that may include bradycardia, hypotension, or sudden pulseless electrical activity cardiac arrest. If auto-PEEP occurs, remove the BVM or ventilator circuit and allow the patient to exhale fully. It may be necessary to physically push on the patient's chest to force exhalation. The clinician should assess for pneumothorax and perform tube or finger thoracostomy if suspected.[39]

Pulmonary Embolism

Patients who are in extremis due to a pulmonary embolism present a unique challenge regarding respiratory support. These patients have increased pulmonary artery pressures, leading to increased right ventricular (RV) afterload and, often, a dilated and hypokinetic RV. In these patients, intubation and/or positive pressure should be avoided if possible. Delivering positive-pressure ventilation will decrease venous return to the right heart and increase RV afterload, which may precipitate severe hemodynamic compromise including cardiac arrest.

If intubation is indicated, it is almost always due to the hemodynamic effects of the failing RV.[40] As such, strongly consider tissue plasminogen activator or mechanical thrombectomy in addition to circulatory support with extracorporeal membrane oxygenation (ECMO) before converting the patient to positive-pressure ventilation. Fully resuscitate the patient before intubation by maintaining mean arterial pressure with norepinephrine or low-dose vasopressin, followed by inodilators, such as dobutamine or milrinone. It is important to avoid excessive tachycardia and volume overload. High-flow NC may be beneficial by decreasing hypoxemia-induced pulmonary vasoconstriction and reducing the patient's work of breathing. Inhaled nitric oxide[41] or inhaled epoprostenol also may be beneficial by increasing pulmonary vasodilation. For the failing RV, no intubation is almost always better than intubation; however, if intubation becomes necessary, an awake approach using only topical lidocaine is the safest. If an awake technique is not possible, then a ketamine-only breathing intubation with a DL/VL device would be an alternative option.[10] After intubation, care should be taken to deliver the lowest amount of end-expiratory and mean airway pressure possible. In addition, consider transferring the patient to an ECMO center.

Sepsis

Patients with sepsis often have respiratory compromise. Septic patients are at increased risk of suffering hemodynamic deterioration during intubation as a result of their venodilation and frequently encountered hypovolemia. Vasoactive agents must be immediately available before RSI and crystalloid boluses should be given before induction. Ketamine at half the typical dose (0.5–1 mg/kg) is the induction agent of choice in this patient population due to its increased hemodynamic safety.[42] Ketamine should be administered slowly over 30 to 60 seconds, rather than pushing the entire dose at once, to mitigate the likelihood of hypotension and apnea.

Hemorrhagic Shock

As in septic patients, when managing the airway of patients in hemorrhagic shock, vasoactive agents must be ready, and ketamine administered at a reduced rate and dose. The most salient differences between the two are that blood products are the volume expanders of choice and large-suction catheters should be available when managing massive airway or gastrointestinal hemorrhages.

Exposure to Fire/Heat

Patients who are exposed to smoke, fire, or high-temperature gases often require airway intervention. These patients may be conscious and talking but have potential to deteriorate as a result of ongoing airway swelling and inflammation. Early intervention is critical if airway burns are suspected. Signs of possible airway compromise include hoarseness, sore throat, soot in mouth or pharynx, singed nose or facial hair, respiratory distress, cough, hypoxia, and tachypnea.[43,44] When planning to intubate, the provider always should be prepared to perform a surgical airway, as laryngeal or subglottic swelling may prevent passage of an endotracheal tube.

Angioedema

Patients with angioedema should be kept as upright as possible to optimize airway patency. Except in rare cases, the airway should be secured via the nasal route using an awake technique.[45] Paralytics should not be administered, unless a surgical airway must be performed, as loss of tone can lead to airway collapse and cardiac arrest.[45] Importantly, if awake techniques fail, one must be mentally and physically prepared to perform a surgical cricothyrotomy every time a patient with angioedema is being intubated.[45] Patients with respiratory distress, or any need for airway involvement, should be admitted to the intensive care unit for close monitoring of the airway and rapid intervention if needed (**Fig. 9**).[45]

Ludwig Angina

Management of Ludwig angina must begin with securing the airway, as loss of airway is the primary cause of mortality. Where available, experienced anesthesia

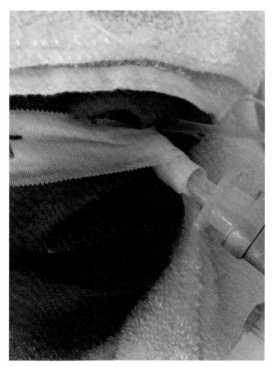

Fig. 9. Patient intubated nasally for angioedema.

and ear, nose, and throat providers should be consulted to assist with management. A select few of the patients with Ludwig angina can be monitored closely with frequent nasal flexible endoscopic evaluation. In most cases, patients will need a definitive airway, ideally performed in the operating room.[46,47] Initial approach to the management of the airway in Ludwig angina is controversial.[48,49] In general, standard endotracheal intubation is less than ideal and typically leads to increased morbidity and mortality. The patient should be maintained in an upright sitting position with nebulized humidified air administered. If airway protection is immediately needed, an awake endoscopic intubation should be performed similarly to the patient with angioedema. Preparations for a surgical airway should be performed simultaneously.[48]

POSTINTUBATION ANALGESIA AND SEDATION

Both analgesia and sedation are important parts to postintubation management. In general, while a patient is still paralyzed, deep sedation and analgesia must be used. In addition, patients who required emergent surgical airway, or those with angioedema or Ludwig angina, should be deeply sedated for patient safety. Once paralytics wear off, analgesia should be used only when able with the addition of the lowest dose sedative as needed (**Table 3**). We, in general, advocate use of propofol for sedation and fentanyl for analgesia, as these are widely available and have significant literature behind them. In patients with profound hemodynamic compromise, we advocate the use of midazolam in place of propofol. When available, ketamine is an alternative agent that includes both analgesia and sedation.

DISCUSSION

The emergent airway is always high risk, and may be further complicated by difficult anatomy or physiology during airway management. The contents of the toolbox for the high-risk airway will vary based on setting, operator experience, and resources. We are confident that with careful consideration of the clinical pearls written herein, along with deliberate practice and integration of those pearls, tomorrow's high-risk airway will be approached with greater comfort.

Table 3
Postintubation sedation and analgesia

Agent	Dosage	Considerations
Sedation		
Propofol[50]	5–50 µg/kg per min titrated every 10 min	• Caution in profound hemodynamic compromise
Midazolam[50]	0.02–0.1 mg/kg per h titrated hourly	• Second-line agent • Caution in renal failure
Analgesia		
Fentanyl[50]	0.7–10 µg/kg per h titrated every 20 min	
Sedative and Analgesic		
Ketamine[10]	1–5 mg/kg per h titrated every 20 min	

Data from Refs.[10,50]

DISCLOSURE

The authors have nothing to disclose.

SUPPLEMENTARY DATA

Supplementary data related to this article can be found online at https://doi.org/10.1016/j.emc.2020.01.008.

REFERENCES

1. Heffner AC, Swords DS, Neale MN, et al. Incidence and factors associated with cardiac arrest complicating emergency airway management. Resuscitation 2013; 84(11):1500–4.
2. Mosier JM, Joshi R, Hypes C, et al. The physiologically difficult airway. West J Emerg Med 2015;16(7):1109–17.
3. Ko BS, Ahn R, Ryoo SM, et al. Prevalence and outcomes of endotracheal intubation–related cardiac arrest in the ED. Am J Emerg Med 2015;33(11):1642–5.
4. Weingart SD, Levitan RM. Preoxygenation and prevention of desaturation during emergency airway management. Ann Emerg Med 2012;59(3):165–75.e1.
5. Gleason J, Christian B, Barton E. Nasal cannula apneic oxygenation prevents desaturation during endotracheal intubation: an integrative literature review. West J Emerg Med 2018;19(2):403–11.
6. Casey JD, Janz DR, Russell DW, et al. Bag-mask ventilation during tracheal intubation of critically ill adults. N Engl J Med 2019. https://doi.org/10.1056/NEJMoa1812405.
7. Mort TC. Complications of emergency tracheal intubation: hemodynamic alterations - part I. J Intensive Care Med 2007;22(3):157–65.
8. Walls R, Murphy M. Manual of emergency airway management. Philadelphia: Lippincott Williams & Wilkins; 2012.
9. Weingart S. Push-dose pressors for immediate blood pressure control. Clin Exp Emerg Med 2015;2(2):131–2.
10. Merelman A, Perlmutter M, Strayer R. Alternatives to rapid sequence intubation: contemporary airway management with ketamine. West J Emerg Med 2019; 20(3):466–71.
11. Khandelwal N, Khorsand S, Mitchell SH, et al. Head-elevated patient positioning decreases complications of emergent tracheal intubation in the ward and intensive care unit. Anesth Analg 2016;122(4):1101–7.
12. Lane S, Saunders D, Schofield A, et al. A prospective, randomised controlled trial comparing the efficacy of pre-oxygenation in the 20° head-up vs supine position. Anaesthesia 2005;60(11):1064–7.
13. Lee BJ, Kang JM, Kim DO. Laryngeal exposure during laryngoscopy is better in the 25° back-up position than in the supine position. Br J Anaesth 2007;99(4):581–6.
14. Melo LC, Silva MA, Calles AC. Obesity and lung function: a systematic review. Einstein (São Paulo). 2014;12(1):120–5.
15. De Jong A, Chanques G, Jaber S. Mechanical ventilation in obese ICU patients: from intubation to extubation. Crit Care 2017;21(1):1–8.
16. Driver BE, Prekker ME, Klein LR, et al. Effect of use of a bougie vs endotracheal tube and stylet on first-attempt intubation success among patients with difficult

airways undergoing emergency intubation a randomized clinical trial. JAMA 2018;319(21):2179–89.

17. Kidd J, Dyson A, Latto I. Successful difficult intubation: use of the gum elastic bougie. Anaesthesia 1988;43(6):437–8.

18. Rezaie S. Dosing sedatives low and paralytics high in shock patients requiring RSI. REBEL EM. Available at: https://rebelem.com/dosing-sedatives-low-and-paralytics-high-in-shock-patients-requiring-rsi/. Accessed August 10, 2019.

19. Marland S, Ellerton J, Andolfatto G, et al. Ketamine: use in anesthesia. CNS Neurosci Ther 2013;19(6):381–9.

20. Rosenbaum S, Palacios J. Ketamine. StatPearls. Available at: https://www.ncbi.nlm.nih.gov/books/NBK470357/. Accessed August 10, 2019.

21. Oglesby AJ. Should etomidate be the induction agent of choice for rapid sequence intubation in the emergency department? Emerg Med J 2004;21(6):655–9.

22. Bergen JM, Smith DC. A review of etomidate for RSI in the emergency department. J Emerg Med 1996;15. https://doi.org/10.1016/S0736-4679(96)00350-2.

23. Stollings JL, Diedrich DA, Oyen LJ, et al. Rapid-sequence intubation: a review of the process and considerations when choosing medications. Ann Pharmacother 2014;48(1):62–76.

24. Patanwala AE, Stahle SA, Sakles JC, et al. Comparison of succinylcholine and rocuronium for first-attempt intubation success in the emergency department. Acad Emerg Med 2011;18(1):11–4.

25. Alvarellos ML, McDonagh EM, Patel S, et al. PharmGKB summary: succinylcholine pathway, pharmacokinetics/pharmacodynamics. Pharmacogenet Genomics 2015;25(12):622–30.

26. Patanwala AE, Sakles JC. Effect of patient weight on first pass success and neuromuscular blocking agent dosing for rapid sequence intubation in the emergency department. Emerg Med J 2017;34(11):739–43.

27. Bhat R, Mazer-Amirshahi M, Sun C, et al. Accuracy of rapid sequence intubation medication dosing in obese patients intubated in the ED. Am J Emerg Med 2016; 34(12):2423–5.

28. Rosenberg P, Veering B, Urmey W. Maximum recommended doses of local anesthetics: a multifactorial concept. Reg Anesth Pain Med 2004;29(6):564–74.

29. El-Boghdadly K, Pawa A, Chin KJ. Local anesthetic systemic toxicity: current perspectives. Local Reg Anesth 2018;11:35–44.

30. Braude D, Webb H, Stafford J, et al. The bougie-aided cricothyrotomy. Air Med J 2009;28(4):191–4.

31. Henlin T, Michalek P, Tyll T, et al. A randomized comparison of bougie-assisted and tracheoquick plus cricothyrotomies on a live porcine model. Biomed Res Int 2017;2017:1–6.

32. Chang SS, Tong QJ, Beh ZY, et al. A bench study comparing between scalpel-bougie technique and cannula-to-Melker technique in emergency cricothyroidotomy in a porcine model. Korean J Anesthesiol 2018;71(4):289–95.

33. Warner KJ, Cuschieri J, Copass MK, et al. Emergency department ventilation effects outcome in severe traumatic brain injury. J Trauma 2008;64(2):341–7.

34. Dumont TM, Visioni AJ, Rughani AI, et al. Inappropriate prehospital ventilation in severe traumatic brain injury increases in-hospital mortality. J Neurotrauma 2010; 27(7):1233–41.

35. Godoy DA, Seifi A, Garza D, et al. Hyperventilation therapy for control of posttraumatic intracranial hypertension. Front Neurol 2017;8:1–13.

36. Bar-Joseph G, Guilburd Y, Tamir A, et al. Effectiveness of ketamine in decreasingintracranial pressure in children with intracranial hypertension. J Neurosurg Pediatr. 2009;4(1):40–6. https://doi.org/10.3171/2009.1.peds08319.
37. Zeiler FA, Teitelbaum J, West M, et al. The ketamine effect on ICP in traumatic brain injury. Neurocrit Care 2014;21(1):163–73.
38. Austin N, Krishnamoorthy V, Dagal A. Airway management in cervical spine injury. Int J Crit Illn Inj Sci 2014;4(1):50.
39. Leatherman J. Mechanical ventilation for severe asthma. Chest 2015;147(6): 1671–80.
40. Lualdi JC, Goldhaber SZ. Right ventricular dysfunction after acute pulmonary embolism: pathophysiologic factors, detection, and therapeutic implications. Am Heart J 1995;130(6):1276–82.
41. Kline JA, Puskarich MA, Jones AE, et al. Inhaled nitric oxide to treat intermediate risk pulmonary embolism: a multicenter randomized controlled trial. Nitric Oxide 2019;84:60–8.
42. Morris C, Perris A, Klein J, et al. Anaesthesia in haemodynamically compromised emergency patients: does ketamine represent the best choice of induction agent? Anaesthesia 2009;64(5):532–9.
43. Jones SW, Carolina N, Burn J, et al. Inhalational injury: pathophysiology, diagnosis, and treatment. Clin Plast Surg 2018;44(3):505–11.
44. Sabri A, Dabbous H, Dowli A, et al. The airway in inhalational injury: diagnosis and management inhalation. De Fumées Et Voies Aériennes: Diagnostic Et Prise En Charge. Ann Burns Fire Disasters 2017;30:24–9.
45. Moellman J, Bernstein J, Lindsell C. A consensus parameter for the evaluation and management of angioedema in the emergency department. Acad Emerg Med 2015;21(4):469–84.
46. Saifeldeen K. Ludwig's angina. Emerg Med J 2004;21(2):242–3.
47. Candamourty R, Venkatachalam S, Babu M, et al. Ludwig's angina - an emergency: a case report with literature review. J Nat Sci Biol Med 2012;3(2):206.
48. Johnson J, Rosen C. Ludwig angina. In: Bailey's head and neck surgery-otolaryngology, vol. 2. Philadelphia; 2014. p. 770–81.
49. Hartman N. Neck and upper airway. In: Judith E, Tintinalli, editors. Tintinalli's emergency medicine: a comprehensive study guide. 8th edition. New York: McGraw-Hill; 2016. p. 1613–8.
50. Barr J, Fraser GL, Puntillo K, et al. Clinical practice guidelines for the management of pain, agitation, and delirium in adult patients in the intensive care unit. Crit Care Med 2013;41(1):263–306.

Emergency Department Evaluation of the Adult Psychiatric Patient

Lauren M. Nentwich, MD[a],*, Curtis W. Wittmann, MD[b]

KEYWORDS

- Psychiatric emergencies • Risk assessment • Medical evaluation

KEY POINTS

- Psychiatric patients presenting to the emergency department should be triaged based on evaluation of risk to self or others.
- The initial medical evaluation is an important part of the psychiatric patient's care and should evaluate whether a medical illness is causing or exacerbating psychiatric symptoms.
- The emergency physician must evaluate for high-risk medical conditions in all patients presenting with acute psychiatric symptoms.
- Risk assessment for suicide or violence is a dynamic process that requires an appropriate psychiatric assessment and clinical judgment using patient factors, social supports, and community resources.
- Psychiatric patients boarding in the emergency department should have ongoing psychiatric care for their psychiatric disorder and continued medical care for their chronic and newly diagnosed medical needs.

INTRODUCTION

In 2014, there were an estimated 43.6 million adults, representing 18.1% of the adult population, living in the United States with a mental, behavioral, or emotional disorder. Substantial declines in psychiatric services and mental health resources have greatly burdened emergency departments (ED) with increased numbers of patients with psychiatric issues.[1,2] Approximately, 1 in 8 patient visits to an ED involves a mental health and/or substance use disorder.[3] From 2006 to 2014, the ED visit rate for mental health and substance use disorder diagnoses increased 44.1% from 14.1 to 20.3 visits per 1000 population,[4] and the numbers of patients who require help for their acute psychiatric illnesses continues to increase each year.

[a] Department of Emergency Medicine, Boston University Medical Center, One Boston Medical Center Place, BCD Building, Boston, MA 02118, USA; [b] Department of Psychiatry, Massachusetts General Hospital, Founders 826, 55 Fruit Street, Boston, MA 02114, USA
* Corresponding author.
E-mail address: lauren.nentwich@bmc.org

Emerg Med Clin N Am 38 (2020) 419–435
https://doi.org/10.1016/j.emc.2020.02.001
0733-8627/20/© 2020 Elsevier Inc. All rights reserved.

The ED is often the primary entry point for many patients suffering from acute psychiatric emergencies, including patients who are in the midst of an acute psychiatric crisis and those who have nowhere left to turn. These psychiatric patients are high-risk medical patients.

This article focuses on risk management in the ED care of the adult psychiatric patient, 18 years of age or older. Pediatric patients with psychiatric complaints carry their own challenges and requirements for care and their care is not covered in this article.

EMERGENCY DEPARTMENT IDENTIFICATION AND TRIAGE

The ED often serves as the primary entrance to the mental health care system for patients, and patients with psychiatric complaints present to the ED in a number of different ways:

- Self-referral (ie, walk-in) for psychiatric evaluation
- Referred in from psychiatric provider or other primary medical provider
- Brought in by police or emergency medical services for suicidality, acute agitation, or presumed intoxication
- Identified during ED evaluation for another medical complaint

On arrival, psychiatric patients should be triaged based on an initial evaluation of risk and a question of safety for the patient and others. Patients should undergo priority triage if they are identified to have an increased risk (**Box 1**). These patients should be immediately evaluated by a provider and not be left alone or allowed to leave the ED before assessment. These patients should also be offered or given medications (eg, antipsychotics, anxiolytics) early to decrease the risk of restraints and injury, as well as to offer relief from what are often debilitating symptoms.

Psychiatric patients without an increased risk of harm to self and others may undergo standard triage. This standard assessment includes patients presenting with depression without suicidality or stable psychiatric patients seeking medication refills or outpatient referral. These patients represent a lower risk group and can often proceed through the standard triage and evaluation process.

Many patients with psychiatric complaints that require urgent high priority triage may lack the capacity to consent to or refuse medical care based on the presence of suicidality, intoxication, or acute psychosis. Additionally, in most states, danger to self or others or an inability to provide for one's basic needs is sufficient cause for involuntary treatment. Emergency physicians should be aware of the laws governing involuntary psychiatric treatment in their state or jurisdiction that may govern some of these situations and have a low threshold for obtaining psychiatric consultation on these patients. A full review of the capacity of patients to make medical decisions to consent to or refuse medical care is reviewed in detail in Joseph H. Kahn's article,

---

Box 1
Psychiatric patient with high priority triage

- Active suicidal ideation
- Acute psychosis
- Violent or homicidal patient
- Acute mania
- Acutely agitated or combative patient

"Confidentiality and Capacity," elsewhere in this issue, including the 4 primary components required to have capacity.

EMERGENCY DEPARTMENT MEDICAL EVALUATION

All patients who present to the ED with an acute psychiatric emergency require a medical evaluation before their psychiatric evaluation. The primary purpose of the medical evaluation is to determine whether a medical illness is causing or exacerbating the psychiatric condition. The secondary purpose of the medical evaluation is to identify acute medical or surgical conditions identified that are co-occurring with the psychiatric issue and require immediate medical treatment.

Long known as medical clearance, this term has become problematic because it implies different things to the psychiatrist and the emergency physician, and there is no standard definition or process for performing a medical clearance. In addition, it is a misnomer, because the completion of the ED evaluation does not clear the patient of all possible medical conditions. The American College of Emergency Physicians (ACEP) recommends a focused medical assessment for all acute psychiatric ED patients during which a medical etiology for the patients' symptoms is excluded and other illness or injury in need of acute care is detected and treated.[5]

This medical evaluation by the emergency physician is an important part of the psychiatric patient's overall care. Patients requiring acute psychiatric treatment often have active and important coexisting organic disease,[6,7] and the rate of comorbid medical illness that may cause, contribute to, or exacerbate a patient's psychiatric symptoms ranges from 19% to 80%.[8] In addition, psychiatric facilities often have limited resources for further evaluation and treatment of acute and chronic medical conditions, and at times, the initial ED assessment is the only nonpsychiatric medical evaluation the patient will receive.[5] As such, it is important for the emergency physician to perform a thorough history and examination with focused testing as clinically indicated, and document that no acute organic cause for the patient's current psychiatric illness had been identified[9] and there is no further need for acute medical intervention before psychiatric treatment and/or hospitalization. For acute psychiatric patients who do not need inpatient medical care and are safe for disposition to psychiatric care, a detailed account of any medical abnormalities should be explained, as well as directions for care including necessary medications and outpatient follow-up.

Although we review the high-risk areas of the ED medical evaluation of patients presenting with psychiatric symptoms in this article, emergency physicians should be aware that a task force of the American Association for Emergency Psychiatry consisting of physicians from emergency medicine and psychiatry and a psychologist developed a consensus recommendation advocating for further medical evaluation of specific patients presenting with psychiatric complaints to US EDs (**Box 2**).[10]

History

Taking a thorough history on a psychiatric patient in the ED poses unique challenges to the clinician. Often times, patients are unable to provide a thorough and accurate history owing to their underlying psychiatric disease or alterations in their mental status. Owing to fear of psychiatric hospitalization or secondary gain, patients may not be truthful and may minimize or accentuate the severity of symptoms. Additionally, the busy and chaotic nature of the ED adds to this complexity, because patients are often interviewed in hallways or curtained rooms that do not allow for privacy or a focused interview free of distraction.

Box 2
Recommendations from the American Association for Emergency Psychiatry for ED psychiatric patients who should be considered for further medical workup

1. New-onset psychiatric symptoms in patients with an age of greater than 45 years

2. Advance age (age ≥65 years)

3. Cognitive deficits or delirium

4. Positive review of systems indicative of a physical etiology

5. Focal neurologic findings or evidence of a head injury

6. Substance intoxication, withdrawal, or exposure to toxins or drugs

7. Decreased level of awareness

8. Other indications, such as abnormal vital signs that direct further assessment

Adapted from Wilson MP, Nordstrom K, Anderson EL, et al. American Association for Emergency Psychiatry Task Force on Medical Clearance of Adult Psychiatric Patients. Part II: Controversies over Medical Assessment, and Consensus Recommendations. *West J Emerg Med.* 2017;18(4):640-646. https://doi.org/10.5811/westjem.2017.3.32259

If able, patients should have their history taken in a quiet and secluded area of the ED or in a private room. The psychiatric evaluation often requires patients to share personal details of their history, which may invoke shame, fear of legal consequence, or guilt.[11] Questions should be open ended and focus on critical signs and symptoms of major psychiatric or medical illness. Every effort should be made to obtain collateral information from other providers, family, friends, police, or emergency medical services personnel when possible.

Because patients presenting with psychiatric complaints can have medical issues, the emergency physician should perform a thorough history and review of systems to investigate for evidence of other medical conditions. Any history of recent trauma or injury should be elicited. A past medical and surgical history should be obtained, including prescribed medications and patient adherence. A complete alcohol and illegal drug history should be obtained, including last use and history of prior or current withdrawal.

Physical Examination

Like all patients presenting to the emergency department, the initial evaluation should focus on stabilization of the patient including a primary survey and focus on airway, breathing, and circulation. Patients who are acutely agitated should be rapidly evaluated and attempts at deescalation should be the first line in the management of the agitated patient. If deescalation is unsuccessful, the patient should undergo treatment with physical restraint and medication treatment, for the safety of the patient and staff. The requirements and procedure for restraints and sedation in the acutely agitated patient, including clinical details on medication choice, is described in Pilar Guerrero and Mark B. Mycyk's article, "Physical and Chemical Restraints (An Update)," elsewhere in this issue.

On presentation of the acute psychiatric patient, vital signs should be obtained and abnormal vital signs immediately addressed. Vital sign abnormalities may signify an organic cause for the patient's presentation, including such medical issues as infection, toxidromes, withdrawals, endocrine abnormalities, autoimmune dysfunction, or central nervous system disease.[12] Hypoxia and hypotension are not caused by psychiatric illness and can cause agitation and altered mental status owing to an organic cause that must be investigated and corrected. Hypertension may be due to stress, agitation, or an underlying diagnosis of primary hypertension, but may also be due to intoxication, withdrawal, an acute neurologic event, or other serious acute medical condition. Tachycardia may be caused by agitation or anxiety, but also may be a sign of an underlying medical disorder and should raise the clinicians' suspicion for other organic causes, such as infection, intoxication, withdrawal, cardiac disease, or overdose. Hyperthermia or hypothermia should illicit a full workup of potential causes of abnormal temperature such as life-threatening psychiatric conditions (see High-risk Diagnoses), sepsis, infection, intracranial abnormality, or other acute causes of temporal dysregulation.

A head to toe physical examination, including a thorough neurologic examination, should be performed on all patients to look for and exclude any acute medical or surgical illness. Although this examination should be a complete screening examination evaluating for acute pathology, there are a number of notable findings that should prompt a further workup (**Table 1**). The neurologic examination should include an assessment of orientation, language, memory, cranial nerves, motor system (including gait), reflexes, sensation, and cerebellar function. Patients found to have a new focal neurologic deficit on examination should undergo further testing to evaluate for acute neurologic causes of their presentation. In addition to the general screening examination, patients with specific complaints may require a further focused examination

Table 1 Notable findings on physical examination that should prompt a further workup	
System	**Notable Findings on Physical Examination**
Head, eyes, ears, nose, and throat	Evidence of head trauma (including raccoon eyes, hemotympanum, Battle's sign, cerebral spinal fluid, otorrhea, and rhinorrhea) Evidence of prior neurosurgical surgery, including shunt or prior craniotomy Pupillary examination showing anisocoria or abnormal constriction or dilation Neck palpated for thyroid enlargement/nodularity and tested for signs of meningitis (eg, nuchal rigidity)
Heart	Abnormal rhythms New cardiac murmurs
Lungs	Abnormal lung sounds consistent with pneumothorax, pneumonia, asthma or chronic obstructive pulmonary disease, or pulmonary congestion Evidence of trauma to chest wall
Abdomen	Abdominal pain indicative of intra-abdominal or surgical pathology Stigmata of liver disease including ascites, hepatomegaly, or caput medusa Suprapubic tenderness and mass, which could signify urinary retention or infection
Skin	Rashes, including cellulitis or scabies Signs of trauma or injury Abscesses Jaundice Signs of intravenous drug use, including track marks
Neurologic	New focal deficits, including gait and cranial nerve abnormalities Muscle tone abnormalities Involuntary movements, such as tremors or dystonia Cognitive deficits or delirium
Psychiatric	Visual hallucinations

based on the complaint, including examination of the genitourinary system in patients with testicular pain, vaginal discharge, or sexual assault. Furthermore, atypical features of psychiatric illness, such as visual hallucinations or prominent physical findings, should suggest etiologies other than a primary psychiatric illness.

A mental status examination should be conducted. Pay attention to the patient's appearance (grooming and hygiene), general behaviors, mood and affect, thought process, speech pattern, evidence of perpetual disturbances, and unusual thought content, particularly suicidal or violent ideation, attention, and memory function. The mental status examination can be time consuming in a busy ED. This detailed evaluation may be performed by clinicians, such as a mental health consultant or allied health staff, who are trained in mental health testing, but the decision for further testing should be based on the emergency physician's full assessment.[10]

Routine Laboratory Testing

The question often arises as to whether or not routine laboratory tests are necessary for adult patients presenting with psychiatric symptoms without other signs or symptoms of medical illness. There have been multiple studies that show that ordering routine laboratory screening on psychiatric patients is expensive and provides minimal to no use in the evaluation of the stable ED patient without medical complaints, and it is likely safe to forgo routine testing in these patients.[13-15] However, patients with higher rates of disease, including those who are elderly, immunosuppressed, newly psychotic, or acutely intoxicated, have not been well-studied, and these patients may benefit from routine laboratory testing.

The 2017 ACEP clinical policy guidelines offers a level C recommendation that the alert adult patient presenting with acute psychiatric symptoms should not undergo routine laboratory testing, but have laboratory testing guided by medical history, previous psychiatric diagnoses, and physical examination.[16]

An important caveat is that often psychiatric facilities will strongly request general laboratory screening for admission to their facility, including a complete blood count, comprehensive metabolic panel, toxicology screening for recreational drugs, and a pregnancy test in women of childbearing age. ED providers should work with their mental health colleagues to determine necessary testing to facilitate and expedite admission to regional psychiatric facilities.

Neuroimaging

Often when patients present to the ED with acute psychiatric complaints, the question arises of whether neuroimaging of the brain via computed tomography (CT) or MRI is necessary to evaluate for or exclude organic causes of acute psychiatric illness. For patients presenting with acute psychiatric complaints whose physical examination is positive for focal neurologic deficits, trauma, new-onset seizures, possible encephalitis or meningitis, or excessive cognitive impairment or altered mental status of unknown etiology, neuroimaging is appropriate to evaluate for potential organic brain pathology.[17] Typically, owing to cost and access issues, a noncontrast brain CT is the first imaging modality to be obtained, with a contrast-enhanced CT or MRI subsequently performed if indicated clinically.

Traditionally, a brain CT has been recommended in patients with new-onset psychosis without focal neurologic deficits to exclude medical pathology, such as a mass lesion, as an organic cause of symptoms. This question was recently reviewed by ACEP clinical policy committee, and the committee found an absence of adequate published literature to formulate a recommendation. The committee released a Level C consensus recommendation stating that emergency providers, "Use individual assessment of risk factors to guide brain imaging in the ED for patients with new-onset psychosis without focal neurologic deficits."[16] It is uncommon for new-onset psychosis owing to schizophrenia to be diagnosed in a person younger than 12 or older than 40 years of age.[18] As such, in adults older than 40 years of age who present with new-onset psychosis, it would be reasonable to obtain neuroimaging to evaluate for possible organic intracranial cause. Additionally, in patients with new onset psychosis who present with fever without a clear cause, immunosuppression, history of intravenous (IV) drug use, trauma, headache, or who are unable to participate in a full neurologic examination, it may be reasonable to obtain a brain CT to exclude organic causes based on clinical examination and suspicion.

Additional Testing

Additional testing for the medical evaluation in the ED should be based on the overall clinical picture and prior ED workup. Electrocardiography may be considered in patients with concerns for cardiac arrhythmia or ischemia based on risk factors, history, and examination. In addition, a prolonged QT interval may be seen in patients taking various antipsychotic (eg, neuroleptic agents and atypical antipsychotics) and antidepressant (eg, amitriptyline, desipramine, imipramine, maprotiline, doxepin, and fluoxetine) medications, as well as with methadone. Excessive QT prolongation carries a risk of sudden death owing to a polymorphic tachycardia known as torsades de pointes.[19] It is prudent to check an electrocardiogram on patients who are on these medications and being given repeated doses of these medications in the ED or psychiatric unit to monitor the QT interval.

The differential diagnosis for new-onset psychosis is broad and includes neurologic causes such as meningitis, seizure (including nonconvulsive status, temporal lobe seizure), and encephalitis (including limbic encephalitis). A lumbar puncture is indicated to rule out meningitis or encephalitis if there is evidence of fever or leukocytosis (without an obvious cause), delirium, or change in level of consciousness. A neurology consult and possibly an electroencephalogram may be considered in patients with known seizure disorder or seizure before arrival in the ED.

HIGH-RISK DIAGNOSES
Intoxication or Withdrawal

Patients who present with acute psychiatric symptoms may be suffering from acute intoxication or withdrawal from recreational drugs. Acute intoxication with cocaine, amphetamines, lysergic acid diethylamide, phencyclidine, 3,4-methylenedioxymethamphetamine can result in a sympathomimetic toxidrome with tachycardia, tachypnea, hypertension, hyperthermia, psychosis, mania, hallucinations, and paranoia. Alcohol intoxication and withdrawal can induce a state of agitation, psychosis, and confusion. Severe alcohol and benzodiazepine withdrawal can progress to delirium tremens with resulting confusion, agitation, and psychosis. Sedative hypnotics and opioid intoxication can present with decreased level of consciousness. Opioid withdrawal can result in anxiety, irritability, restlessness, and tremor.

In patients with suspected intoxication or withdrawal of recreational drugs, it is important to obtain a thorough history from the patient and/or collateral sources. Toxicology screens may assist in determining the presence or absence of recreational drugs. Benzodiazepines treat alcohol and benzodiazepine withdrawal, as well as the severe agitation and psychosis of the sympathomimetic toxidrome. Opioid withdrawal may treated with buprenorphine or methadone. Given that many patients with substance use disorders have concurrent mental health issues, it is important to perform a risk assessment on these patients once they are clinically stabilized and no longer experiencing the effects of substance use.

Although a full review on the treatment of substance use disorder is beyond the scope of the article, the current opioid epidemic has made the treatment of patients with opioid use disorder a high-risk area. Opiate overdose survivors are at increased risk of death and it has been shown that initiation of medication-assisted therapy with methadone or buprenorphine is associated with decreased all-cause and opioid-related mortality.[20] The ED is often the initial point of contact for many patients with opioid use disorder, and EDs should have protocols and be equipped to offer patients who present with an opiate overdose or opioid use disorder treatment with medication for addiction and referral into treatment.

Delirium

According to the fifth edition of the *Diagnostic and Statistical Manual of Mental Disorders* (DSM-5), delirium is defined as a disturbance in attention and awareness that develops acutely and tends to fluctuate in severity and cannot be better explained by preexisting dementia. It should have at least one additional disturbance in cognition and have evidence of an underlying organic cause(s) (**Box 3**).[21–23] Delirium is traditionally classified into 3 subtypes:[24,25]

- Hypoactive – decreased psychomotor activity with hypoarousal and lethargy
- Hyperactive – increased psychomotor activity with restlessness, hyperarousal, hypervigilance, and agitation
- Mixed – Fluctuating levels of psychomotor activity

Delirium has a prevalence of 10% to 15% in elderly adults in the ED and is a high-risk diagnosis because it is associated with high morbidity and mortality, increased admission rates, prolonged hospital stays, and cognitive deterioration.[21,25,26] In addition, delirium is missed by ED physicians in 57% to 83% of cases and is often not screened for in the chaotic busy nature of the ED.[27]

Box 3
DSM-5 criteria for delirium

A. A disturbance in attention (ie, decreased ability to direct, focus, sustain, and shift attention) and awareness (decreased orientation to the environment).

B. The disturbance develops over a short period of time (usually hours to a few days), represents a change from baseline attention and awareness, and tends to fluctuate in severity during the course of a day.

C. An additional disturbance in cognition is present (eg, memory deficit, disorientation, language, visuospatial ability, or perception).

D. The disturbances in criteria A and C are not explained by another preexisting, established, or evolving neurocognitive disorder and do not occur in the context of a severely reduced level of arousal, such as coma.

E. There is evidence from the history, physical examination, or laboratory findings that the disturbance is a direct physiologic consequence of another medical condition, substance intoxication or withdrawal (ie, owing to a drug of abuse or to a medication), or exposure to a toxin, or is due to multiple etiologies.

From European Delirium Association; American Delirium Society. The DSM-5 criteria, level of arousal and delirium diagnosis: inclusiveness is safer. BMC Med. 2014;12:141. Published 2014 Oct 8. https://doi.org/10.1186/s12916-014-0141-2

Dementia, depression, and psychiatric disorders are all on the differential diagnosis for acute delirium and can co-occur with delirium. Systematic reviews support the Confusion Assessment Method as a useful bedside assessment for delirium and is worth reviewing.[21] The Confusion Assessment Method criteria for the presence of delirium requires (1) the presence of an acute change in mental status with fluctuating course and inattention plus (2) either disorganized thinking or an altered level of consciousness.[28] There are multiple other tools that can be used to establish a diagnosis of delirium and a full review is outside the scope of this article. However, the emergency physician should keep delirium on his or her differential, especially when assessing elderly patients presenting with acute psychiatric complaints.

Newly diagnosed delirium can signify an impending life-threatening condition, and patients should undergo prompt evaluation for the cause of their delirium. The common reversible contributors can be recalled via the DELIRIUM mnemonic (**Box 4**).[21,25]

Treatment of delirium is performed by eliminating and correcting the underlying causes.[25] If removing deliriogenic factors does not result in clinical improvement, antipsychotic medications are the initial pharmacologic treatment of choice. Haloperidol may be initiated in the range of 1 to 2 mg every 2 to 4 hours as needed (0.25–0.5 mg every 4 hours as needed for elderly patients).[25,29]

Given the high morbidity and mortality of delirium, it is important to screen for this disorder in patients presenting with psychiatric complaints, especially in the elderly, so as to rapidly identify and treat one of the potential causes of behavioral disorder.

Neuroleptic Malignant Syndrome

Neuroleptic malignant syndrome (NMS) is a hyperpyrexic, life-threatening syndrome associated with the use of dopamine-receptor antagonist or rapid withdrawal of

---

Box 4
Modifiable contributors to delirium: The DELIRIUM mnemonic

*D*rugs – New medications, increased doses of medications, overdose, poisons, medication interactions, alcohol, sedative-hypnotic drugs, steroids, anticholinergics, dissociative anesthetics, and illegal drugs

*E*lectrolyte or endocrine disturbances – Hypoglycemia, diabetic coma, dehydration, sodium imbalance, thyroid abnormalities, and severe electrolyte or acid–base disturbances

*L*ack of drugs – Withdrawal from sedatives or alcohol, poorly controlled pain

*I*nfection – Sepsis, urinary infection, respiratory infection, soft tissue infections, meningitis, encephalitis, and endocarditis

*R*educed sensory input – Issues involving decreased vision (lack of glasses) and hearing

*I*ntracranial disorders – Stroke, intracerebral hemorrhage, intracranial infection, seizures, postictal state, intracranial mass, Wernicke's encephalopathy, and normal pressure hydrocephalus

*U*rinary and gastrointestinal disorders – Renal failure, uremia, urinary retention, and fecal impaction

*M*yocardial and pulmonary disorders – Myocardia infarction, cardiac arrest, arrhythmia, heart failure, hypotension, shock, hypertensive encephalopathy, anemia, chronic obstructive pulmonary disease exacerbation, carbon monoxide poisoning, hypoxia, and hypercarbia

Adapted from Marcantonio ER. Delirium in Hospitalized Older Adults. Solomon CG, ed. N Engl J Med. 2017;377(15):1456-1466. https://doi.org/10.1056/NEJMcp1605501 and Fricchione GL, Nejad SH, Esses JA, et al. Postoperative Delirium. Am J Psychiatry. 2008;165(7):803-812. https://doi.org/10.1176/appi.ajp.2008.08020181

dopaminergic medications.[30,31] Although it has been associated with every neuroleptic agent, it is most commonly reported with the high-potency typical antipsychotics, such as haloperidol and fluphenazine.[31] The core clinical features of NMS are hyperthermia, hypertonicity of skeletal muscles, fluctuating consciousness, and autonomic instability.[30] Although uncommon, NMS remains a high-risk diagnosis to look for in patients with fever and mental status changes who are on dopamine receptor antagonist or dopaminergic medications. Treatment of this disorder is discontinuing the offending agent and supportive therapy, including cooling and correction of dehydration and electrolyte imbalances. In cases where NMS is due to dopaminergic withdrawal, restarting those medications may ameliorate the symptoms. In severe cases, treatment with bromocriptine (a dopamine agonist), dantrolene (a muscle relaxant), and benzodiazepines (to help with agitation) may be given.[31] Electroconvulsive therapy has been used to treat patients with NMS refractory to pharmacotherapy.[32] Given its high morbidity and mortality, these patients should be admitted to the intensive care unit. Early reports of NMS had mortality rates of 30% or higher,[30] but increased awareness and earlier diagnosis have decreased the mortality rate to less than 10%.[31] Delayed diagnosis and treatment of this disorder has a high morbidity and mortality rate, making this a high-risk diagnosis to make in patients with psychiatric disease.

Serotonin Syndrome

Serotonin syndrome is a life-threatening adverse drug reaction owing to excess serotonergic agonism of the central and peripheral receptors. It can result from therapeutic drug use, intentional overdose, or inadvertent medication reactions. A remarkable number of drugs from many different classes has been implicated in serotonin syndrome,[33] and serotonin syndrome has been found to occur in 14% of overdoses with selective serotonin reuptake inhibitors.[34] Patients present with a triad of symptoms (altered mental status, neuromuscular abnormalities, and autonomic hyperactivity) that range in severity.[35] Mild cases typically present afebrile with mild hypertension, tachycardia, mydriasis, diaphoresis, shivering, tremor, myoclonus, and hyper-reflexia. Patients with moderate syndrome have these symptoms plus hyperthermia, horizontal ocular clonus, mild agitation, hypervigilance, and pressured speech. In severe cases, patients have all of the previous listed symptoms, as well as hyperthermia of greater than 41.1°C, autonomic instability, delirium, and muscle rigidity. To make the diagnosis, the Hunter Serotonin Toxicity Criteria is recommended with an 84% specificity and 97% sensitivity for serotonin syndrome (**Box 5**).[36] Serotonin syndrome is a high-risk diagnosis because it often goes undetected by providers and, left untreated, it can progress to seizures, rhabdomyolysis, myoglobinuria, metabolic acidosis, renal failure, respiratory failure, diffuse intravascular clotting, coma, and death. Treatment of serotonin syndrome includes removal of the precipitating drugs and initiation of supportive therapy to control autonomic instability, hyperthermia, and agitation. The control of agitation with benzodiazepines is essential. Moderate to severely ill patients may benefit from the addition of a serotonin 2A antagonist, such as cyproheptadine. Hyperthermic patients with a temperature of greater than 41.1°C are severely ill and should receive the earlier therapies mentioned, as well as immediate sedation, paralysis, and intubation.[33] When treated, most patients with serotonin syndrome have good outcomes. However, this diagnosis remains high risk owing to its varied presentation and difficulty in diagnosing. Owing to the extensive use of serotonergic medications, emergency physicians must maintain a high clinical suspicion for serotonin syndrome, because early recognition and treatment can prevent significant morbidity and mortality.

Box 5
Hunter serotonin toxicity criteria

A serotonergic agent has been administered in the past 5 weeks

and

One of the following combinations of symptoms are present:
- Tremor and hyperreflexia
- Spontaneous clonus
- Muscle rigidity, temperature of greater than 38°C, and either ocular clonus or inducible clonus
- Ocular clonus and either agitation or diaphoresis
- Inducible clonus and either agitation or diaphoresis

Adapted from Dunkley EJC, Isbister GK, Sibbritt D, Dawson AH, Whyte IM. The Hunter Serotonin Toxicity Criteria: simple and accurate diagnostic decision rules for serotonin toxicity. QJM Int J Med. 2003;96(9):635-642.

Catatonia

Catatonia is a neuropsychiatric syndrome characterized by psychomotor abnormalities and is observed in a variety of medical, neurologic, and psychiatric disorders.[37] It is a high-risk diagnosis because it is ubiquitous, with a prevalence of 7% to 45% in differing clinical situations,[37] is difficult to identify and diagnose in a busy ED, and has high morbidity and mortality if not treated appropriately. There are 2 subtypes of catatonia: retarded and excited. Retarded catatonia is the more frequently observed subtype; it is associated with signs reflecting a paucity of movement, including stupor, mutism, staring, rigidity, immobility, negativism, cataplexy, waxy flexibility, posturing, echophenomena, stereotypy, and automatic obedience. Excited catatonia is marked by psychomotor agitation with excitement, aggressiveness, and impulsivity.[37,38] Both clinical forms can occur in the same patient during the same episode. Catatonia can also become a life-threatening type called malignant catatonia when it is associated with hyperthermia, tachycardia, labile blood pressures, diaphoresis, and alternating excitement versus stuporous mental status. Malignant catatonia is life threatening and should be treated emergently.[37] In the DSM-5, the diagnosis of catatonia is defined as the presence of 3 or more of the following: catalepsy, waxy flexibility, stupor, agitation, mutism, negativism, posturing, mannerisms, stereotypies, grimacing, echolalia, or echopraxia.[22,39] A lorazepam trial, via the IV route if possible, is the treatment of choice for catatonia and can help to make the diagnosis, especially in the retarded subtype. A positive response typically confirms the diagnosis of catatonia and helps to predict a sustained treatment plan; these patients should be started on standing lorazepam as initiation of treatment. Electroconvulsive therapy may be attempted in patients with catatonia who do not respond to lorazepam.[38] Patients with catatonia often have an organic cause to their symptoms and, once diagnosed, should undergo an evaluation for possible etiologies of catatonia, including neurologic, infectious, metabolic, and pharmacologic causes.[37] Malignant catatonia is a medical emergency and should be treated with supportive therapy, IV lorazepam, and possible electroconvulsive therapy.

Central Nervous System Diseases

Brain dysfunction associated with certain central nervous system pathology may produce psychiatric symptoms.[17] **Box 6** lists central nervous system diseases that may present with acute psychiatric symptoms.

Box 6
Central nervous system diseases that can masquerade as psychiatric disorders

- Traumatic brain injury
- Stroke (ischemic, hemorrhagic)
- Intracranial hemorrhage (subdural hematoma, epidural hematoma, subarachnoid hemorrhage)
- Intracranial mass (tumor, abscess, infection, aneurysm)
- Encephalitis (especially limbic encephalitis – infectious, autoimmune [paraneoplastic, nonparaneoplastic])
- Meningitis
- Seizures
- Multiple sclerosis
- Parkinson disease
- Dementia

A history or evidence of acute trauma as well as patients predisposed to falls and/or intracranial hemorrhage (eg, chronic anticoagulation or alcohol use) should prompt brain imaging to look for traumatic brain injury or intracranial hemorrhage. A patient with an abnormal neurologic examination should undergo brain imaging and a workup to assess for stroke, mass, or multiple sclerosis. Patients who present with headache with or without focal neurologic deficits and who are immunosuppressed or have a history of IV drug use or endocarditis should undergo brain imaging to look for a brain abscess. Seizures, including partial seizures and nonconvulsive status epilepticus, may also present with acute psychiatric symptoms and emergency physicians should consider this diagnosis in patients with a known seizure disorder or other risk factors for seizure. Parkinson disease and dementia should be on the differential for elderly patients presenting with psychiatric symptoms.

Meningitis and encephalitis can present with psychiatric symptoms and should be considered in patients with fever, headache, altered mental status, and/or meningeal signs on examination. Of note, limbic encephalitis in particular can present with psychiatric symptoms. Limbic encephalitis is an inflammation in the limbic region of the brain and can be infectious or autoimmune.[40] Patients typically present with behavioral and psychiatric symptoms such as anxiety, depression, irritability, personality change, acute confusional state, hallucinations, psychosis, and seizures.[41] They may have a history of a virus-like prodrome with headaches, lethargy, and fever followed by the psychiatric symptoms within 2 weeks.[42] The limbic encephalitis most closely associated with psychiatric presentations is N-methyl-D-aspartate receptor antibody encephalitis, which can be either paraneoplastic or nonparaneoplastic.[17] Delayed diagnosis of limbic encephalitis is common, but it should be high on the differential for patients who present with new-onset psychosis with findings as listed because the symptoms may improve with early diagnosis and treatment.[41] Patients in whom meningitis or encephalitis is clinically suspected should undergo brain imaging and lumbar puncture.

RISK ASSESSMENT

Models of static risk factors for suicide or violence poorly predict current risk, and a tool to determine the level of risk for suicidal patients has not been found. Suicide and violence are complex disease processes with fluctuating thoughts of self-harm or aggression, changes in psychiatric conditions over time, changes in social supports, and contribution from substance use and stressors.[16]

As such, a dynamic risk assessment performed at the time of presentation is essential for safely assessing a patient's risk. In a busy ED setting, using a structured tool to guide clinicians through this process, such as the Columbia-Suicide Severity Rating Scale,[43,44] can aid in protocolizing an approach to risk for the ED patient. The risk assessment should include an assessment of a patient's ability to meaningfully participate in their own assessment, specifically the likelihood that their answers are truthful, that they are cognitively able to participate, and that they are not experiencing the effects of substance use. The assessment should focus on the presence of psychiatric symptoms or conditions, recent psychosocial changes (particularly major losses), individual psychological factors, and a history of self-harm or harming others. It is imperative that patients are asked directly about their thoughts of suicide or self-harm and if they are having violent ideation, even when clinical suspicion may be low. If a person discloses active thoughts of self-harm or harming others, a more detailed interview should focus on details of a plan and access to intended methods, preparatory behavior or acts of furtherance (eg, rehearsing behaviors, writing a suicide note), and intention to act, as well as protective factors that may keep someone from acting. In addition, the evaluation should take into account collateral information from outside providers, family, friends, emergency medical services personnel, and the police, and every effort should be attempted to obtain this outside information.

ACEP clinical policies provides a Level C recommendation to the question of whether risk assessment tools in ED identify the patient presenting with suicidal ideation as safe for discharge. Per the ACEP, "In patients presenting to the ED with suicidal ideation, physicians should not use currently available risk-assessment tools in isolation to identify low-risk patients who are safe for discharge. The best approach to determine risk is an appropriate psychiatric assessment and good clinical judgment, taking patient, family, and community factors into account."[16]

Patients who exhibit an increased risk require consultation with a mental health specialist for appropriate management and disposition. Mental health consultants (eg, psychiatrists, psychologists, social workers) generally have more training and more time to spend with patients and can help to identify the level of risk and recommend an appropriate ultimate disposition. Consultations may occur in person or by electronic communication and often depend on the ED environment and resources. It is important to remember that, although specialist consultation is useful in these patients, ED physicians ultimately retain the final authority and responsibility for discharging these patients.[45] As such, although suicide is a rare event, the risk of litigation is high if a patient completes suicide soon after leaving the ED. If there is any doubt regarding a patient's risk of self-harm, the emergency physician should have a low threshold for obtaining psychiatric specialty consultation. For patients who are discharged, emergency physicians must thoroughly document a risk assessment, thought process, and any related consultation.

PSYCHIATRIC PATIENT EMERGENCY DEPARTMENT BOARDING

The closure of many US public psychiatric hospital beds and decrease in acute general psychiatric beds over recent decades has led to a mental health crisis; the overall inpatient mental health capacity is inadequate to treat the needs of patients with psychiatric disorders.[1,2] The total number of psychiatric beds in the United States had decreased from 31 beds per 100,000 population in 2000 to 21 beds per 100,000 population in 2016, a decrease of 32%.[46] This decrease in psychiatric beds coupled with increased numbers of patients with acute psychiatric needs presenting to EDs has resulted in prolonged ED stays for patients with psychiatric illness who require hospitalization and increased psychiatric patient boarding rates. Owing to the chaotic nature of the ED coupled with crowding and large numbers of all patients in the ED at any one point in time, psychiatric patients boarding in the ED are often ignored and do not receive the medical or psychiatric care that they require, which may result in worsening of their clinical condition.[47]

The ACEP Emergency Medicine Practice Committee created a review of best practices to reduce ED boarding of psychiatric patients, including[48]:

- *Psychiatric consultations live or via telemedicine* to decrease the need for admission or to start a treatment regimen.
- *Telemedicine in psychiatry* when an on-site psychiatrist is not readily available.
- *Treatment protocols* to be initiated until psychiatry is available and to help decrease lengths of stay.
- *Psychiatry ED observation unit* to keep psychiatric patients in a quiet environment separate from the chaotic nature of the main ED.
- *ED case management* to find appropriate inpatient beds and outpatient treatment follow-up.
- *Mobile crisis intervention team and crisis management prevention* to communicate between EDs and mental health services and facilitate faster placement of patients.
- *Developing statewide patient dashboards* to allow EDs to place patients in available inpatient beds more quickly by allowing ED staff to view all available beds simultaneously and eliminate the need for individual calls.
- *Changing billing and reimbursement guidelines* to increase reimbursement for psychiatric services to encourage providers to increase supply.

Psychiatric patients boarding in the ED should have ongoing psychiatric care for their psychiatric disorder and medical care for their chronic and ongoing medical needs. Patient should undergo daily psychiatric assessment by a mental health professional with initiation and adjustment of medications as appropriate and reassessment of correct level of care for disposition. In addition, it is important not to forget the medical needs of this high-risk subset of patients, and they should be continued on their home medications for their chronic medical conditions as well as undergo continued treatment and reassessment for any new medical conditions identified during the medical assessment. The management of patients' medical conditions can be performed by the emergency physician or an inpatient medical team that manages patients boarding in the ED.

DISCLOSURE

The authors (L.M. Nentwich, C.W. Wittmann) have nothing to disclose.

REFERENCES

1. Increase in US suicide rates and the critical decline in psychiatric beds | psychiatry | JAMA | JAMA Network. Available at: https://jamanetwork.com/journals/jama/fullarticle/2580183. Accessed January 4, 2020.
2. Sharfstein SS, Dickerson FB. Hospital psychiatry for the twenty-first century. Health Aff (Millwood) 2009;28(3):685–8.

3. Trends in emergency department visits involving mental and substance use disorders, 2006-2013 #216. Available at: https://www.hcup-us.ahrq.gov/reports/statbriefs/sb216-Mental-Substance-Use-Disorder-ED-Visit-Trends.jsp?utm_source=AHRQ&utm_medium=EN1&utm_term=&utm_content=1&utm_campaign=AHRQ_EN1_10_2017. Accessed January 4, 2020.

4. Trends in emergency department visits, 2006-2014 #227. Available at: https://hcup-us.ahrq.gov/reports/statbriefs/sb227-Emergency-Department-Visit-Trends.jsp. Accessed January 4, 2020.

5. Lukens TW, Wolf SJ, Edlow JA, et al. Clinical policy: critical issues in the diagnosis and management of the adult psychiatric patient in the emergency department. Ann Emerg Med 2006;47(1):79–99.

6. Koran LM, Sheline Y, Imai K, et al. Medical disorders among patients admitted to a public-sector psychiatric inpatient unit. Psychiatr Serv 2002;53(12):1623–5.

7. Carlson RJ, Nayar N, Suh M. Physical disorders among emergency psychiatric patients. Can J Psychiatry 1981;26(1):65–7.

8. Anderson EL, Nordstrom K, Wilson MP, et al. American Association for emergency psychiatry task force on medical clearance of adults part I: introduction, review and evidence-based guidelines. West J Emerg Med 2017;18(2):235–42.

9. Good B, Walsh RM, Alexander G, et al. Assessment of the acute psychiatric patient in the emergency department: legal cases and caveats. West J Emerg Med 2014;15(3):312–7.

10. Wilson MP, Nordstrom K, Anderson EL, et al. American Association for emergency psychiatry task force on medical clearance of adult psychiatric patients. Part II: controversies over medical assessment, and consensus recommendations. West J Emerg Med 2017;18(4):640–6.

11. Sood TR, Mcstay CM. Evaluation of the psychiatric patient. Emerg Med Clin North Am 2009;27(4):669–83, ix.

12. Tucci VT, Moukaddam N, Alam A, et al. Emergency department medical clearance of patients with psychiatric or behavioral emergencies, Part 1. Psychiatr Clin North Am 2017;40(3):411–23.

13. Olshaker JS, Browne B, Jerrard DA, et al. Medical clearance and screening of psychiatric patients in the emergency department. Acad Emerg Med 1997;4(2):124–8.

14. Janiak BD, Atteberry S. Medical clearance of the psychiatric patient in the emergency department. J Emerg Med 2012;43(5):866–70.

15. Parmar P, Goolsby CA, Udompanyanan K, et al. Value of mandatory screening studies in emergency department patients cleared for psychiatric admission. West J Emerg Med 2012;13(5):388–93.

16. Brown MD, Byyny R, Diercks DB, et al. Clinical policy: critical issues in the diagnosis and management of the adult psychiatric patient in the emergency department. Ann Emerg Med 2017;69(4):480–98.

17. Welch KA, Carson AJ. When psychiatric symptoms reflect medical conditions. Clin Med 2018;18(1):80–7.

18. What is schizophrenia? NAMI: National Alliance on Mental Illness. Available at: https://www.nami.org/learn-more/mental-health-conditions/schizophrenia. Accessed January 28, 2020.

19. Nachimuthu S, Assar MD, Schussler JM. Drug-induced QT interval prolongation: mechanisms and clinical management. Ther Adv Drug Saf 2012;3(5):241–53.

20. Larochelle MR, Bernson D, Land T, et al. Medication for opioid use disorder after nonfatal opioid overdose and association with mortality: a cohort study. Ann Intern Med 2018;169(3):137.
21. Marcantonio ER. Delirium in hospitalized older adults. Solomon CG, ed. N Engl J Med 2017;377(15):1456–66.
22. American Psychiatric Association. Diagnostic and statistical manual of mental disorders: diagnostic and statistical manual of mental disorders. 5th edition. Arlington (VA): American Psychiatric Association; 2013.
23. European Delirium Association, American Delirium Society. The DSM-5 criteria, level of arousal and delirium diagnosis: inclusiveness is safer. BMC Med 2014; 12. https://doi.org/10.1186/s12916-014-0141-2.
24. Meagher DJ, Trzepacz PT. Motoric subtypes of delirium. Semin Clin Neuropsychiatry 2000;5(2):75–85.
25. Fricchione GL, Nejad SH, Esses JA, et al. Postoperative delirium. Am J Psychiatry 2008;165(7):803–12.
26. Kennedy M, Enander RA, Tadiri SP, et al. Delirium risk prediction, healthcare use and mortality of elderly adults in the emergency department. J Am Geriatr Soc 2014;62(3):462–9.
27. Han JH, Zimmerman EE, Cutler N, et al. Delirium in older emergency department patients: recognition, risk factors, and psychomotor subtypes. Acad Emerg Med 2009;16(3):193–200.
28. Inouye SK, van Dyck CH, Alessi CA, et al. Clarifying confusion: the confusion assessment method. A new method for detection of delirium. Ann Intern Med 1990;113(12):941–8.
29. Trzepacz PT, Breitbart W, Franklin J, Levenson J, Richard Martini D, Wang P. Treatment of patients with delirium. In: Practice Guideline for the treatment of patients with delirium. Trzepacz PT, cheir. American Psychiatric Association, APA Press; 2010. https://doi.org/10.1176/appi.books.9780890423363.42494.
30. Guzé BH, Baxter LR. Neuroleptic malignant syndrome. N Engl J Med 1985; 313(3):163–6.
31. Simon LV, Hashmi MF, Callahan AL. Neuroleptic malignant syndrome. In: StatPearls. Treasure Island (FL): StatPearls Publishing; 2020. Available at: http://www.ncbi.nlm.nih.gov/books/NBK482282/. Accessed January 28, 2020.
32. Morcos N, Rosinski A, Maixner DF. Electroconvulsive therapy for neuroleptic malignant syndrome: a case series. J ECT 2019;35(4):225–30.
33. The Serotonin syndrome | NEJM. Available at: https://www.nejm.org/doi/full/10.1056/NEJMra041867. Accessed January 28, 2020.
34. Isbister GK, Bowe SJ, Dawson A, et al. Relative toxicity of selective serotonin reuptake inhibitors (SSRIs) in overdose. J Toxicol Clin Toxicol 2004;42(3):277–85.
35. Volpi-Abadie J, Kaye AM, Kaye AD. Serotonin syndrome. Ochsner J 2013;13(4): 533–40.
36. Dunkley EJC, Isbister GK, Sibbritt D, et al. The Hunter Serotonin Toxicity Criteria: simple and accurate diagnostic decision rules for serotonin toxicity. QJM 2003; 96(9):635–42.
37. Jaimes-Albornoz W, Serra-Mestres J. Catatonia in the emergency department. Emerg Med J 2012;29(11):863–7.
38. Rasmussen SA, Mazurek MF, Rosebush PI. Catatonia: our current understanding of its diagnosis, treatment and pathophysiology. World J Psychiatry 2016;6(4): 391–8.
39. Tandon R, Heckers S, Bustillo J, et al. Catatonia in DSM-5. Schizophr Res 2013; 150(1):26–30.

40. Limbic encephalitis. The Encephalitis Society. Available at: https://www. encephalitis.info/limbic-encephalitis. Accessed January 29, 2020.
41. Anderson NE, Barber PA. Limbic encephalitis – a review. J Clin Neurosci 2008; 15(9):961–71.
42. Hermetter C, Fazekas F, Hochmeister S. Systematic review: syndromes, early diagnosis, and treatment in autoimmune encephalitis. Front Neurol 2018;9. https://doi.org/10.3389/fneur.2018.00706.
43. C-SSRS_Pediatric-SLC_11.14.16.pdf. Available at: https://cssrs.columbia.edu/ wp-content/uploads/C-SSRS_Pediatric-SLC_11.14.16.pdf. Accessed January 29, 2020.
44. Posner K, Brown GK, Stanley B, et al. The Columbia–Suicide Severity Rating Scale: initial validity and internal consistency findings from three multisite studies with adolescents and adults. Am J Psychiatry 2011;168(12):1266–77.
45. Betz ME, Boudreaux ED. Managing suicidal patients in the emergency department. Ann Emerg Med 2016;67(2):276–82.
46. Health care utilisation. Available at: https://stats.oecd.org/Index.aspx?Query Id=30144. Accessed January 4, 2020.
47. Zun L. Care of psychiatric patients: the challenge to emergency physicians. West J Emerg Med 2016;17(2):173–6.
48. psychiatric-patient-care-in-the-ed-2014.pdf. Available at: https://www.acep.org/ globalassets/uploads/uploaded-files/acep/clinical-and-practice-management/res ources/mental-health-and-substance-abuse/psychiatric-patient-care-in-the-ed-2014. pdf. Accessed January 29, 2020.

Physical and Chemical Restraints (an Update)

Pilar Guerrero, MD, Mark B. Mycyk, MD*

KEYWORDS

• Physical restraint • Chemical restraint • Workplace violence • Safety • Sedation

KEY POINTS

- Safety of patients and staff is a priority for any emergency department.
- The use of physical or chemical restraints may need to be used when challenged by a combative, agitated, or cognitively impaired patient who poses a threat to self or others.
- Physical or chemical restraints should be used in the most safe and ethical manner when indicated.

INTRODUCTION

Emergency department (ED) staff have the challenge of triaging, evaluating, diagnosing, treating and providing safe, ethical, and competent care to all who present to the department. Patients with altered mental status, agitation, and aggression add complexity to an already stressful and chaotic environment that is open 24 hours each day. The etiology of altered mental status may be multifactorial and include but not limited to medical illness, trauma, psychiatric disorders, cognitive dysfunction and drug use. These patients may elicit behavior that put them at risk of harming themselves, other patients, staff, or causing significant damage to the surrounding environment.[1-4] Abnormal behavior can be an obstacle to providing the medical care needed, and when de-escalation strategies fail, then restraint modalities need to be considered.[5] Hospital and departmental protocols should be written and updated as needed based on standards of care as well as the policies and regulations from the Centers for Medicare and Medicaid Services (CMS) and The Joint Commission (TJC).[6,7] The American College of Emergency Physicians (ACEP) also provides guidelines for the management of agitated patients and appropriate use of restraints in alignment with these regulatory agencies.[8] De-escalation techniques, physical and chemical restraints, and special circumstances presented by the pediatric and geriatric populations are discussed.

Department of Emergency Medicine, Cook County Health, 1950 West Polk, 7th Floor EM Admin, Chicago, IL 60612, USA
* Corresponding author. 1950 West Polk, 7th Floor EM Admin, Chicago, IL 60612.
E-mail address: mmycyk@cookcountyhhs.org

Emerg Med Clin N Am 38 (2020) 437–451
https://doi.org/10.1016/j.emc.2020.02.002
0733-8627/20/© 2020 Elsevier Inc. All rights reserved.
emed.theclinics.com

EPIDEMIOLOGY

Violence is prevalent in our society, and health care workers are at a high risk of workplace violence. According to the Bureau of Labor Statistics in 2016, health care workers sustained 70% of the workplace nonfatal injuries in private industries, and nearly 20% required 3 to 5 days away from work and 21% required 31 or more days away from work to recover.[9] Workplace violence and injuries are often underreported, especially in the ED environment. High stress, fragmented communication, long waiting times, overcrowding, staff shortages, financial issues, and confusion can provoke violent behavior in predisposed individuals.[1,10–12] A recent study also showed most emergency medical services (EMS) providers reported experiencing assault at some point in their line of duty.[13]

PATHOPHYSIOLOGY

It is helpful for the emergency physician to be familiar with the characteristics that predispose patients to violent or aggressive behavior in the ED.[14] Positive predictors of potential violent behavior are male gender, having a prior history of violence, arriving in the custody of the police, being a victim of violence, and having a history of alcohol or drug abuse.[15,16] Psychiatric illness (especially schizophrenia, personality disorders, mania, and psychotic depression) also has been identified as a significant risk for violent behavior in the ED.[15] Agitation can have an organic cause, such as delirium, dementia, traumatic brain injury, neurologic disease, metabolic disturbance, infection, vascular or circulatory issues, renal or hepatic insufficiency, and endocrine dysfunction. Intoxication or withdrawal from alcohol or other recreational drugs can lead to out-of-control behavior. It is important to differentiate between functional and organic causes for a patient's agitated behavior and carefully rule out organic causes even in patients with a history of psychiatric illness or substance abuse problems. When ruling out an organic cause, a medical workup should be performed as clinically indicated.[17,18]

RECOGNIZING AND PREPARING FOR THE VIOLENT PATIENT

Violence is not usually the initial response of a patient in the ED, but is the result of increasing tension and frustration. In addition to the risks mentioned earlier, certain cues from the patient can predict the possibility of violent behavior. If these cues are noticed, a situation may be diffused with de-escalation techniques. The American Association for Emergency Psychiatry has promoted Project BETA (Best Practices in Evaluation and Treatment of Agitation) to help organizations understand that changes in culture, training, environment, resources, behavioral consulting teams, and other de-escalation strategies may lead to a decrease in use of restraints and seclusion.[19–21] This would lead to improvements in safety, length of stay, medical costs, patient-physician relationship, and enhance the overall patient experience.

When EMS is transporting a violent patient to a hospital, ideally a call should be made to alert ED staff to prepare and mobilize appropriate resources. Having response teams, adequate resources, and properly trained staff, as well as using a multidisciplinary simulation training will aid in the immediate proper management of these challenging patients.[8,22–24] Furthermore, CMS requires that facilities provide staff with training to deal with a combative, uncooperative patient.[6,7] These situations are stressful to staff and it is important to have debriefing sessions with the staff after the event.[19] Proper documentation from the time of patient arrival through discharge should identify team members, de-escalation strategies attempted, reason for use of restraints, and any adverse events.[6–8,25] TJC also requires all deaths related to use of restraints be reported within 24 hours.[26]

DE-ESCALATION

Before ordering any physical or chemical restraints for the agitated patient, de-escalation strategies should be attempted first, including offering reassurance, simplifying communication, demonstrating empathy, ignoring challenging arguments, adjusting the environment with dim lights, offering oral medication, and even offering food.[21] When trying to de-escalate the agitated patient, it is paramount to prioritize the safety of the patient and the treating staff, assist the patient with managing emotions, and avoid coercive interventions that may exacerbate agitation.[27,28] It may be necessary to have hospital security or police nearby in case de-escalation techniques are not successful and provider needs to implement physical and/or chemical restraints.

A previous review found that cultural bias, role perceptions, and attitude by staff were associated with the frequency of seclusion and restraint use.[19] As our country becomes more diverse, these are factors that need to be considered in using de-escalation strategies and then proper use of physical or chemical restraints if de-escalation fails.

PHYSICAL RESTRAINTS

When verbal and nonverbal de-escalation modifications have failed and the patient continues to be a threat to self or others, or their agitation prevents delivery of medical care needed, the use of physical restraints may need to be implemented. Risk factors associated with use of physical restraints in the ED include arrival by prehospital staff already in restraints, brought in by law enforcement, bipolar mania or psychosis, and insight impairment.[29]

In 2 recent studies, patients needing restraints during their ED visit were most often young patients under the influence of psychoactive substances who were eventually discharged, and confused older patients who were eventually hospitalized.[30,31]

The decision to order physical restraints is difficult because it can be perceived as coercion or punishment instead of a last resort to ensure safety, and complications may occur.[19,32,33]

ACEP has established the principles shown in **Box 1** regarding physical restraint use.[34]

Although restraining patients can be risky, appropriate use of restraints may be necessary rather than allowing the patient's out-of-control behavior to progress, which may lead to delayed treatment of the patient and/or injury to self, ED staff or others.

Every institution should have a detailed protocol for the use of restraints.[7] This protocol should identify the members of a restraint team and how to activate the team. All members of the restraint team should be appropriately trained and familiar with the restraining procedure. The team should have at least 5 members, including a designated leader who explains the process to the patient in clear language. Although not always possible, every attempt should be made to have a woman on the restraint team, especially if a woman patient is being restrained.[25] This show of force of a large, organized team alone can sometimes de-escalate the patient and avoid eventual use of restraints.

Before entering a patient's room and initiating the restraining procedure, all personal belongings that could potentially be used as a weapon or cause injury should be removed, including necklaces, lanyards with IDs, stethoscopes around the neck, neckties, and hanging earrings.[35]

Box 1
ACEP's Established Principles for Physical Restraint Use

- Use only after verbal de-escalation attempted
- Maintain privacy and dignity of patients
- Restraint should be the least restrictive
- Staff should be properly trained in usage of restraints and monitoring of patients
- Protocols should be developed on safety, monitoring, and periodic evaluations of continuing need for physical restraints
- Proper documentation should include reasons for restraints, alternative methods tried, monitoring, and periodic assessment of need for restraints
- Federal standards, rules, and laws should be followed

Data from Use of Patient Restraints. ACEP; revised 2014, approved 1991. Retrieved from https://www.acep.org/patient-care/policy-statements/use-of-patient-restraints. Accessed July 2, 2019.

During the restraining procedure, the team leader maintains the safety of the patient's head while each of the other members takes control of a preassigned extremity. Each extremity should be controlled at the major joint (elbow, knee), and the restraint should be tied to the frame of the bed, not the handrails. All restraint positions carry certain risks, and careful monitoring of the restrained patient is essential. If aspiration is a risk, or the patent is pregnant, the patient should be restrained on the left lateral side, otherwise restraint in the supine position may facilitate the medical examination and be more comfortable for the patient. Sentinel event tracking by TJC indicates that restraining patients on their side reduces adverse restraint events.[7] Restraining a patient in the prone position predisposes them to suffocation and aspiration. If a patient requires restraint in the prone position for medical or significant safety issues, specific attention should be paid to the patient's airway and breathing. The airway must remain unobstructed at all times, the head be able to rotate side to side, the head of bed should be elevated if not contraindicated, and the expansion of the lungs must not be restricted by excessive pressure on the patient's back.[36] If 4-point restraints are used, the arms should be restrained so that one arm is up and one down. This position makes it difficult for the patient to generate enough force to overturn the stretcher. If additional restraint is needed, a sheet can be placed around the chest and tied to the stretcher, taking care that the sheet is not so tight that it prevents adequate chest expansion.[1] If the patient is semi-cooperative, or if going from 4-point to 2-point restraints, the contralateral arm and leg should be restrained. Soft restraints also can be used in semi-cooperative patients, but for patients who are combative and trying to escape, leather or nylon restraints are preferred. Soft restraints can tighten and cause circulatory compromise as a patient struggles, whereas leather restraints rarely compromise distal circulation but are more difficult to cut and remove in an emergency.[37] While restrained, patients should be under continuous observation and close monitoring. Change in position is important to prevent rhabdomyolysis, pressure sores, and paresthesias.

The treating physician should not be involved in the actual restraint process to preserve the doctor-patient relationship.[4] However, a member of the medical team should be present during the restraining process to monitor the patient. The order for implementation of restraints when a threat of imminent harm to self or staff is evident can be initiated by a physician or other licensed independent practitioner, or as a verbal order by a nurse; however, the physician is required to conduct a face-to-face evaluation of the patient within an hour.[26] Orders must be rewritten, for they are time limited as follows: 4 hours for adults, 2 hours for children and adolescents ages 9 to 17, and 1 hour for patients younger than 9 years. The restraint procedure requires careful documentation by the physician and the nurse. Physician documentation should cite that verbal techniques failed to calm the patient, the specific indication for the restraining procedure, the time the restraints were applied, the time-limited duration of the restraining procedure, the planned medical workup or treatment, and the patient's decision-making capacity.[33] Nursing documentation should include frequent assessment of the patient's vital signs, nutrition and hydration status, circulation, range-of-motion of extremities, hygiene and elimination, physical and psychological status, comfort, and readiness for discontinuation of restraints. The patient must also be reassessed by a physician at the end of predefined time limits. When clinically appropriate, restraints should be removed 1 at a time in 5-minute intervals until 2 are left. If the patient remains cooperative, the last 2 can be removed (**Box 2**).

TJC lists patient injury or death under restraint as 1 of the top 10 sentinel events in the ED.[7] There are many issues that can lead to patient injury or death from use of restraints, including miscommunication among staff or between staff and patient, procedural noncompliance, inadequate patient assessment, and restraint of a patient in a room not under continuous observation. During TJC inspections, failure to document and practice safe use of restraints is one of the leading citations for hospitals.[7] Any complication from the use of physical restraints should be documented, with abrasions and bruising being the most common complications.[38] Positional asphyxia has been reported to occur if the patient is restrained in the prone position.[39] Death can occur if the restraints are not applied properly or the patient is not carefully

---

Box 2
The Joint Commission Standards on Restraint and Seclusion

1. The [organization] uses restraint or seclusion only when it can be clinically justified or when warranted by patient behavior that threatens the physical safety of the patient, staff, or others.

2. The [organization] uses restraint or seclusion safely.

3. The [organization] initiates restraint or seclusion based on an individual order.

4. The [organization] monitors patients who are restrained or secluded.

5. The [organization] has written policies and procedures that guide the use of restraint or seclusion.

6. The [organization] evaluates and reevaluates the patient who is restrained or secluded.

7. The [organization] continually monitors patients who are simultaneously restrained and secluded.

8. The [organization] documents the use of restraint or seclusion.

9. The [organization] trains staff to safely implement the use of restraint or seclusion.

10. The [organization] reports deaths associated with the use of restraint and seclusion.

Data from Crisis Prevention Institute. Joint Commission Standards on Restraint and Seclusion/ Nonviolent Crisis Intervention Training Program. Available at: https://www.crisisprevention. com/CPI/media/Media/Resources/alignments/Joint-Commission-Restraint-Seclusion-Alignment-2011.pdf Accessed July 13, 2019; with permission.

monitored.[36] Other known complications of restraints are deep vein thrombosis, rhabdomyolysis, hyperthermia, increased sympathetic tone with vasoconstriction, metabolic acidosis due to lactic acid release from prolonged isotonic muscle contractions, and negative psychological impact. Cardiovascular collapse from metabolic acidosis has been found in many restraint-associated deaths, especially in those with acute agitation related to sympathomimetic drug use such as cocaine and methamphetamine.[36,38–42]

Physical restraints should be used for the least amount of time needed, and reevaluation for readiness of discontinuing physical restraints should be done following predefined institutional policies. Often, these may be removed once the use of chemical restraints have been successful at calming the patient. Some experts suggest that physicians are more likely to use more pharmacologic restraints or other informal restraint methods in place of physical restraints in settings with computerized forcing functions that limit their choices or require additional documentation steps to meet an institutional regulatory requirement.[43] Careful, consistent, thorough, and standardized documentation minimizes the risk of miscommunication, adverse events, and other complications from physical restraints.[33,44]

CHEMICAL RESTRAINTS

Chemical or pharmaceutical restraints, called "rapid tranquilization" in older literature, should also be considered in conjunction with or in place of physical restraints. Physical restraints can be counterproductive because struggling against restraints may prevent obtaining a history or completing a thorough physical examination.[45] Chemical restraints can help gain better control of the agitated patient, allow evaluation and treatment, and even hasten removal of physical restraints.[46] Complications associated with struggling against physical restraints, such as hyperthermia, dehydration, rhabdomyolysis, or lactic acidosis, can all be minimized with the early use of chemical sedation.[45]

Antipsychotics/Neuroleptics

Because so many patients with violent behavior in the ED have an underlying psychiatric illness, antipsychotic medications, either alone or combined with benzodiazepines, are used commonly in the ED setting.[47,48] Antipsychotics have a high therapeutic index and a lack of addictive potential. This class of medication has a high affinity for the dopamine-2 receptor. Contraindications to these medications include an allergy to the class, Parkinson disease, and anticholinergic drug intoxication. Relative contraindications include pregnancy, lactation, and hypovolemia.

First-Generation Antipsychotics

Haloperidol, a butyrophenone, is classified as a first-generation antipsychotic.[49] It is easily given intramuscularly (IM) at doses of 2.5 to 10 mg. The time of onset is 2 to 6 hours for oral and 30 to 60 minutes for IM/intravenous (IV). Repeat doses can be given at 30-minute to 60-minute intervals, and the desired effect is usually obtained within 3 doses. The half-life of haloperidol is 10 to 19 hours. IV administration has not been approved by the US Food and Drug Administration (FDA), but it is frequently given via this route. Extrapyramidal syndrome (EPS) is a potential side effect of haloperidol and, in rare cases, has been reported to occur days after administration, even after only 1 dose. This risk may be reduced with the concomitant use of an anticholinergic agent or benzodiazepine.[14] Occurrence of EPS is easily treated with diphenhydramine or benztropine.[50] Haloperidol can be safely given in the same syringe as lorazepam, thus facilitating administration, hastening onset of sedation, and resulting in fewer EPS episodes than when haloperidol is given alone.[47] Combinations of halo-peridol with a benzodiazepine have been suggested to be superior to either drug alone with no difference in adverse events.[51,52] Caution must be taken if using antipsy-chotics such as droperidol or haloperidol, as there is a risk of QT prolongation and resultant torsades de pointes.[53]

Neuroleptic malignant syndrome (NMS) is an idiosyncratic adverse effect that can occurs in 1% of patients receiving antipsychotics, and this is more common in those receiving a first-generation antipsychotic. NMS is recognized by autonomic instability, hyperthermia, altered mental status, and muscle rigidity. Creatine phospho-kinase levels may be elevated.[54] Treatment is supportive, with aggressive cooling measures and cessation of all neuroleptics. In some cases, dantrolene is indicated for treatment of extreme muscle rigidity.

Second-Generation Antipsychotics

Second-generation (previously known as "atypical") antipsychotic medications, have a similar efficacy to first-generation antipsychotics and a better side-effect profile.[14] Risperidone, olanzapine, quetiapine, and ziprasidone are the most commonly used atypical antipsychotics in the ED. Second-generation antipsychotics inhibit dopamine-2 and serotonin receptors and thus provide more tranquilization and less sedation. An important benefit of these atypical antipsychotics is the lower incidence of EPS from the serotonergic activity.[55] This generation of antipsychotic medications has also been found to be particularly useful in cases of acute agitation from metham-phetamine use.

Risperidone (Risperdal) may be given IM or orally by elixir or a recently available dis-integrating tablet. Studies have shown risperidone to be as effective as IM haloperidol and less sedating than in the acute treatment of psychosis.[50] Convincing an out-of-control patient to take risperidone orally can be challenging, but onset is rapid with the orally dissolving tablets, so this option is safer and potentially more convenient for nursing staff.

Olanzapine, available IM or in orally dissolving tablets, has been found to be com-parable in efficacy to either lorazepam or haloperidol in many well-controlled studies assessing its use for the treatment of agitated elderly patients with Alzheimer disease, patients with bipolar disorder with mania, and schizophrenic patients in acute agita-tion.[56,57] Occurrence of dystonia and akathisia are less common than with haloper-idol.[58,59] Mild hypotension is a common side effect and olanzapine has significant anticholinergic properties, which could exacerbate an agitated patient who overdosed on an anticholinergic agent such as diphenhydramine or jimsonweed. Quetiapine, similar to olanzapine, can have higher sedative effects due to high affinity for antihis-taminic receptors, but is available only in oral tablets.

Ziprasidone has been approved by the FDA for the treatment of acute agitation in pa-tients with schizophrenia and patients with bipolar disorder with mania. Studies have shown IM ziprasidone has a higher affinity to serotonin receptor compared with D2 re-ceptors and to be superior to haloperidol with fewer extrapyramidal symptoms.

Inhaled loxapine has been studied for use in the ED because of its rapid onset for treatment of agitation, peaking within 2 minutes after administration, and has been approved for acute agitation associated with schizophrenia or bipolar I disorder. It is associated with less frequent occurrence of EPS, but may cause bronchospasm.[60] An additional benefit to this drug is that it lacks sedative effects, so one can still attempt verbal de-escalation and potentially avoid additional sedation or physical restraints.

Benzodiazepines

This class of drugs are central nervous system depressants because they augment activity at gaba-aminobutyric acid (GABA) receptors. Because benzodiazepines enhance sedation and restore inhibition, they are particularly useful in cases of agitation secondary to acute sympathomimetic drug use, such as cocaine and methamphetamine. Lorazepam is one of the more frequently used benzodiazepines for the treatment of agitation in the ED setting. It is a favorable medication because of its rapid onset, lack of active metabolites, effectiveness in patients intoxicated with a sympathomimetic agent such as cocaine, and availability in oral, IM, and IV formulations. Of all the benzodiazepines, it is the one most reliably absorbed when administered IM, so it is especially useful in the agitated patient without IV access.[46–48] Time of onset is 30 to 60 minutes orally, 10 to 20 minutes IM, and 5 to 15 minutes IV. It has a half-life of 10 to 20 hours. It is also particularly useful in patients with alcohol dependence or cirrhosis because its inactivation is preserved in the setting of liver disease.[49] Most common side effects include sedation, confusion, nausea, and ataxia. Patients must be closely monitored for respiratory depression. It is a class D agent in pregnancy and should also be avoiding in lactating women. As mentioned earlier, studies by Battaglia and colleagues have shown that the sedative effect from the combination of lorazepam and haloperidol is superior to higher doses of either medication alone. In addition, occurrence of EPS is less common in those given lorazepam and haloperidol together compared with those given haloperidol alone.[47]

Midazolam is a water-soluble short-acting benzodiazepine that has become popular because it can be administered IM or IV, intranasal, rectal, and oral. It has a rapid time to onset (18 minutes) and a time to arousal of 30 to 120 minutes (average 82 minutes). When administered IV, midazolam may result in significant hypotension, whereas IM administration has little effect on the cardiopulmonary system.[61] Some studies confirm midazolam had similar efficacy to haloperidol or lorazepam but was superior to both in that time to arousal was significantly quicker for midazolam.[62–64] A shorter time to arousal is a useful quality in the ED in that it allows these patients' evaluations to be completed more rapidly, allowing for faster determination of the appropriate disposition of the patient. Midazolam has recently become a favorable benzodiazepine option for use in agitated patients by prehospital staff.[63]

Ketamine

Ketamine, previously used most commonly for procedural sedation in the ED, has recently become a first-line agent to treat agitation in the prehospital and ED setting.[65,66] It interacts with several receptors, including N-methyl-D-aspartate, nitric oxide synthase, and multiple opioid receptors. It has a quick onset of action (2–3 minutes) and a duration of 5 to 30 minutes.[14,66] When compared with haloperidol, in the prehospital setting, it is noted to cause a higher rate of complications, including the need for intubations.[67–69] Some have recommended it be avoided in schizophrenia, as it can exacerbate the symptoms.[20] Studies of ketamine for sedation of agitated patients in the ED are limited to date, but prehospital studies and early data in the ED are promising. Ketamine has been shown to have faster onset to sedation and no significant changes in re-dosing, or in adverse effects, compared with other agents.[66] Due to variation in dosing and use of additional sedative agents, the need for airway management and rates of intubation vary in different studies on ketamine.

Special Populations

Restraints in the geriatric patients

In the past decade, we have seen an increase in the population 65 years and older and this growth is expected to continue for the next several decades. This group has grown by 30% since 2010, and in 2018, people older than 65 years comprised 16% of the US population.[70] In 2015, there were 47.8 million and it is projected that by 2060, this number will reach 98.2 million.[70] As this segment of the population grows, so will the number of elderly patients presenting to the ED with acute agitation and psychiatric disorders. The elderly also often have multiple comorbidities, use of polypharmacy, dementia, Alzheimer disease, and other cognitive impairments. As our country becomes more culturally and linguistically diverse, so will this segment of the population, and communication may add another challenge. There also will be an increase in alternative living arrangements (ie, nursing homes, assigned living), where historically restraints are used more often.[71]

The agitated, confused, suicidal, delusional, or aggressive geriatric patient poses a unique challenge to the ED physician and staff.[72] Studies looking at the use of restraints in the elderly presenting to the ED are limited.[31,72–74] Proper de-escalation techniques, including use of family to calm the agitated patient, should be attempted before any chemical or physical restraint is used. The use of chemical or physical restraints has been associated with prolonged length of stay in the ED for elderly patients who present with behavioral complaints, and this puts them more at risk for adverse events.[71,75] If chemical restraints are ordered, the physician needs to be cognizant that the elderly may metabolize medications differently because of age and other medical conditions and are often on multiple medications that may increase their risk of an adverse event when combined with sedatives or antipsychotics.[76] Elderly patients may already be on medications that cause QT prolongation or sedation, and the use of certain antipsychotics or anxiolytics may exacerbate symptoms and lead to serious complications. Documentation should include reasons for chemical sedation, use of screening agitation scales, as well as reason for agent and dosage chosen.[23] As with adults and children, little is known of the psychological adverse outcomes of restraint use in the geriatric population,[72] and providers should minimize duration of restraining whenever possible.

Restraints in the pediatric population

The pediatric patient may present agitated or violent as a result of a medical or psychiatric illness, psychological trauma, delirium, substance use, developmental/behavioral/cognitive disorders (attention-deficit/hyperactivity disorder, hyperactive, autism, impulsivity, intellectual disability), fear, pain, or from the stress of the ED environmental stimuli.[77,78] This population presents unique challenges to the ED staff, as they may be of nonverbal age, or not able to communicate their feelings of fear, anxiety, or even pain. They also may not comprehend explanations from the staff.[77] The number of mental health–related visits to the ED has increased, accounting for approximately 5.0% to 6.8% of all pediatric ED visits.[79,80] Although a large proportion of ED visits in the pediatric population are young adults (17–24 years old), the biggest increase from 2011 to 2015 was seen in the adolescent and nonwhite youth. There has been a 2.5-fold increase seen in self-injury and suicide-related visits in the adolescent age.[80]

Clinicians need to be aware of specific standards from CMS and TJC related to this group of patients, because they include different parameters from those used in adults requiring restraints.[81,82] The American Academy of Pediatrics and ACEP developed a joint policy statement based on federal regulations to provide guidelines for clinicians caring for pediatric mental health emergencies.[78] Restraints used are to be the least-restrictive, age-appropriate methods, and not as a punishment or staff convenience.[8,27] There is a paucity of rigorous studies evaluating risks, efficacy, adverse events, of verbal, chemical, or physical restraints. Staff training; use of a family member to calm the patient; use of child psychologist, social worker, or other specially trained staff; child-life specialist; environmental adaptations; verbal restraints; and age-appropriate de-escalation strategies have shown to be helpful in calming patients.[80,81,83,84] Restraint and seclusion can result in significant long-term psychological trauma, which has not been well studied.[77] The use of a child-life specialist, child psychiatrist, or mental health social worker have shown to aid in the management of pediatric patients with mental health presentation.[77,84]

PREVENTIVE MEASURES

Various environmental, administrative, and behavioral preventive measures can be implemented to help make the ED a safer environment.[85–87] Certain environmental designs can strategically minimize violence in hospitals. Monitoring systems, such as metal detectors and security cameras, have been found to discourage aggressive behavior in the ED and other industries.[88] Waiting rooms should be designed to accommodate and assist visitors and patients who may have a delay in service. The triage area, waiting rooms, and reception areas should have heavy furniture that cannot be lifted and used as weapons.

Uniformed security available 24 hours a day is one of the best ways to increase the safety of a department and hospital. Alarm systems and other ways of emergency signaling should be in place in all EDs. A panic button in patient rooms, bathrooms, and hallways can be helpful. A verbal alarm system to get the attention of other staff, such as a code like "Dr Armstrong to room 8," is another effective way to mobilize appropriate staff without upsetting other patients.[33]

Administrative controls to help reduce patient violence include designing staffing patterns to minimize patient waiting times and to prevent staff from working alone. Restricting the movement of the public throughout the hospital or various sections of the ED by card-controlled ID access has also been recommended. Behavioral prevention strategies include continually educating and training all staff to recognize and manage violent events and assaults, resolve conflicts when dealing with patients, and maintain situational awareness. Training should prioritize a patient-centric approach, de-stigmatize illnesses, collaborate in management, and be a part of other institutional and societal activities that can improve the patient experience.[19,27,89]

SUMMARY

As EDs continue to become more crowded, safely managing violent or aggressive patients will continue to be challenging. Appropriately trained personnel in verbal de-escalation and behavioral/environmental modifications, adherence to protocol, careful attention to documentation, and good common sense will minimize complications and ensure safe use of physical or chemical restraints when indicated.

REFERENCES

1. Lavoie FW, Carter GL, Danzi DF, et al. Emergency department violence in United States teaching hospitals. Ann Emerg Med 1988;17(11):1227–33.

2. Al-Sahlawi KS, Zahid MA, Shahid AA, et al. Violence against doctors: 1. A study of violence against doctors in accident and emergency departments. Eur J Emerg Med 1999;6:301.

3. Roca RP, Charen B, Bonow J. Ensuring staff safety when treating potentially violent patients. JAMA 2016;316:2669.

4. Tadros A, Kiefer C. Violence in the emergency department: a global problem. Psychiatr Clin North Am 2017;40(3):575–84.

5. Ziaei M, Massoudifar A, Rajabpour-Sanati A, et al. Management of violence and aggression in emergency environment; a narrative review of 200 related articles. Adv J Emerg Med 2019;3(1):e7.

6. Available at: https://www.cms.gov/Regulations-and-Guidance/Guidance/.../ R37SOMA.pdf. Accessed July 7, 2019.

7. Joint Commission Standards on Restraint and Seclusion/Nonviolent. Available at: https://www.crisisprevention.com/.../Joint-Commission-Restraint-Seclusion-Alignment. Accessed July 13, 2019.

8. Use of patient restraints. Policy statement. Ann Emerg Med 2014;64(5):574.

9. Centers for Disease Control and Prevention/National Institute for Occupational Safety and Health 2016. Accessed July 3, 2019. Available at: https://www.cdc. gov/niosh.

10. Behnam M, Tillotson RD, Davis SM, et al. Violence in the emergency department: a national survey of emergency medicine residents and attending physicians. J Emerg Med 2011;40:565–79.

11. McAneney CM, Shaw KN. Violence in the pediatric emergency department. Ann Emerg Med 1994;23(6):1248–51.

12. Kansagra SM, Rao SR, Sullivan AF, et al. A survey of workplace violence across 65 US emergency departments. Acad Emerg Med 2008;15:1268.

13. Furin M, Eliseo LJ, Langlois B, et al. Self-reported provider safety in an urban emergency medical system. West J Emerg Med 2015;16(3):459–64.

14. Gottlieb M, Long B, Koyfman A. Approach to the agitated emergency department patient. J Emerg Med 2018;54(4):447–57.

15. Citrome L, Volavka J. Violent patients in the emergency setting. Psychiatr Clin North Am 1999;22(4):789–801.

16. Tardiff K. Diagnosis and management of violent patients. In: Michels R, Cavener JD, Cooper AM, et al, editors. Psychiatry, vol. 3. Philadelphia: Lippincott-Raven; 1997. p. 1–17.

17. Regier DA, Farmer ME, Rae DS, et al. Comorbidity of mental disorders with alcohol and other drug abuse. Results from the Epidemiologic Catchment Area (ECA) Study. JAMA 1990;264(19):2511–8.

18. Tardiff K. Unusual diagnoses among violent patients. Psychiatr Clin North Am 1998;21(3):567–76.

19. Knox DK, Holloman GH Jr. Use and avoidance of seclusion and restraint: consensus statement of the american association for emergency psychiatry project Beta seclusion and restraint workgroup. West J Emerg Med 2012;13(1): 35–40.

20. New A, Tucci VT, Rios J. A modern-day fight club? The stabilization and management of acutely agitated patients in the emergency department. Psychiatr Clin North Am 2017;40(3):397–410.

21. Zeller SL, Citrome L. Managing agitation associated with schizophrenia and bipolar disorder in the emergency setting. West J Emerg Med 2016;17(2):165–72.

22. Hill S, Petit J. The violent patient. Emerg Med Clin North Am 2000;18:301–15.

23. Simpkins D, Peisah C, Boyatzis I. Behavioral emergency in the elderly: a descriptive study of patients referred to an Aggression Response Team in an acute hospital. Clin Interv Aging 2016;11:1559–65.

24. Wong AH, Wing L, Weiss B, et al. Coordinating a team response to behavioral emergencies in the emergency department: a simulation-enhanced interprofessional curriculum. West J Emerg Med 2015;16(6):859–65.

25. Thomas J, Moore G. Medical-legal issues in the agitated patient: cases and caveats. West J Emerg Med 2013;14:559–65.

26. Available at: https://www.jointcommission.org/mobile/search/?keywords=restraint+deaths&f=sitename&sitename=Joint+Commission. Accessed July 2, 2019.

27. Richmond JS, Berlin JS, Fishkind AB, et al. Verbal de-escalation of the agitated patient: consensus statement of the American Association for Emergency Psychiatry Project BETA De-escalation Workgroup. West J Emerg Med 2012;13(1):17–25.

28. Downey LV, Zun LS, Gonzales SJ. Frequency of alternative to restraints and seclusion and uses of agitation reduction techniques in the emergency department. Gen Hosp Psychiatry 2007;29(6):470–4.

29. Simpson SA, Joesch JM, West II, et al. Risk for physical restraint or seclusion in the psychiatric emergency service (PES). Gen Hosp Psychiatry 2014;36(1):113–8.

30. Beysard N, Yersin B, Carron PN. Mechanical restraint in an emergency department: a consecutive series of 593 cases. Intern Emerg Med 2018;13(4):575–83.

31. Wong AH, Taylor RA, Ray JM, et al. Physical restraint use in adult patients presenting to a general emergency department. Ann Emerg Med 2019;73(2):183–92.

32. Annas GJ. The last resort–the use of physical restraints in medical emergencies. N Engl J Med 1999;341(18):1408–12.

33. Rice MM, Moore GP. Management of the violent patient: therapeutic and legal considerations. Emerg Med Clin North Am 1991;9(1):13–30.

34. https://www.acep.org/patient-care/policy-statements/use-of-patient-restraints. Accessed July 2, 2019.

35. Kuhn W. Violence in the emergency department: managing aggressive patients in a high-stress environment. Postgrad Med 1999;105(1):143–8.

36. Chan TC, Vilke GM, Neuman T, et al. Restraint position and positional asphyxia. Ann Emerg Med 1997;30(5):578–86.

37. Isaacs E. The violent patient. In: Adams JG, Barton ED, Collins JL, editors. Emergency medicine: clinical essentials. 2nd edition. Philadelphia: Elsevier Saunders; 2013. p. 1630–8.

38. Zun LS. A prospective study of the complication rate of the use of patient restraint in the emergency department. J Emerg Med 2003;24(2):119–24.

39. Hick JL, Smith SW, Lynch MT. Metabolic acidosis in restraint associated cardiac arrest: a case series. Acad Emerg Med 1999;6(3):239–43.

40. Ishida T, Katagiri T, Uchida H, et al. Incidence of deep vein thrombosis in restrained psychiatric patients. Psychosomatics 2014;55(1):69–75.

41. Stratton SJ, Roger C, Brickett K, et al. Factors associated with sudden death of individuals requiring restraint for excited delirium. Am J Emerg Med 2001;19:187–91.

42. Pollanen MS, Chiasson DA, Cairns JT, et al. Unexpected death related to restraint for excited delirium: a retrospective study of deaths in police custody and in the community. CMAJ 1998;158:1603–7.

43. Bisantz A, Wears R. Forcing functions: the need for restraint. Ann Emerg Med 2009;53(4):477–9.
44. Griffey RT, Wittels K, Gilboy N, et al. Use of computerized forcing function improves performance in ordering restraints. Ann Emerg Med 2009;53(4):469–76.
45. Diaz JE. Chemical restraint. J Emerg Med 2000;19(3):289–91.
46. Wilson MP, Pepper D, Currier GW, et al. The psychopharmacology of agitation: consensus statement of the American Association for Emergency Psychiatry project BETA psychopharmacoogy workgroup. West J Emerg Med 2012;13:26–34.
47. Battaglia J, Moss S, Rush J, et al. Haloperidol, lorazepam or both for psychotic agitation? A multicenter, prospective, double blind, emergency department study. Am J Emerg Med 1997;15(4):335–40.
48. Seitz DP, Gill SS, van Zyl LT. Antipsychotics in the treatment of delirium: a systematic review. J Clin Psychiatry 2007;68:11–21.
49. Clinton JE, Sterner S, Stelachers Z, et al. Haloperidol for sedation of disruptive emergency patients. Ann Emerg Med 1987;16:319–22.
50. Currier GW, Trenton A. Pharmacologic treatment of psychotic agitation. CNS Drugs 2002;16(14):219–28.
51. Zun LS. Evidence-based review of pharmacotherapy for acute agitation. Part 1: onset of efficacy. J Emerg Med 2018;54(3):364–74.
52. Korczak V, Kirby A, Gunja N. Chemical agents for the sedation of agitated patients in the ED: a systematic review. Am J Emerg Med 2016;34(12):2426–31.
53. Kao LW, Kirk MA, Evers SJ, et al. Droperidol, QT prolongation and sudden death: what is the evidence? Ann Emerg Med 2003;41(4):546–58.
54. Dubin WR, Weiss KJ. Emergency psychiatry. In: Michels R, Caverner JD, Cooper AM, et al, editors. Psychiatry, vol. 2. Philadelphia: Lippincott-Raven; 1997. p. 1–15.
55. Rund DA, Ewing JD, Mitzel K, et al. The use of intramuscular benzodiazepines and antipsychotic agents in the treatment of acute agitation or violence in the emergency department. J Emerg Med 2006;31(3):317–24.
56. Meehan KM, Wang H, David SR, et al. Comparison of rapidly acting intramuscular olanzapine, lorazepam and placebo: a double blind randomized study in acutely agitated patients with dementia. Neuropsychopharmacology 2002; 26(4):494–504.
57. Meehan K, Zhang F, David S, et al. A double blind, randomized comparison of the efficacy and safety of intramuscular injections of olanzapine, lorazepam or placebo in treating acutely agitated patients diagnosed with bipolar mania. J Clin Psychopharmacol 2001;21(4):389–97.
58. Breier A, Meehan K, Birkett M, et al. A double blind, placebo controlled dose response comparison of intramuscular olanzapine and haloperidol in the treatment of acute agitation in schizophrenia. Arch Gen Psychiatry 2002;59(5):441–8.
59. Wright P, Birkett M, David SR, et al. Double blind, placebo controlled comparison of intramuscular olanzapine and intramuscular haloperidol in the treatment of acute agitation in schizophrenia. Am J Psychiatry 2001;158(7):1149–51.
60. McDowell M, Nitti K, Kulstad E, et al. Clinical outcomes in patients taking inhaled loxapine, haloperidol, or ziprasidone in the emergency department. Clin Neuropharmacol 2019;42(2):23–6.
61. Gerecke M. Chemical structure and properties of midazolam compared with other benzodiazepines. Br J Clin Pharmacol 1983;16(Supp 1):11S–6S.
62. Nobay F, Simon B, Levitt A, et al. A prospective double-blind, randomized trial of midazolam versus haloperidol versus lorazepam in the chemical restraint of violent and severely agitated patients. Acad Emerg Med 2004;11(7):744–9.

63. Isenberg DL, Jacobs D. Prehospital Agitation and Sedation Trial (PhAST): a randomized control trial of intramuscular haloperidol versus intramuscular midazolam for the sedation of the agitated or violent patient in the prehospital environment. Prehosp Disaster Med 2015;30(5):491–5.

64. Klein LR, Driver BE, Miner JR, et al. Intramuscular midazolam, olanzapine, ziprasidone, or haloperidol for treating acute agitation in the emergency department. Ann Emerg Med 2018;72:374–85.

65. Isbister GK, Calver LA, Downes MA, et al. Ketamine as rescue treatment for difficult-to-sedate severe acute behavioral disturbance in the emergency department. Ann Emerg Med 2016;67:581–7.

66. Riddell J, Tran A, Bengiamin R, et al. Ketamine as a first-line treatment for severely agitated emergency department patients. Am J Emerg Med 2017; 35(7):1000–4.

67. Cole JB, Moore JC, Nystrom OC, et al. A prospective study of ketamine versus haloperidol for severe prehospital agitation. Clin Toxicol (Phila) 2016;54(7): 556–62.

68. Cole JB, Klein LR, Nystrom PC, et al. A prospective study of ketamine as primary therapy for prehospital profound agitation. Am J Emerg Med 2018;36(5):789–96.

69. Mankowitz SL, Regenberg P, Kaldan J, et al. Ketamine for rapid sedation of agitated patients in the prehospital and emergency department settings: a systematic review and proportional meta-analysis. J Emerg Med 2018;55(5):670–81.

70. Available at: https://www.census.gov/newsroom/press.../cb18-41-population-projections.html. Accessed July 21, 2019.

71. Rhodes SM, Patanwala AE, Cremer JK, et al. Predictors of prolonged length of stay and adverse events among older adults with behavioral health–related emergency department visits: a systematic medical record review. J Emerg Med 2016; 50:143–52.

72. Swickhamer C, Colvig C, Chan SB. Restraint use in the elderly emergency department patient. J Emerg Med 2013;44:869–74.

73. Peisah C, Chan DK, McKay R, et al. Practical guidelines for the acute emergency sedation of the severely agitated older patient. Intern Med J 2011;41:651–7.

74. Calver L, Isbister GK. Parenteral sedation of elderly patients with acute behavioral disturbance in the ED. Am J Emerg Med 2013;31:970–3.

75. Warren MB, Campbell RL, Nestler DM, et al. Prolonged length of stay in ED psychiatric patients: a multivariable predictive model. Am J Emerg Med 2016;34(2): 133–9.

76. Welker K, Mycyk MB. Pharmacology in the geriatric patient. Emerg Med Clin North Am 2016;34(3):469–81.

77. Gerson R, Malas N, Mroczkowski MM. Crisis in the emergency department: the evaluation and management of acute agitation in children and adolescents. Child Adolesc Psychiatr Clin N Am 2018;27(3):367–86.

78. Chun TH, Katz ER, Duffy SJ. Pediatric mental health emergencies and special health care needs. Pediatr Clin North Am 2013;60(5):1185–201.

79. Dorfman DH, Mehta SD. Restraint use for psychiatric patients in the pediatric emergency department. Pediatr Emerg Care 2006;22(1):7–12.

80. Kalb LG, Stapp EK, Ballard ED, et al. Trends in psychiatric emergency department visits among youth and young adults in the US. Pediatrics 2019;143(4) [pii:e20182192].

81. Chun TH, Mace SE, Katz ER. Evaluation and management of children and adolescents with acute mental health or behavioral problems. Part I: common clinical

challenges of patients with mental health and/or behavioral emergencies. Pediatrics 2016;138(3) [pii:e20161570].

82. Chun TH, Mace SE, Katz ER. Evaluation and management of children with acute mental health or behavioral problems. Part II: recognition of clinically challenging mental health related conditions presenting with medical or uncertain symptoms. Pediatrics 2016;138(3) [pii:e20161573].

83. Masters KJ, Bellonci C, Bernet W, et al. Practice parameter for the prevention and management of aggressive behavior in child and adolescent psychiatric institutions with special reference to seclusion and restraint. J Am Acad Child Adolesc Psychiatry 2002;41(2):4S–25S.

84. Hamm MP, Osmond M, Curran J, et al. A systematic review of crisis interventions used in the emergency department: recommendations for pediatric care and research. Pediatr Emerg Care 2010;26(12):952–62.

85. Sheridan DC, Sheridan J, Johnson KP, et al. The effect of a dedicated psychiatric team to pediatric emergency mental health care. J Emerg Med 2016;50(3): e121–8.

86. Rankins RC, Hendey GW. Effect of a security system on violent incidents and hidden weapons in the emergency department. Ann Emerg Med 1999;33(6):676–9.

87. Blanchard JC, Curtis KM. Violence in the emergency department. Emerg Med Clin North Am 1999;17(3):717–31.

88. Mattox EA, Wright SW, Bracikowski AC. Metal detectors in the pediatric emergency department: patron attitudes and national prevalence. Pediatr Emerg Care 2000;16(3):163–5.

89. Gerson R, Malas N, Feuer V, et al. Best Practices for Evaluation and Treatment of Agitated Children and Adolescents (BETA) in the emergency department: consensus statement of the American Association for Emergency Psychiatry. West J Emerg Med 2019;20(2):409–18.

High-Risk Chief Complaints I
Chest Pain—The Big Three (an Update)

Benjamin Bautz, MD[a], Jeffrey I. Schneider, MD[a,b],*

KEYWORDS

- Chest pain • Myocardial infarction • Thoracic aortic dissection
- Pulmonary embolism • Tension pneumothorax • Esophageal rupture
- Cardiac tamponade • Risk management

KEY POINTS

- Acute coronary syndromes present particularly high medico-legal risk. A high index of suspicion is required in all patients with chest pain, even in those with "atypical" presentations or without traditional risk factors. Validated diagnostic tools such as the History, ECG, Age, Risk Factors, Troponin score may allow safe identification of patients suitable for emergency department discharge.
- Thoracic aortic dissection, although rare, portends tremendous and time-sensitive mortality and is frequently missed or misdiagnosed. No decision pathway is sufficiently sensitive to identify all patients with the disease, and careful history, examination, and investigation of risk factors are paramount.
- Pulmonary embolism is difficult to diagnose clinically due to its spectrum of disease and nonspecific symptoms. Clinicians should document risk stratification using the Wells or Geneva score, Pulmonary Embolism Rule-out Criteria rule, and age-adjusted D-dimer testing and have a low threshold for testing in high-risk patients.

INTRODUCTION

For the emergency physician, chest pain presents a familiar yet vexing challenge. As one of the most common chief complaints, it is responsible for approximately 10 million emergency department (ED) visits each year[1] at an estimated cost of $10 billion annually.[2] Consequently, emergency medicine literature is filled with research seeking to improve the diagnostic accuracy, efficiency, and cost-effectiveness of the tools available for the evaluation of this complaint. The differential diagnosis of ED patients with chest pain includes entirely benign conditions and those that may be an immediate life threat, often with little differentiation in presentation between the two. In

[a] Department of Emergency Medicine, Boston Medical Center, 1 Boston Medical Center Place, Boston, MA 02118, USA; [b] Department of Emergency Medicine, Boston University School of Medicine, Boston, MA, USA
* Corresponding author. Department of Emergency Medicine, Boston Medical Center, 1 Boston Medical Center Place, Boston, MA 02118.
E-mail address: jeffrey.schneider@bmc.org

Emerg Med Clin N Am 38 (2020) 453–498
https://doi.org/10.1016/j.emc.2020.01.009
0733-8627/20/© 2020 Elsevier Inc. All rights reserved.
emed.theclinics.com

particular, acute coronary syndromes (ACSs), aortic dissection, and pulmonary embolism are sources of high morbidity and mortality and as a group represent a significant threat to public health. Although most of the patients seeking care for chest pain are not experiencing an acutely life-threatening event, the symptom holds a unique place in public consciousness, perhaps in part due to successful public health campaigns against cardiovascular disease. Chest pain and related diagnoses sit at the top of the list of most common sources of ED malpractice claims,[3] as the combination of relatively low prevalence and high morbidity/mortality of missed or delayed diagnoses pose significant clinical risk to the patient and medico-legal risk to the provider. Accordingly, the emergency physician must strike a difficult balance between resource utilization, risk management, and patient satisfaction. Here we review the clinical features and diagnostic challenges presented by each of these "big three" diagnoses with an eye toward approaches physicians can take to achieve this challenging balance. Tension pneumothorax, esophageal rupture, and cardiac tamponade are also discussed in brief.

ACUTE CORONARY SYNDROME

Ischemic heart disease is the leading cause of death in the United States,[4,5] with 1 in 6 deaths in 2010 attributed to coronary heart disease.[6] Identification of life-threatening coronary disease accordingly represents a diagnostic imperative for the emergency clinician. Nevertheless, historica ldata suggest that a small but significant percentage of patients discharged from EDs with presumed "noncardiac chest pain" are ultimately diagnosed with ACSs. Although data from the 1970s and 80s demonstrated the rate of mistakenly discharged acute myocardial infarctions (AMIs) to range between 2% and 8%,[7,8] findings from the last several decades indicate that approximately 2% of patients with ACS—either unstable angina (UA) or MI—are inappropriately discharged from the ED.[9-12] Not surprisingly, these discharged patients have nearly twice the mortality of those who are appropriately admitted.[10] This misdiagnosed population accounts for 20% of medical malpractice litigation against ED physicians,[13] with AMI remaining the most frequently alleged missed diagnosis and the one with the highest payout rate in all malpractice claims.[3] As a result, attempts to obviate this source of significant liability, morbidity, and mortality have been at the forefront of risk management strategies for decades. Concern over missing a case of ACS has resulted in increased admission rates for suspected cardiac ischemia, resulting in higher diagnostic sensitivity at the expense of specificity.[14,15] Conversely, rising health care costs and an increasingly litigious environment[16] have spurred a movement toward attempting to identify a low-risk population who might be safely discharged from the ED, and recent data provide reason for some optimism in this regard.[17,18]

Clinical Presentations of Acute Coronary Syndrome

The classic patient with ACS is a white man, aged 60 years or older, with multiple coronary artery disease (CAD) risk factors, who presents with left-sided chest pressure radiating to the arm with some combination of associated dyspnea, nausea, lightheadedness, or diaphoresis. The classically *missed* patient is quite different; the patient is more likely to be woman, nonwhite, younger (age <55 years), and without a previous history of CAD.[10] The patient is also less likely to identify chest pain as their chief complaint and may not report other classically associated symptoms of acute cardiac ischemia. Suprisingly, diabetics and the elderly are not among the most frequently misdiagnosed patients, perhaps as a result of heightened awareness in this population that has been classically thought to present atypically. Characteristics of those patients most at risk for missed ACS are presented here.

Atypical presentations

When the Framingham researchers discovered that 25% of the MIs in their cohort of patients had been diagnosed by routine office electrocardiograms (ECGs) *after* the actual event had long been completed, they postulated that these MIs were missed as a result of being "silent" or atypical.[19] Inconsistent methods of defining atypical presentations, however, have resulted in widely varying estimates of their incidence, ranging from 6% to 52%.[20–26] Nevertheless, these studies have identified several populations that are consistently more likely to present in an atypical fashion: women, the elderly, and nonwhite minorities.[4,20,27] Painless presentations in particular are associated with diabetes, dementia, and heart failure.[20,23] Those with a history of hyperlipidemia, tobacco use, and strong family history seem to be *less* likely to present atypically.[24]

An analysis of more than 20,000 patients with suspected ACS found that the most commonly reported symptoms in those who had complaints other than chest pain included (from most to least common) dyspnea, diaphoresis, nausea/vomiting, and syncope/presyncope.[22] These patients often take longer to present to the ED and are more likely to experience delay in diagnosis and initiation of adequate medical therapies and interventions when compared with those who report chest pain.[20,22,26] Not surprisingly, those with atypical presentations tend to have a higher mortality rate.[22,23,26] As the population ages, some have postulated that the incidence of atypical symptoms in those with ACS is likely to increase.

Gender

Women who are ultimately confirmed to have ACS tend to be older, are more likely to have a history of hypertension, and are more likely to delay their presentation to medical providers after symptom onset.[25] At the same time, they are generally less likely to have undergone prior revascularization despite similar rates of prior MIs or positive stress tests.[28] Although chest pain is still a common chief complaint in women with ACS, it is less common than in men, a disparity that may in part be explained by women's older age and higher prevalence of diabetes on presentation. When present, the chest pain described by women is more likely to radiate to the right arm or shoulder, front neck, or back.[29] Left arm pain and diaphoresis is more common in men, whereas women are more prone to gastrointestinal symptoms such as nausea, vomiting, and indigestion.[29,30] Women are also more likely to report dizziness, fatigue, loss of appetite, and syncope during an acute MI.[29] Multiple studies have demonstrated that women—in particularly those older than 65 years—are less likely to receive percutaneous coronary intervention (PCI), and when they do it is more likely to be delayed.[31–33] These findings highlight the need for a high degree of suspicion for ACS in the elderly woman with nonspecific symptoms and the importance of recognition of the potential impact of implicit biases.

Race

African Americans who present to the ED with chest pain tend to be younger, are more likely women, and are less likely to have had a history of CAD than their white counterparts, features that may lead clinicians to have a lower index of suspicion for ACS.[34,35] African Americans also tend to delay their presentations to health care providers.[27,36] Despite some initial smaller studies to the contrary however, robust data now suggest that once they do seek care, African Americans tend to present similarly to white patients (ie, with similar propensity to present with typical vs atypical symptoms and a similar descriptions of symptoms).[34,35] Their ECGs are more frequently complicated by left ventricular hypertrophy (LVH), presumably stemming from a higher incidence of hypertension.[37] Unfortunately, the literature reports significant race-related disparities regarding the evaluation of patients with chest pain in the ED: nonwhite patients presenting with chest pain are less likely to be triaged as emergent,[35] are likely to experience longer wait times,[38] and several large studies report lower rates of ordered ECGs, chest radiographs, cardiac monitoring,[35,39] and cardiac enzymes[35] in nonwhite patients when compared with white patients. Pope and colleagues[10] found that nonwhite patients with ACS were more than twice as likely as white patients to be discharged from the ED and among those with acute MI, 4 times as likely to be sent home. Although most data suggest that these racial disparities have been stable over time, there is perhaps some reason for guarded optimism: in one recent study of ED patients with chest pain, Musey and Kline report that although nonwhite patients were consistently rated by providers as less likely than their white counterparts to have ACS (before any testing was completed), they had similar evaluations and rates of ACS diagnoses.[40] Although the persistent implicit bias this study reports is distressing, the results are encouraging in that they suggest that improved awareness of racial disparities (or perhaps just increased use of testing algorithms) has decreased the impact of this bias on decisions to order diagnostic testing. Additional large-population studies are needed to fully understand the complex socioeconomic, cultural, and biological factors influencing race-related differences. Nevertheless, from a risk-management perspective, clinicians should keep these racial disparities—and the subconscious or systemic biases of which they are likely evidence—in mind when caring for nonwhite patients.

Younger patients

Although many population-based studies of missed ACS exclude adults younger than 30 years, there is literature suggesting that misdiagnosed patients tend to be younger. This finding is especially true for women younger than 55 years. With increasing rates of obesity, insulin resistance, and metabolic syndrome in today's youth, the prevalence of CAD in younger age groups is expected to increase.[41] Although younger patients with ACS are more likely to present with features that are classically associated with ischemic chest pain, their presentations often lack the forewarning of previous angina symptoms,[42] they are at higher risk of being misclassified as noncardiac chest pain, and they may be recipients of greater damage payments in the event of a bad outcome due to potential lost wages. With respect to CAD risk factors, family history of premature CAD, smoking, and hyperlipidemia (specifically higher triglycerides or lower high-density lipoprotein levels) are significantly more prevalent in patients with early onset CAD when contrasted to their older-age counterparts, who are more likely hypertensive and diabetic.[42] Younger patients should also be queried regarding recreational drug use and the presence of congenital heart vascular abnormalities or hypercoagulable syndromes. In a potential approach to risk-stratify younger adults, one group reported an overall 5% incidence of ACS in adults younger than 40 years who received an ECG for noncocaine-related chest pain.[43] This risk decreased to 1.0% if the patient had no previous cardiac history, a normal ECG, and no conventional CAD risk factors and further dropped to 0.14% if initial cardiac enzymes were negative.

Diagnostic Tests and Their Limitations

History

Numerous studies and meta-analyses have tried to identify which aspects of a patient's history are most critical in determining whether their chest pain is cardiac in origin. Altogether, few elements of the "typical" ACS symptomatology have borne out as reliable indicators of cardiac ischemia. For example, although ACS-related chest pain is classically described as "pressure," this descriptor turns out to have minimal utility for predicting true ACS.[44–46] Thankfully, several historical features have demonstrated some utility: pain described as similar to or worse than a previous MI should heighten the clinician's concern, as multiple studies have shown that it carries a positive likelihood ratio (LR) of approximately 2 for ACS.[47–50] Similarly, radiation of chest pain to one or especially both shoulders/arms (LR 1.5–7.7)[44,46,51–53] or pain produced by exertion (LR 1.5–2.8)[44,48,49] also predicts ACS. Some data also suggest that vomiting and diaphoresis in the ED carry positive LRs (3.09 and 6.39, respectively) for ACS.[53,54] In contrast, pain that is described as sharp, stabbing, pleuritic, or positional is less likely cardiac in nature, with an LR of MI from 0.2 to 0.4.[48,51] Chest wall tenderness carries a similar LR of 0.17 to 0.3 for ACS.[51,52] These descriptors should be used cautiously, however; ischemia is nevertheless diagnosed in 22% of patients who present with sharp or stabbing pain, 13% of patients with pleuritic pain, and 7% of patients whose pain is reproducible with palpation.[47,55,56]

Pain lasting longer than 30 minutes, if ischemic in origin, is more likely to evolve into MI. However, pain from esophageal pathology may also persist for prolonged periods, for example, in gastroesophageal reflux disease. Brief episodes of pain, lasting a few seconds, are generally considered nonischemic but have not been confirmed in the literature as such. Finally, any clinical suspicion of angina or its equivalents should elicit a brief assessment of the patient's functional status. Doing so may elicit a history that is consistent with unstable angina and prevent one from inadvertently missing such patients.

Although risk factors for the development of CAD have been clearly identified by longitudinal studies such as the Framingham Study,[57] these same risk factors not always predict *acute* ischemia in the ED setting, especially when compared with presenting features of chest pain or ECG changes. One large prospective cohort study of patients presenting with suspected cardiac chest pain demonstrated no significant relationship between cardiovascular risk factors and likelihood of AMI with an area under the receiver-operating curve of 0.49.[58] Another even larger study[59] of more than 5000 patients showed no statistically significant associations between traditional risk factors (ie, hypertension, hypercholesterolemia, smoking) and acute ischemia, with the exception of diabetes and family history of CAD in men only (with relative risk [RR] of 2.4 and 2.1, respectively). Family history of early CAD (age <55 years in male and <65 years in female relatives) was also found to have an odds ratio of 1.62 for ACS or cardiovascular death in a study of more than 28,000 ED patients with chest pain in Sweden.[60] Nevertheless, these risks pale in comparison to the RR of 12 to 25 for chest pain and 2.2 to 22 for specific ECG changes.[59] Interestingly, a large post hoc analysis suggests that traditional ACS risk factors can be predictive of acute ischemia in patients younger than 40 years, having no risk factors conferred a negative LR of 0.17, whereas more than 4 risk factors was associated with a positive LR of 7.39; this effect weakened in those aged 40 to 65 years and was absent in the elderly.[61] In summary, although risk factors *are* correlated with worse prognosis and necessitate more aggressive treatments once ACS is diagnosed,[62] one should use caution when relying exclusively on the presence or absence of conventional risk factors in the diagnosis of ACS in ED patients.

Altogether, the data suggest that although some features of the patient's history may point toward or away from ischemic heart disease, clinicians should not rely solely on any of these features alone, especially as newer evidence suggests that the characteristics discussed here may not hold true across all cultural/ethnic groups[54] and, furthermore, that perhaps clinician gestalt is not as discriminatory as previously believed.[4]

Response to therapy
Medication response has also demonstrated a poor ability to discriminate between cardiac and noncardiac causes of chest pain. For example, nitroglycerin, a hallmark of antianginal therapy, has been shown to provide symptom relief in those with cardiac chest pain as well as in those with esophageal spasm. Multiple studies have demonstrated the lack of utility in assessing response to nitroglycerin in determining the cause of chest pain, with, in fact, a trend toward high response rates from *non*cardiac versus cardiac causes of chest pain.[49,63–65]

Physician reliance on patient's response to a "gastrointestinal (GI) cocktail" can similarly be misleading. Numerous case reports have documented patients who responded to a GI cocktail and were subsequently diagnosed with an MI.[66,67] It has been demonstrated physiologically that instillation of hydrochloric acid into the distal esophagus of patients with known CAD significantly reduces coronary blood flow.[68] When patients with known CAD were continuously monitored for both ECG and esophageal pH changes, the frequency and duration of ST depressions correlated with the number of reflux episodes, *all* of which were subsequently improved by omeprazole therapy.[69] Similar reductions in the frequency of angina episodes and ST depressions were seen in patients with CAD subjected to treadmill testing after randomization to omeprazole (vs placebo) therapy.[70] So-called linked angina[71] may be related to a postulated neural reflex mechanism, as heart transplant patients do not exhibit the same symptoms,[72] and illustrates the danger of relying on a GI cocktail to "rule out" ACS.

Electrocardiogram
Although the ECG remains the critical diagnostic tool in the evaluation of chest pain, with ischemic findings conferring markedly increased likelihood of ACS,[49] it should be interpreted with several caveats in mind. Of importance from a risk management perspective, as many as 53% of missed acute MI and 62% of missed UA cases have a normal or nondiagnostic ECG on presentation. An ECG provides only a single snapshot of a potentially dynamic process, and comparison with a patient's baseline ECG, whenever available, is crucial for identifying new abnormalities. Serial ECG monitoring has been shown to identify an additional 16% of acute MIs not seen on initial presenting ECGs,[73] and as a result, some suggest that a repeat ECG be obtained between 15 and 60 minutes later for symptoms potentially consistent with ongoing ischemia.[74] The ECG is also known to underappreciate damage in the right ventricle or posterior basal or lateral walls unless additional leads are requested. The frequent presence of patterns such as left bundle branch blocks (LBBBs), LVH, and paced rhythms can confound interpretation. Moreover, the emerging recognition of ECG patterns that do not meet traditional ST-elevation MI (STEMI) criteria but that may represent coronary occlusion requiring emergent intervention (termed STEMI equivalents)[75,76] further increases the possibility for interpretation error. Finally, the ECG has a highly variable sensitivity and specificity based on how stringently any abnormal findings, many of which may be nondiagnostic for new ischemia, are analyzed and appreciated. These findings must be taken in the context of a patient's level of risk for acute ischemia.

ED physicians are susceptible to ECG misclassification (although at similar rates to cardiologists and other physicians[77]); it has been reported that as many as 1 in 4 missed MIs might have been prevented by correct ECG interpretation.[9] One retrospective study of admitted patients with acute MI found that 1 in 8 ECGs had demonstrated high-risk abnormalities (defined as at least 2 contiguous leads with ST-segment elevation of 0.1 mV or greater, ST-segment depression of 0.05 mV or greater, or T-weave inversions of 0.2 mV or greater) that were missed in the ED.[78] Missed patients tended to be older, less likely to present with chest pain, and more likely to have a history of heart failure or other cardiac disease (and thus more likely to have confounding patterns on ECG). Although ST elevations were less commonly missed than ST depressions or T-wave inversions, they were significantly more likely to be missed when chest pain was not the presenting symptom. Other studies have analyzed disagreements in ST elevations, reporting a 6% to 8% rate of discrepancy between ED attending readings when interpreting whether ST elevations were due to LVF, LBBB, benign early repolarization, or acute MI, particularly when the degree of elevation was less than 2 mm or when there was an absence of reciprocal ST changes.[79–81] Of note, inferior lead MIs were found to have a higher rate of misinterpretation. These data indicate that the ECG should not be used as the sole test for MI; the physician should have a low threshold for ordering repeat ECG testing. Reassuringly, several large studies reviewing emergency physician ECG interpretation suggest that the rate of clinically significant errors is very low.[82,83]

Cardiac enzymes

The last decade has seen considerable research effort devoted to the development and use of cardiac biomarkers and associated protocols allowing rapid but sensitive discrimination between patients with and without ACS. Early studies indicated poor sensitivity (<50%) for cardiac enzymes drawn at presentation in ruling out ACS,[84] with a reported 30-day adverse event rate greater than 2% even in patients with low-risk chest pain with a single negative initial conventional troponin.[85] These findings are perhaps unsurprising, given the natural history of cardiac enzyme release in AMI, understanding that patients present at varying time points in their disease course. The sensitivity of a single conventional troponin for MI increases from 10% to 45% (depending on cutoff used) within the first hour to 90% at 8 or more hours from symptom onset.[86] Accordingly, in order to increase sensitivity, some physicians prefer to check for any change (or "delta") between 2 cardiac biomarker levels, obtained at least 6 hours apart[1] when evaluating patients with potential MI. A retrospective study of 588 low-risk patients (either without CAD risk factors or with CAD risk factors but presenting atypically) with nondiagnostic ECGs and negative troponins drawn 6 to 9 hours after symptom onset reported a 0.3% rate of adverse events and no deaths at 30 days.[87] In addition, a large body of research has developed in recent years combining troponin testing with other clinical features with the goal of accelerating this 6-hour time period while still identifying truly low-risk patients. These systems are discussed later (see "Risk Stratification Tools").

In part related to a need to shorten ED length of stay while also increasing diagnostic accuracy for ACS, newer assays have been developed, which are capable of quantifying even smaller concentrations of cardiac troponin I, termed "high-sensitivity troponin" (hsTn) assays. A large meta-analysis including more than 22,000 patients demonstrated a negative predictive value of 99.5% for the primary outcome of MI or cardiac death at 30 days in patients with suspected ACS and cardiac troponin I concentrations less than 5 ng/L at presentation.[88] Another prospective study of 1600 patients with suspected ACS showed a negative predictive value for AMI of 99.4% with a single hsTnT less than 6 ng/L, with 0- and 3-hour hsTnT levels less than 19 ng/L providing negative predictive value of 99.3% for 30-day major adverse cardiac events (MACE, defined as mortality, MI, or need for PCI).[89] With increased sensitivity comes decreased specificity, however, with the possibility that use of these high-sensitivity assays leads to misidentification of patients with noncoronary causes of myocardial injury as having ACS.[90] There are also concerns that decreased specificity will result in increased downstream testing and cost. Nevertheless, it should be emphasized that, regardless of specificity for MI related to coronary thrombus, elevated troponin consistently portends a worse prognosis across the spectrum or patient populations and disease entities.[90,91]

From a risk management perspective, recent developments in cardiac enzyme testing may facilitate the identification of those patients at risk of morbidity and mortality due to missed or delayed diagnosis of ACS. However, further prospective studies are needed to understand the full implications of such testing for our health system. At present, the American College of Emergency Physicians (ACEP) makes an "expert consensus-level" recommendation that conventional troponin testing at 0 and 3 hours among patients with low-risk ACS (defined by the History, ECG, Age, Risk Factors, Troponin [HEART] score[92] of 0–3 [**Table 1**]) can predict an acceptably low rate of 30-day MACE (which ACEP defines as between 1% and 2%).[1] ACEP also recommends with expert consensus level certainty that either a single negative hsTn or negative serial hsTn results at 0 and 2 hours can predict a low rate of 30-day MACE in low-risk patients.

Point-of-care ultrasound

Although resting echocardiography is not sufficiently sensitive to rule out cardiac ischemia in patients with chest pain,[93] point-of-care ultrasound (POCUS) has benefit for the emergency physician in the evaluation for ACS. Although the core applications of emergency bedsides echocardiography consist of evaluation for pericardial effusion, global reduction in ejection fraction, and dilation of the right ventricle,[94,95] more advanced applications are rapidly evolving. In particular, animal data suggest that

Table 1
The history, electrocardiogram, age, risk factors, troponin score for patients with chest pain in the emergency department

Variable	Features	Points
History	Highly suspicious	0
	Moderately suspicious	1
	Slightly or nonsuspicious	2
ECG	Significant ST-depressions	0
	Nonspecific repolarization abnormality	1
	Normal	2
Age	$\geq$64 y	0
	>45 to <65 y	1
	$\leq$45 y	2
Risk Factors[a]	$\geq$3 risk factors or known atherosclerotic disease	0
	1 or 2 risk factors	1
	No risk factors	2
Troponin	$\geq$3x normal limit	0
	>1 to <3x normal limit	1
	$\leq$ Normal limit	2

[a] Diabetes mellitus, hypertension, hypercholesterolemia, family history of coronary artery disease, obesity, smoking, or known atherosclerotic disease.

Adapted from Backus BE, Six AJ, Kelder JC, et al. A prospective validation of the HEART score for chest pain patients at the emergency department. Int J Cardiol 2013;168(3):2153-8.

coronary occlusion reliably induces regional wall-motion abnormalities (RWMA) on echocardiography,[96] and early studies demonstrated that such abnormalities can be identified in most of the patients with acute MI.[97,98] Emerging data suggest that with proper training emergency physicians can accurately detect RWMA on POCUS,[95] and several investigators report that identification of RWMA may help identify high-risk patients who do not otherwise meet criteria for aggressive intervention.[99,100] Larger, prospective studies are needed to confirm these findings and to elucidate the appropriate evidence-based role for POCUS in the currently accepted diagnostic pathways for ACS, however, and use of bedside echocardiography in diagnosis of ACS is not presently endorsed by ACEP. Conversely, in a patient with undifferentiated chest pain, POCUS may immediately identify an alternative diagnosis such as cardiac tamponade, aortic dissection, or pneumothorax, and it may also identify complications of MI including septal defects, ventricular aneurysm or rupture, and mitral regurgitation.[93] Accordingly, for those physicians with proper training it is an indispensable tool, and where ACS is concerned, it may offer the clinician further reason for heightened concern and may help drive additional diagnostics, treatment, and disposition.

Stress testing

Most of the individuals presenting to EDs with chest pain do not have ACS. In one large study of more than 10,000 patients presenting to the ED with symptoms suggestive of ACS, only 8% were ultimately diagnosed with MI and 15% with UA.[101] Many subsequent observational trials have confirmed an overall MACE rate of 10% to 15% in ED patients with chest pain.[89,102,103] The use of provocative testing in low- to intermediate-risk patients—either in the ED or observation unit—to identify those that may safely be discharged without further testing has become commonplace. Early data from the 1990s and early 2000s suggested that the use of risk stratification protocols that incorporated stress testing along with standard clinical evaluation was safe and effective in establishing which patients have truly low 30-day risk.[104–107] Indeed, current 2014 American heart Association (AHA)/American College of Cardiology (ACC) guidelines recommend (as class IIa) that "it is reasonable for patients with possible ACS who have normal serial ECGs and cardiac troponins to have a treadmill ECG (level of evidence A), stress myocardial perfusion imaging, or stress echocardiography before discharge or within 72 hours of discharge (level of evidence B)".[108] The safety of this recommendation was evaluated in a study of 979 largely insured low-risk patients.[109] Ninety-two percent of these patients completed their stress tests as scheduled and 68% were within the 72-hour window. At 6-month follow-up there were no deaths, 0.2% had had MIs, and 2% required coronary intervention. Thus, in a low-risk patient in whom timely follow-up can be assured, outpatient testing may be a feasible option.

Despite the widespread adoption of these types of clinical protocols however, newer research has called into the question the utility of stress testing in low-risk patients. In particular, ACEP 2018 guidelines recommend, with moderate clinical certainty, *against* the routine use of stress testing before discharge "in low risk patients in whom MI has been ruled out."[1] This recommendation stems from several small studies finding that stress testing in low-risk patients (defined as either modified HEART score of 0–3 or negative 6-hour serial troponin testing) does not alter 30-day MACE risk.[110,111] Furthermore, several investigators have reported high false-positive rates—near 50%—of stress testing,[1,112,113] raising concerns about associated costs and potential for harm. Accordingly, although larger studies are needed, it may be appropriate to eschew stress testing in appropriately risk-stratified low-risk patients.

The emergency clinician must also remain cautious when incorporating patients' previous stress testing results in assessing risk. Although most of the aforementioned studies support a less than 2% risk for acute MI for at least 6 months following a negative diagnostic stress testing and mortality rate approaching 0%, most of these were in already low-risk patients. Importantly, even when diagnostic (a sufficient elevation of heart rate is reached), stress test results must be interpreted in the context of a patient's pretest probability of CAD.[114] Although a true negative test has high negative predictive value in truly low-risk patients, this negative predictive value decreases with increasing pretest probability of CAD. As a result, the provider should not be falsely reassured simply because a patient has had a recent negative stress test. For example, one retrospective study examined all patients presenting to the ED with chest pain who had a recent negative stress test with imaging; 6% of patients had an MI within 3 years of their testing, one-third of which had been sustained in the first year.[115] Another retrospective chart review of patients presenting with chest pain with a negative or "normal" indeterminate stress testing in the last 3 years found that 20.7% of patients were subsequently found to have CAD in the next 30 days, and 7.9% had an AMI.[116] Most remarkably, 23.5% of these patients diagnosed with significant CAD had had their stress test within 1 month of presentation.

Computed tomography coronary angiography

In the early 2000s, enthusiasm developed for using computed tomography angiography (CTCA) to risk stratify patients with chest pain in the ED. CTCA allows for the noninvasive evaluation of the extent of calcium deposits and degree of stenosis in the coronary arteries, and interest in its use stemmed from data demonstrating a high level of diagnostic accuracy compared with invasive coronary angiography.[117] Studies evaluating its use in ED patients with chest pain consistently reported a negative predictive value for the presence of CAD between 97% and 100%[118–122] and an accuracy comparable to stress testing in the identification of CAD.[123,124] Moreover, 2 large randomized trials of 1000[125] and 1370[126] patients comparing use of CTCA to standard care in patients with low- to intermediate-risk chest pain both described this excellent negative predictive value as well as improved time to discharge and frequency of discharge from the ED. Indeed, current 2014 ACC/AHA guidelines make class IIa recommendations that "In patients with possible ACS and a normal ECG, normal cardiac troponins, and no history of CAD, it is reasonable to initially perform (without serial ECGs and troponins) coronary CT angiography to assess coronary artery anatomy (level A evidence)".[108]

Enthusiasm for CTCA has waned in recent years, however, likely for several reasons. CTCA may be harder to interpret in patients with known CAD or in older patients who naturally accumulate more coronary calcium over time.[127] Moreover, CTCA cannot identify vulnerable plaques without calcifications nor can it determine the physiologic significance of "intermediate" lesions. Concerns raised initially that the resultant lower specificity of CTCA could lead to increased unnecessary downstream testing have indeed been borne out by the literature.[125,128] Most importantly of all, the lessons learned from experience with stress testing are applicable here, too: modern cardiac biomarker testing in conjunction with risk stratification tools allows selection of such a low-risk population that there is little to be gained—and potential for harm (in the form of radiation, incidental findings, and unnecessary follow-up testing)—from further advanced diagnostic testing of these groups. A retrospective matched cohort analysis of 1788 ED patients with chest pain comparing CTCA and standard care found no difference in MACE at 1 month (both<1%) and no deaths in either group.[129] Accordingly, ACEP 2018 guidelines recommend, with moderate certainty, *against* the use of coronary CT angiography before discharge in low-risk patients in whom acute MI has been ruled out.[1]

Risk Stratification Tools

Clinicians are able to use patient history and physical examination findings in combination with ECG and biomarker results in their evaluation of patients with chest pain. Various predictive models have been proposed, which attempt to quantify the importance of these variables and assist physicians with decisions concerning the management and disposition of these patients, taking into account short- and long-term risks. The last decade has seen considerable progress in the development and validation of such models in the ED setting, with newer scoring systems such as the HEART score largely supplanting older ones (eg, the Agency for Health Care Policy and Research guidelines[130] and Acute Cardiac Ischemic Time-Insensitive Predictive Instrument[131]) The validity, use in the ED setting, and impact of several of these commonly discussed models are briefly explored here. Detailed descriptions of these models are discussed elsewhere.

History, electrocardiogram, age, risk factors, troponinscore

The HEART score, first developed from retrospective review of chest pain patients in one Netherlands ED,[132] assigns between 0 and 2 points to increasingly concerning features of each of a patient's history, ECG, age, number of risk factors, and troponin level. An initial validation study[92] of 2440 chest pain patients across 10 Netherlands EDs reported rate of MACE at 6 weeks of 1.7% in patients with HEART scores of 0 to 3, which compared favorably to the rate of 2.8% among patients with a low Thrombolysis in Myocardial Infarction (TIMI) score (0–1). Similarly, a retrospective analysis of more than 8000 patients across 8 Netherlands EDs confirmed a negative predictive value of 98.2% for 30-day MACE for a HEART score of 0 to 3.[133]

However, some more recent data have dampened the initial excitement around the HEART score. One study randomizing 3648 Dutch ED patients to use of HEART score–guided treatment versus standard care reported a rate of 6-week MACE of 2% for low-risk patients (HEART score 0–3).[134] A large meta-analysis of 9 studies with 11,217 patients (total 15.4% MACE rate) reported incidence of missed MACE in patients with HEART score 0 to 3 of just 1.6%.[135] However, the pooled sensitivity analysis found a sensitivity of just 96.7% for a "low-risk" cutoff of 3 points, although this was improved to 99.4% with use of a cutoff at 2 points. The disparity in these numbers—MACE incidence of 1.6% but sensitivity of 96.7%—may be related to the fact that the prevalence of disease was variable between studies, and the investigators accordingly present sensitivity as the better test measure. They consequently urge caution in use of the HEART score with a single troponin value in determining patients to be truly low risk. Another caveat in the use of the HEART score comes from its incorporation of a patient's history: point values are assigned based on patients having "highly," "moderately," or "slightly or nonsuspicious" history of presenting illness. In one sense this is beneficial, as it allows the incorporation of some amount of subjective provider gestalt into risk stratification. On the other hand, this introduces the potential for interuser variability, undermining the scoring system's value as an objective tool.

The creators of the HEART score subsequently developed the "HEART pathway"— use of the HEART score with conventional troponin testing at 0 and 3 hours—which retrospective analyses suggest may have improved sensitivity.[136] A randomized trial of 282 patients comparing the HEART pathway with usual care showed that no patients identified as low risk had MACE within 30 days, providing a sensitivity of

100%[137] (although the overall MACE rate in the study was only 6%). These are encouraging data, and although further study is needed, the HEART score has earned ACEP's level B recommendation for use as a clinical prediction instrument for risk stratification.[1]

Thrombolysis in myocardial infarction risk score

Despite its initial derivation as a risk-stratification tool in patients already diagnosed with UA or non-ST elevation MI,[62] the TIMI score has shown predictive value for 30-day rates of death, acute MI, and revascularization in ED patients, with a TIMI score of zero demonstrating 2% risk of 30-day adverse events and a score of 6 or 7 predicting 33% to 100% risk.[138–141] Although initial data supported the use of a TIMI score of 0 as a cutoff to define low-risk patients, this threshold missed approximately 2% of patients with 30-day adverse events.[138,139] Several more robust trials reported sensitivity of a TIMI score of 0 to have a sensitivity of 96.7% to 97%, with confidence intervals as low as 94%.[102,103] Given that the TIMI score assigns a point for age of 65 years or older (meaning no patient aged 65 years or older can be stratified as low risk), and the fact that newer scoring systems designed specifically for ED use have been developed, it is not surprising that the TIMI score is largely being supplanted and earns only an expert-consensus level recommendation from ACEP for use in risk stratification.

Alternative scoring systems

There are several other scoring systems and risk stratification tools in the literature, although none have been widely accepted or incorporated into standard practice due to suboptimal performance. For example, the North American Chest Pain Rule[48] in its derivation study of 2718 ED patients showed 100% sensitivity for 30-day MACE, although specificity was low at 20.9%. When combined with a negative ECG and troponin testing at 0 and 2 hours, the Emergency Department Assessment of Chest pain Score in its derivation and validation cohorts of 1974 and 608 ED patients respectively showed a sensitivity of 99% to 100% for 30-day MACE.[142] These characteristics were not supported by a reproducibility study, however,[143] which found a sensitivity of only 88%. Several other scoring systems (eg, Vancouver Chest Pain Rule, GRACE score, Manchester Acute Coronary Syndromes score, ADAPT protocol) have been developed, although at present none have yet to withstand rigorous reproducibility and reliability testing; accordingly no scoring systems beyond the HEART score and TIMI score are recommended or endorsed by ACEP at this time.

Pitfalls and Risk Management Strategies

Critical analyses of malpractice claims for missed MIs yield valuable insights into some factors that might contribute to misdiagnosis or inappropriate discharge. A retrospective examination of 65 closed claim cases of missed MIs revealed that those patients who were misclassified were more likely to be younger and presented with symptoms other than classically described angina. Misdiagnosed patients had fewer ECGs ordered, and these ECGs had higher rates of misinterpretation. Providers for these patients were more likely to have fewer years of ED experience and were found to have documented less thorough histories and physical examinations.[144] When the Physician Insurers Association of America performed a similar analysis of missed MI cases,[145] they reported that 70% of misdiagnosed MIs had never had a previous history of CAD, that almost half of these patients were younger than 50 years, and that 1 in 6 patients were younger than 40 years. These patients were most commonly discharged with a diagnosis of a GI disorder (26%) or costochondritis (21%). These disturbing trends seem to be confirmed in the later and wider-based population studies of missed MIs and ACS.

The ED physician should perform a thorough history but should not be falsely reassured if the patient has no prior history of CAD or any of the other conventionally associated risk factors. A strong index of suspicion for atypical presentations should be maintained, especially in women, nonwhite individuals, elderly patients, and those with a history of diabetes or congestive heart failure. Other high-risk groups include psychiatric patients, "frequent flyers," and intoxicated patients.[146] The ED physician should have a low threshold for obtaining an ECG, even in younger adults with chest-related complaints or patients with chest wall tenderness. Although a normal ECG does not rule out ACS, 1 in 4 cases of misdiagnosed acute MIs may be averted by improved ECG interpretations.[9] As with all strategies aimed at mitigating risk, the ED physician must carefully weigh a patient's clinical presentation in the setting of any diagnostic testing obtained. Although no single test is able to rule out the presence of ACS, the presence of multiple data points that suggest a noncardiac cause of pain, in combination with careful and meticulous charting that clearly explains the thought process of the clinician, will likely be of help in defending cases of missed ACS.

In addition to missed diagnoses, an increasing number of lawsuits are now citing failure to provide treatment in a timely manner as a reason for litigation,[147,148] with damages not only for death but also reduced viable myocardium as a result of delayed therapy. A recent analysis reported a higher rate of judgments against defendants in disputes alleging delay in diagnosis rather than misdiagnosis.[148] Failure to comply with the standard of care in the treatment of ACS can result in significant damages. It is incumbent on ED physicians to ensure that guidelines are followed, that consultants see patients within an appropriate timeframe, and that patients are transferred for definitive care when needed. Failure to do so can expose ED practitioners to significant liability.

Lastly, it is important to keep these risk management strategies in perspective. Although emergency physicians are often subject to a cultural and legal expectation of diagnostic perfection, this is neither feasible nor constructive. A review of 122 closed malpractice claims involving missed or delayed diagnosis suggests that such diagnostic breakdowns are often multifactorial in nature, involving both cognitive and systems errors,[149] suggesting that even a perfectly performing clinician may be subject to error in an imperfect health care system. Not only is a 0% miss rate likely unattainable, striving for this goal is likely to further drive up already skyrocketing health care costs. For example, one case-based survey of emergency physicians suggests that when "allowed" a miss rate of 1% to 2%, they might admit as many as 29% fewer patients.[150] Although no diagnostic pathway is without misses, the best risk management strategy likely involves forthright and thorough (and documented) communication with patients. A recent study of 898 patients with chest pain being considered for observation admission who were randomized to usual care or a decision aid—based shared decision-making discussion showed a 15% reduction in admissions and no change in clinical outcomes.[151] Moreover, patient communication is more closely associated with legal risk than the nature or magnitude of adverse outcomes,[152] with most of the plaintiffs citing an adverse relationship with their health care provider as a driver toward filing a suit.[153] Documented reassessment of patients before discharge, discharge diagnoses that reflect the possibility of severe illness (ie, "chest pain" instead of "costochondritis"), clear discharge instructions, and good communication with patients are all important for risk management and patient care perspectives.[152]

THORACIC AORTIC DISSECTION
Introduction

Famously described in 1760 when King George II of England died while straining on the commode, thoracic aortic dissection (TAD) presents a particular challenge for the emergency physician. As William Osler remarked, "There is no disease more conducive to clinical humility than aneurysm of the aorta" c 1900.[154] Although the incidence of aortic dissection is low—just 3 to 6 per 100,000 patient years in the general population[155,156]—it is likely to increase as the population ages. Without treatment, nearly 75% of patients with ascending aortic dissections can be expected to die within 2 weeks,[157] and 90% of all patients with untreated dissections will die within a year.[158] Moreover, the disease presents an acutely time-sensitive diagnostic challenge, with a mortality of at least 1% per hour in the first 48 hours.[158,159] In contrast, with rapid diagnosis and definitive therapy, 30-day survival rates as high as 90% have been reported.[154,160,161] Men are affected more often than women,[155,162] and most of those afflicted are aged between 50 and 70 years, with a median age of 61years.[155,163] African Americans have a higher incidence of aortic dissection than whites, potentially related to a higher incidence of hypertension.[164] The most common comorbidity reported in cases of TAD is hypertension, but several other risk factors have been described including male gender, advanced age, pregnancy, connective tissue disorders (such as Marfan syndrome or cystic medial necrosis), presence of a bicuspid aortic valve or previous aortic valve replacement, Turner syndrome, weight-lifting, and cocaine or methylenedioxymethamphetamine ("ecstasy") use.[155,165–169]

Clinical Presentations of Thoracic Aortic Dissection

The diagnosis of TAD is unfortunately often a difficult one to make. Retrospective analyses of patients with confirmed dissections suggest that emergency physicians suspected the diagnosis in only 43% to 65% of cases.[170,171] This is perhaps unsurprising, given that data from a database of 9.5 million ED visits identified just one dissection for every 980 patients seen for atraumatic chest pain.[172] However, as with many clinical entities, a careful history and physical examination can point the clinician toward the correct diagnosis.

As part of the Rational Clinical Examination series in the *Journal of the American Medical Association*, data from 16 studies involving 1553 patients were pooled, and sensitivities for various components of the clinical history and physical examination were reported.[154] Most patients presented with pain (pooled sensitivity 90%) of severe intensity (90%) that occurred suddenly (84%). Other symptoms, such as abdominal pain, migrating pain, or syncope, were present in a small to moderate percentage of patients. Although the presence of sudden onset of pain was far from diagnostic (positive LR 1.6; 95% confidence interval [CI] 1.0–2), the absence of this historical feature did decrease the probability that patient had a TAD (negative LR 0.2; 95% CI 0.2–0.5). However, the investigators argue that this likely overrepresents the sensitivity due to inclusion bias in this study of patients with TAD.

The pooled sensitivities of many physical examination findings were also poor in this meta-analysis. When present, however, some findings were highly suggestive of TAD. For example, although a pulse differential had a sensitivity of only 31%, its presence conferred a positive LR of 5.7 (95% CI 1.4–23.0). Focal neurologic deficits, although similarly only present in 17% of those with TAD, should raise one's suspicion for the diagnosis (positive LR 6.6–33.0). However, it should be noted that the specificity of many of these findings is poor: several convenience sampling studies report that as many as 18% to 53% of ED patients may have differences in upper extremity blood pressures greater than 10 mm Hg.[173,174]

More recent data may provide further reason for pessimism regarding the utility of history to make the diagnosis of TAD. Of 141 patients seen in a Hong Kong ED and ultimately diagnosed with aortic dissection, 40% did not report chest pain on presentation[175] and of 98 patients admitted to one Japanese hospital, 17% presented with no pain at all (these are more likely to present with syncope or neurologic symptoms).[176] Data from the International Registry of Acute Aortic Dissection (IRAD) show that presentation without chest pain or without any pain is strongly associated with delay in diagnosis.[177] Lastly, although it is commonly supposed that patients with TAD must seem distressed or ill, caution is advised when making use of acuity of presentation in diagnostic reasoning; ambulatory mode of arrival has been demonstrated to be associated with misdiagnosis of aortic dissection.[178]

There are few, if any, historical features and physical examination findings that, when used in isolation, allow the clinician to positively identify those patients with TAD. Nevertheless, although there is no one historical feature that is pathognomonic for aortic dissection, there is literature that suggests that physicians can improve their diagnostic accuracy by specifically asking about the quality of the patient's pain, the radiation of the pain, and the intensity at its onset. In one retrospective study, only 42% of patients who were found to have a TAD were asked all 3 of these questions. When all 3 questions were asked, the clinician's initial diagnostic impression of TAD was correct in 91% of the cases.[171] Unfortunately, the retrospective nature of this study does not rule out the possibility that clinicians were simply more likely to inquire about additional findings when they already had a strong clinical suspicion. Other combinations of findings, such as the presence of sudden-onset pain that is of tearing or ripping quality, blood pressure or pulse differentials, and mediastinal widening on chest radiography, have been found to have a positive LR of 66.0 (95% CI 4.1–1062.0).[154] Unfortunately, these 3 factors were found in only 27% of patients with TAD.

Diagnostic Tests and Their Limitations

For most ED patients with chest pain, chest radiography and ECG are part of the initial diagnostic evaluation. Unfortunately, the sensitivity for TAD of both of these tests is limited. Data suggest that the ECG is particularly low yield—as many as 9% to 37% of patients with TAD may have normal ECGs.[179,180] However, ischemic changes including T-wave inversions (38%) and Q waves (27%) may be present (although these findings are not specific for TAD).[180] Other nonspecific findings such as LVH and atrial fibrillation have also been reported.[179] Although a traditional teaching has been to use the ECG to distinguish STEMI from TAD, data show that these conditions can coexist. This can occur if the dissection extends proximally to include the coronary ostia, most commonly affecting the right coronary artery causing proximal coronary artery occlusion.[181] To make matters more difficult, a review of 184 TAD patients found that 16% had STEMIs on their initial ECGs, even though in those who underwent coronary angiography, 70% had normal coronary vessels.[180]

Many of those with TAD also do not present with the classically described chest radiograph findings. Again, pooled sensitivities for findings such as an abnormal aortic contour (71%; 95% CI 56%-84%), pleural effusion (16%; 95% CI 12%-21%), displaced intimal calcification (9%; 95% CI 6%-13%), and wide mediastinum (64%; 95% CI 44%-80%) reflect the lack of clinical usefulness of these findings.[154] However, most patients with TAD do have some abnormality on chest radiograph (sensitivity 90%), making the disease less likely in those with an entirely normal chest film.[154,182]

Several imaging modalities, including conventional angiography, ultrasonography (US), computed tomography (CT), and MRI, have been used to diagnose aortic dissection. Although an in-depth discussion of each of these imaging techniques is beyond the scope of this review, there are several factors worth noting. The use of conventional angiography, a time-consuming and invasive procedure that may have limited sensitivity (as low as 88%[183]), has decreased in recent years as the roles of US, CT, and MRI have increased. In one relatively small study in which patients with suspected dissection underwent transesophageal echocardiography (TEE), MRI, and CT, the following sensitivities and specificities were reported (**Table 2**)[183]:

Data from IRAD and other studies have since confirmed excellent sensitivity and specificity (99% and 89% for TEE, 95% and 95% for CT, 95% and 98% and 94% and 98% for MRI) for all 3 modalities.[184] In many institutions, CT is the diagnostic test of choice due to its accessibility, rapid data acquisition, high sensitivity, and ability to simultaneously exclude other morbid causes of chest pain.[185] Present ACEP guidelines issue a level B (moderate clinical certainty) recommendation in favor of the use of CTA to exclude TAD.[186] TEE, although more portable than CT, requires esophageal intubation, may lead to an increase in blood pressure (and a subsequent increase in risk of rupture[187,188]), and may not provide enough anatomic information to surgeons before operative intervention.[188] The usefulness of MRI is limited by the time needed to complete a study (as long as 30 minutes) and its lack of ready availability in many EDs, although it should be considered in stable patients with an equivocal CT or TEE or in patients unable to undergo contrast CT scanning due to allergy.[158]

As point-of-care ultrasound (POCUS) becomes increasingly available in EDs, interest in transthoracic echocardiography (TTE) as a diagnostic modality has heightened. Although TTE is a potentially attractive imaging modality because it can be performed at the bedside of the unstable patient and is less invasive than TEE, there is not yet strong data to support its use for diagnostic purposes, and current ACEP guidelines recommend with moderate certainty *against* reliance on abnormal TTE to establish the diagnosis of TAD, although they also issue an expert consensus-level recommendation in favor of immediate surgical consultation or transfer as appropriate if initial TTE is suggestive of dissection.[186] Accordingly, there may be a role for POCUS in decreasing time to surgery for patients with clear findings, although the modality may face similar barriers to TEE (ie, surgeon hesitancy to operate without cross-sectional imaging).

Given the difficulty of making the diagnosis of TAD by history and examination and the costly and/or invasive nature of testing needed to make the diagnosis by imaging, there has been interest in the use of several biomarkers, including D-dimer, smooth muscle myosin heavy chain, c-reactive protein, and brain natriuretic peptide[189–191] to rule out the disease. Unfortunately, there is not yet robust data to support routine

Table 2		
Sensitivity and specificity for imaging modalities in aortic dissection		
Testing Modality	**Sensitivity (95% CI)**	**Specificity (95% CI)**
CT	100% (89%–100%)	100% (79% –100%)
TEE	100% (89%–100%)	94% (70% –100%)
MRI	100% (89%–100%)	94% (70% –100%)

Data from Sommer T, Fehske W, Holzknecht N, et al. Aortic dissection: A comparative study of diagnosis with spiral CT, multiplanar transesophageal echocardiography, and MR imaging. Radiology 1996;199:347–52.

use of any of these—at least as sole screening tests—to diagnose aortic dissection. D-dimer has received particular attention, perhaps related to the experience using it in conjunction with diagnostic protocols in the diagnosis of pulmonary embolism. Although initial small studies reported sensitivity near 100% for D-dimer testing,[192–195] later work has produced more sobering results. One 2006 study found that younger patients and those with shorter dissection flaps were more likely to have false-negative D-dimer testing, with a total false-negative rate of 8%.[196] Altogether, the D-dimer literature is unconvincing, plagued by small sample sizes, inconsistent methodology, and the use of different assays, and current ACEP guidelines make a level C recommendation against using the D-dimer alone to exclude the diagnosis of TAD.[186] Although there is insufficient evidence to support its use as the *sole* screening test for aortic dissection, it remains to be seen whether a useful diagnostic protocol can be developed using D-dimer in conjunction with other clinical variables.

High-Risk Populations

Although emergency physicians may suspect TAD in a 70-year-old man with hypertension who presents after the acute onset of chest pain radiating to the back, they must also be wary of the diagnosis in patients who do not fit this classic demographic and description. Analysis of patients younger than 40 years in the IRAD database reveals that whereas younger individuals with aortic dissection may have presentations and physical examination findings similar to those of their older counterparts, they vary significantly in their risk factor profile. Younger patients were more likely to have a history of Marfan syndrome, bicuspid aortic valve, and prior aortic valve surgery and were less likely to have hypertension and atherosclerosis.[197] Female gender at any age has also been associated with delay in diagnosis, with multiple linear regression analysis of IRAD data showing women are subject to a 1.73 (95% CI 1.27–2.36) times longer time to diagnosis compared with men.[177] Pregnant women with chest or back pain should also prompt careful clinical consideration, as some data suggest that they are at increased risk of dissection, particularly when the other comorbid conditions such as Marfan syndrome are also present.[168]

Potential Pitfalls

The ED evaluation of chest pain, and in particular the diagnosis of TAD, is fraught with potential pitfalls. There exist no reliable history or physical examination findings that can be trusted to identify those with TAD. Patients with TAD can easily be initially misdiagnosed and are thought to have other potentially life-threatening causes of chest pain (most frequently ACS). Inappropriate treatment with antiplatelet, anticoagulant, and fibrinolytic therapies in patients believed to have ACS but instead found to have TAD can have disastrous consequences. Fibrinolysis in patients eventually found to have TAD has been associated with severe hemorrhagic complications and a fatality rate of 71% (a rate similar to that of untreated TAD and much higher than most studies of current surgical management of the disease). Increasing age and anterior chest pain were highly associated with misdiagnosis, likely reflecting a higher clinician suspicion of ACS.[198]

Risk Management Strategies

The diagnosis of TAD can be a very difficult one to make (in some series the diagnosis is only made at autopsy in as many as 28% of cases).[199] Its presentation can be subtle, and patients may only have symptoms that are a consequence of vascular compromise due to the dissection (such as strokelike complaints, syncope, limb ischemia, GI bleeding, and cardiac ischemia), or may even be entirely pain free.[176,200] As the "classic" presentation of tearing chest pain that radiates to the back may be more uncommon than one would hope,[175,176,201] the emergency physician must be vigilant in the rapid evaluation of any patients with any complaint that might suggest TAD. Although there is significant overlap between the presentation of ACS and TAD, it is incumbent on the emergency physician to differentiate between the two as expeditiously as possible. Recognizing that the incidence of MI is nearly 800 times the estimated incidence of acute aortic dissection in the United States and that STEMI is an uncommon complication of TAD,[202] some investigators have argued that delaying time-dependent therapy (such as anticoagulation or thrombolysis) to rule out dissection in all patients is short sighted and impractical.[203] However, further evaluation in patients with symptoms of concern for aortic dissection (such as those with a classic presentation or those presenting with chest pain in association with a neurologic deficit or complaint) is mandatory, as missing the diagnosis is associated with very high morbidity and mortality. In one series of 33 cases of aortic catastrophes that resulted in litigation, the most common reason for alleged malpractice was failure to diagnose (or delay in diagnosis).[204]

Because of the difficulty in clinically identifying TAD, there has been interest in development of a validated diagnostic pathway that could offer both diagnostic accuracy and some element of medicolegal protection. Unfortunately, despite efforts, at present no such pathway exists. In 2010, the ACC and the AHA released guidelines for the diagnosis and management of thoracic aortic disease, including a diagnostic pathway for the evaluation of potential aortic dissection.[205] These guidelines suggested using the presence or absence of particularly high-risk conditions (Marfan syndrome, connective tissue disease, family history of aortic disease, known aortic valve disease, recent aortic manipulation, known thoracic aortic aneurysm), high-risk pain features (chest, back, or abdominal pain that is abrupt onset, severe in intensity, or ripping/tearing/sharp or stabbing), and high-risk examination features (pulse deficit, systolic blood pressure differential, focal neurologic deficit, new murmur of aortic insufficiency, or hypotension) to stratify patients as low (no high-risk features), intermediate (one high-risk feature), or high (two or more high-risk features) risk. High-risk patients are recommended for immediate surgical consultation, intermediate-risk patients should receive aortic imaging, whereas low-risk patients only require imaging if no diagnosis is found and they are hypotensive or have a widened mediastinum on chest radiograph. Retrospective analysis of IRAD data suggested that this scoring system should have a sensitivity of 95.7%.[206] However, a subsequent large study of 1328 patients with *suspected* TAD—and thus more representative of the ED environment—found the scoring system to have only 91.1% sensitivity (95% CI 87.2%–94.1%) and 39.8% specificity (95% CI 36.8%–42.9%).[207] Accordingly, although the ACC/AHA pathway may have utility in informing clinical decision-making, it is not appropriate as means of ruling out the diagnosis.[158] Indeed, current ACEP clinical guidelines recommend against using existing clinical decision rules alone in attempting to identify patients at very low risk of TAD.[186]

Unfortunately, there are no clear accepted guidelines directing emergency medicine clinicians as to when they should consider the diagnosis of TAD. However, there is evidence suggesting that key aspects of the history and physical examination should lead the physician to at least consider the diagnosis and possibly pursue definitive testing. These critical components include an abrupt onset of pain, pulse or blood pressure differentials, classically described chest radiography findings, or the presence of risk factors such as Marfan syndrome, previous cardiac surgery, stimulant use, or pregnancy. One should also consider the diagnosis of TAD in chest pain patients in whom conventional therapy (nitrates, β-blockers) are ineffective, in those who have chest pain in addition to another complaint (extremity weakness, paresthesias or other neurologic complaints, abdominal pain), or in those who are younger than patients with typical chest pain.

PULMONARY EMBOLISM
Introduction

One of the most common cardiovascular disorders in industrialized countries, venous thromboembolism (VTE), is estimated to occur more than 600,000 times per year in the United States.[208,209] VTE covers a broad spectrum of illness, ranging from asymptomatic deep venous thrombosis to massive pulmonary embolism (PE) causing cardiac arrest. PE in particular carries a high morbidity and mortality, with studies reporting 30-day mortality of anywhere between 6.6% and 12%[210–212] and 3-month and 1-year mortality rates of 17%[212] and 23%,[213] respectively. Altogether, estimates suggest PE is potentially responsible for more than 200,000 deaths yearly[208,214] and for up to 10% of all in-hospital deaths[209] and may be suddenly fatal in as many as one-third of cases.[208] Nevertheless, prompt therapy—either with anticoagulants or, in select patients, fibrinolytics—is effective in reducing mortality.[215,216]

Clinical Presentations of Pulmonary Embolism

As with many other life-threatening disorders, emergency physicians are tasked with distinguishing patients with serious causes of chest pain, such as PE, from the multitude of patients presenting to EDs with less sinister causes of their pain. Unfortunately, the symptoms and signs are highly variable, nonspecific, and are present in many patients with and without PE.[216] In one large, multicenter, prospective study, the most common symptoms were dyspnea at rest or with exertion (73%), pleuritic pain (44%), cough (34%), calf or thigh pain (44%), calf or thigh swelling (41%), and wheezing (21%). Within this same cohort, 54% of patients were tachypneic, 24% were tachycardic, and 17% had decreased breath sounds.[217] The clinical presentation of PE can be as dramatic as cardiovascular collapse and fulminant shock or as subtle as mild dyspnea or pleuritic chest pain. As history and physical examination findings are neither sensitive nor specific, clinicians must rely on ancillary testing to substantiate or confirm the diagnosis of PE.

Diagnostic Tests and Their Limitations

Both the ECG and chest radiograph have limited utility in the diagnosis of PE (other than to perhaps confirm an alternative diagnosis). The classically described ECG finding in PE, S1Q3T3, is rarely seen. More common ECG findings include sinus tachycardia, nonspecific ST- and T-wave changes, or signs of right heart strain, and ECGs are often normal.[218] Initial chest films are normal in as many as 25% of patients who are ultimately found to have a PE. Again classic findings such as Hampton hump and Westermark sign are rarely seen, whereas nonspecific findings such as cardiac enlargement, pleural effusion, and elevated hemi-diaphragm are more common.[219]

D-dimer, released into the bloodstream during fibrinolysis, has been shown to be a marker of endovascular thrombosi, and as a result has been studied for use in the diagnosis of PE. A large body of research indicates that D-dimer may be of use in identifying a population of patients who are at very low risk for PE. Although early reports described variable test characteristics for different assays and cutoff values,[220] several large studies and meta-analyses have since confirmed that quantitative D-dimer testing has excellent sensitivity of 93% to 97%.[221–223] Accordingly, in patients with a low pretest probability of PE (10% or less), a negative test result can be expected to decrease the probability of PE to approximately 1%,[224] and the use of D-dimer testing in evaluation of PE is currently endorsed by both ACEP[224] and American College of Physicians/American Academy of Family Physicians in their guidelines.[225] It should be noted, however, that the specificity of the D-dimer assay for PE is poor (particularly in the elderly[221,226,227]), and it is not sufficiently sensitive to exclude the diagnosis of PE in *all* patients presenting to the ED with pleuritic chest pain.[228] It is important that D-dimer testing should *not* be used as a sole screening tool in anyone other than those who have a low pretest probability of having a PE, as the posttest probability of PE in non–low-risk patients is unacceptably high.[221,229,230] D-dimer values are known to be higher in pregnancy (after 20 weeks' gestation)[231,232] and in those with cancer,[233] which may decrease its utility in these populations. Elderly patients will also have higher D-dimer values,[227] although recent data support the use of "age-adjusted" D-dimer cutoffs in these patients. In particular, Righini and colleagues[234] demonstrated in the ADJUST-PE study that use of an age-adjusted D-dimer cutoff, which they defined as age in years x 10 (using a fibrin equivalent unit assay) based on their own retrospective derivation study, allowed a modest increase in the number of patients deemed low risk without significant increase in missed PEs. These findings have been replicated in several subsequent studies,[235,236] and use of this age-adjusted D-dimer cutoff is currently supported by ACEP guidelines (level B recommendation).[209]

In most EDs, CT pulmonary angiography (CTPA) has become the imaging test of choice in diagnosis of PE. CT is fast, readily available, and interpretation is not complicated by underlying cardiopulmonary disease (as is often a problem with ventilation/perfusion [V/Q] imaging). Moreover, it may identify an alternative diagnosis that explains a patient's symptoms. Rapid advancement in the technology—from slower rotating single-detector imagers to faster multidetector scanners—has allowed for more rapid acquisition of higher-resolution images and ultimately improved diagnostic performance.[224] Indeed, several large meta-analyses with thousands of patients examining the outcomes after negative CTPA report a pooled rate of VTE of just 1.4% (95% CI 1.1%–1.8%),[237] and an overall negative predictive value of 99.1%,[238] both results similar to those reported for conventional pulmonary angiography. Although several robust studies report that PE can be safely excluded by diagnostic protocols using negative CTPA,[239–241] there are some data suggesting caution in use of the test in high-risk patients. Musset and colleagues[242] prospectively studied 1041 inpatients and outpatients with suspected PE and report that 4 of their 76 "high clinical risk" patients with negative CTPA were ultimately diagnosed with PE (either by V/Q scan or angiography), for a false-negative rate of 5.3% (95% CI 1.5%–13.1%). The Prospective Investigation of Pulmonary Embolism Diagnosis II investigators reported that in their cohort of 1090 patients, multidetector CTPA demonstrated negative predictive value of 96% (95% CI 92%–98%) in patients of "low clinical probability," but 6 of their 15 "high clinical probability" patients who had a negative CTPA results were subsequently found to have PE (also by either V/Q scanning or angiography).[243] Based on this finding of an NPV of 60% (95% CI 32%–83%) or false-negative rate of 40% in high-risk patients, the investigators suggest that when clinical probability is inconsistent with imaging results, further testing is warranted. Indeed, ACEP guidelines from 2011 recommend use of negative multidetector CTPA to exclude PE only in patients with low pretest probability for PE (level B recommendation), and additional diagnostic testing (eg, D-dimer, lower extremity imaging, VQ scanning, conventional arteriography) in patients with high pretest probability for PE.[224] Nevertheless, these discouragingly high false-negative rates in high-risk patients reported by Stein and colleagues and Musset and colleagues[242,243] decreased well outside the rates reported in other studies and should be interpreted with caution given the small numbers of patients, wide confidence intervals, and the use of V/Q scanning or angiography as a reference standard. Most of the data suggest that use of modern multidetector CT imaging in concert with validated diagnostic pathways (see section on "Risk Stratification Tools") is safe in ruling out PE, although clinicians should always interpret diagnostic testing results in the context of a patient's symptoms and risk factors, and are encouraged to pursue further testing when test results are discordant with the patient presentation.

Lastly, although point-of-care ultrasound offers neither the sensitivity nor specificity for diagnosis of PE in the undifferentiated patient presenting with chest pain, it may have utility in select patients. Cardiac ultrasound can be used to identify signs of right heart strain, including dilation of the right ventricle (RV), RV hypokinesis (classically with apical sparing), tricuspid regurgitation, and paradoxic motion of the interventricular septum ("septal flattening" in systole or impaired relaxation into the RV in diastole).[93,244] Although these findings can be seen in patients with other causes for RV failure such as chronic obstructive pulmonary disease (COPD), primary pulmonary hypertension, and RV ischemia, in the right clinical scenario, data suggest their specificity for PE is high.[245] Several studies including patients with suspected PE have reported specificities of POCUS for PE of 87% to 90%[246,247] although sensitivities were poor (50%). POCUS may also help identify massive PE in cardiac arrest patients who achieve ROSC.[248] So although the poor sensitivity of POCUS for PE suggests that it may not be useful to exclude the diagnosis of PE, it may have some utility in pointing the clinician toward the diagnosis in the patient with unexplained hypotension or cardiac arrest.

Risk Stratification Tools

As with TAD, it is unreasonable, impractical, and unfeasible to obtain confirmatory testing for PE in all patients who present with chest pain. As a result, several criteria or decision rules have been put forth to aid clinicians in formulating a patient's risk or pretest probability of PE. These include the Geneva score, initially described by Wicki and colleagues,[249] the Wells score, developed by Wells and colleagues,[250] and the Pulmonary Embolism Rule-out Criteria (PERC), developed by Kline and colleagues.[251] A brief discussion of each of these systems and how they may be used to risk stratify patients is presented here.

Although the utility of the original Geneva score[249] in risk stratifying patients has been validated across several studies,[224] its reliance on a variety of parameters including blood gas testing and chest radiography make it somewhat cumbersome to use. As a result, Le Gal and colleagues[252] developed a revised Geneva score omitting these laboratory and imaging parameters in favor of historical and examination features. This system was subsequently prospectively validated in a single-center study.[253] Because of its complicated system of assigning different numbers of points for each risk factor, the revised Geneva score was again modified by Klok and colleagues[254] to produce the simplified revised Geneva score. This scoring system characterizes 36% of patients as "low risk" (8% [95%CI 5.2%–10.8%] risk of PE), 60% of patients as "moderate risk" (29% [95% CI 25.9%–33.1%] risk of PE), and 4% of patients as "high risk" (64% [95%CI 48.0%–78.5%]), performing similarly to the revised Geneva score.

The Wells score was developed by retrospective analysis of 1260 patients at 5 Canadian centers and assigns points to 7 parameters that can be obtained from history and physical examination.[255] This approach was subsequently prospectively validated in 930 patients across 4 Canadian centers, demonstrating a 1.3% (95% CI

0.5%–2.7%) rate of PE in the 57% of patients deemed "low risk," 16% (95% CI 12.5%–20.6%) of the 36% of patients deemed "moderate risk," and in 41% (95% CI 28.7%–53.7%) of the 7% of patients deemed "high risk" (**Table 3**).[256] Since this initial validation study, many others have confirmed the utility of the Wells score in risk stratification.[224] Although the Wells score has seen widespread adoption because of these robust results, it has also been widely criticized due to its inclusion of a subjective variable, "an alternative diagnosis is less likely than PE." In contrast to the Geneva score or PERC rule, Wells' inclusion of this variable introduces clinician judgment, somewhat undermining the purpose of a clinical decision tool.

In 2004, Kline and colleagues[251] described derivation of a clinical rule designed to avoid *all* further testing, termed the PERC rule. Through a retrospective logistic regression analysis of 3148 ED patients being evaluated for PE, they identified 8 variables that when all present could identify patients at very low risk of PE (less than 1.8%) and thus not in need of any further diagnostic testing. Kline and colleagues[257] published a large multicenter prospective validation study with 8138 patients, reporting that in patients in whom clinicians had a low suspicion for PE who were also "PERC negative" (ie, meeting all 8 criteria) (20% of the total study cohort), only 1% (95% CI 0.6%–1.6%) went on to have VTE, resulting in a sensitivity for this combination of findings (low clinical suspicion and PERC negative) of 97.4% (95% CI 95.8%–98.5%) for PE (**Table 4**). Several other validation studies have confirmed similar test characteristics for the PERC rule in otherwise low-risk patients[258,259] including a large meta-analysis of 13,885 patients reporting a pooled sensitivity of 97% (95% CI 96%–98%).[260] Caution is warranted, however, when considering the use of PERC in populations other than those determined to be "low risk," as several studies have demonstrated unacceptably high rates of PE in such patients.[258,261] Accordingly, ACEP guidelines recommend use of PERC only in low-risk patients (level B recommendation).[209]

Altogether, the most sensible evidence-based approach to risk stratification of patients with potential PE is to first establish a sense of pretest probability or risk, using the Wells score, revised Geneva score, or clinical gestalt. It should be noted that presently there are not data to clearly support preference for one of these approaches over another,[224] with several studies reporting similar performance between Wells and Geneva scores[253,262] and others describing similar performance between clinical

Table 3	
Wells score for prediction of pulmonary embolism	
Variable	**Points**
Clinical signs and symptoms of DVT[a]	3
An alternative diagnosis is less likely than PE	3
Heart rate >100 beats/min	1.5
Immobilization or surgery in the previous 4 wk	1.5
Previous DVT/PE	1.5
Hemoptysis	1
Malignancy (treatment within 6 mo or palliative)	1

[a] Minimum of leg swelling and pain with palpation of the deep veins. A score of less than 2 indicates low probability. A score of 2 to 6 indicates moderate probability. A score greater than 6 indicates high probability.

Adapted from Wells PS, Anderson DR, Rodger M, et al. Derivation of a simple clinical model to categorize patients probability of pulmonary embolism: increasing the models utility with the simpleRED d-dimer. Thromb Haemost 2000;83(3):416-20.

Table 4	
Pulmonary embolism rule-out criteria	
Variable	**Points**
Age > 49 y	1
Heart rate > 99 beats/min	1
Pulse oximetry <95% on room air	1
Hemoptysis	1
Exogenous estrogen exposure	1
History of prior VTE	1
Recent trauma or surgery[a]	1
Unilateral leg swelling	1

[a] History of trauma or surgery requiring general anesthesia in the last 4 wk. A score of 0 indicates very low risk of PE. A score of 1 or above indicates non–low risk.

Adapted from Kline JA, Courtney DM, Kabrhel C, et al. Prospective multicenter evaluation of the pulmonary embolism rule-out criteria. J Thromb Haemost 2008;6(5):772-80.

gestalt and Wells score.[263,264] For patients deemed low risk by any of these approaches, subsequent application of the PERC rule allows identification of a very low-risk group in whom no further testing is needed. For patients deemed high risk, diagnostic imaging should be pursued, and further testing should be considered if clinical concern persists even after initial imaging is negative. D-dimer testing (including use of age-adjusted D-dimer test thresholds) should be considered in low-risk patients who are not PERC negative or in intermediate-risk patients, with diagnostic imaging being considered if D-dimer testing is positive in either group. As with other disease processes, but perhaps more critical in the evaluation of patients with suspected PE, clinicians' suspicion regarding likelihood of a disease is important in determining which, if any, definitive testing is performed, and clinical guidelines should never supplant the emergency physician's judgment.

High-Risk Populations

Although presenting symptoms and physical examination findings are unreliable and inconsistent, there are several identifiable risk factors for venous thromboembolism, including recent surgery, trauma, immobility, cancer, neurologic disease with lower extremity paresis, oral contraceptive pills, hormone therapy, and pregnancy.[265,266] It should be noted that older patients with PE are less likely to complain of chest pain, are more likely to be hypoxic, and are more likely to present with syncope.[267]

Potential Pitfalls and Risk Management Strategies

As with several other causes of chest pain, PE presents a diagnostic challenge to ED physicians: its associated symptoms are common and not specific for PE, and both undertreatment (ie, failure to diagnose) and overtreatment (ie, unnecessary anticoagulation) carry significant morbidity. Most patients with symptoms suggestive of the illness do not have PE.[268] This fact must be weighed against the reality that the mortality rate for untreated PE is 18.4%, 7 times greater than that of appropriately treated PE.[269]

As the implementation of specific algorithms and diagnostic tools hinges on the likelihood that a particular patient has a PE, clinicians would be wise to consistently document the absence or presence of risk factors as well as their pretest suspicion that a patient's chest pain is due to PE. Using this pretest probability to determine the diagnostic strategy and rationale for testing is clearly important in cases in which the diagnosis of PE is missed. The related appropriate use of diagnostic tests should be clear. No single test, used in isolation, is sufficiently sensitive to identify all patients with PE in the ED. When there is discordance between clinical probability and the results of objective testing, the posttest probability of PE is neither sufficiently high nor sufficiently low to permit therapeutic decisions.[270] For example, a negative D-dimer in anyone other than a low-risk patient is considered inadequate testing, and in patients with a particularly high probability of having PE, workup should continue even in the presence of a negative CTPA.

Documentation of use of validated decision guidelines—particularly those endorsed by ACEP or other specialty societies—may mitigate medico-legal risk. As with all other potentially life-threatening diseases, maintaining a high index of suspicion for PE is critical (ie, in those with unexplained tachycardia, tachypnea, or hypoxia).[269] Finally, communication with patients—particularly with those in whom the diagnosis of PE is entertained but then "ruled out" by any means—about the possibility of this illness, its potential consequences, the limits of diagnostic testing, and reasons to return to the ED, is paramount.

TENSION PNEUMOTHORAX

The *spontaneous* tension pneumothorax is a less discussed and often later-diagnosed entity than its routinely emphasized traumatic counterpart. Primary spontaneous pneumothoraces classically occur in tall, thin men without previous lung disease. Smoking, a history of Marfan syndrome, and family history of spontaneous pneumothorax are also thought to be risk factors for developing the disease. Secondary spontaneous pneumothoraces are defined as being due to underlying lung disease such as chronic obstructive pulmonary disease, infectious or malignant processes, interstitial lung disease, or unusual causes such as pleural endometriosis (ie, catamenial pneumothoraces).[271] Pneumothoraces may also be iatragonic, typically from central venous catheter placement or due to high pressure mechanical ventilation, and may occur in trauma. Data suggest that all types of pneumothoraces have a 1% to 3% potential to convert from a simple to tension physiology,[272,273] although it should be noted that progression to tension is more likely—and carries higher mortality—in mechanically ventilated patients.[274]

A tension pneumothorax is most accurately defined as a hemodynamically significant increase in pressure within the intrapleural potential space due to a one-way valve effect between the alveolar and pleural borders.[274] The clinical manifestation of this pathology varies, however, from a "hiss" of air and clinical improvement on needle decompression or thoracostomy to mediastinal shift and hypotension with ipsilateral hyperexpansion on chest radiograph. An awake patient may try to compensate by maximizing inspiratory effort to overcome the positive intrapleural pressure as tension develops, and thus may exhibit normal hemodynamics just before suddenly and rapidly decompensating.

A recent systematic review of 183 cases of tension pneumothorax from the literature describes starkly different presentations between mechanically ventilated patients and those breathing unassisted.[275] Of particular note, awake patients do not universally present with classic clinical signs and symptoms. Although the majority (52.3%) reported chest pain, complaints of dyspnea or shortness of breath were present only in the minority (38.4% and 31.4%, respectively). Less than half of patients exhibited tachycardia or tachypnea and fewer than two-thirds were observed to have decreased air entry on the affected side on examination, whereas other classic findings such as thoracic hyper- or hypoexpansion or jugular venous distension were rare. Interestingly, independently breathing patients were more likely to demonstrate tracheal deviation (17.9% vs 2.9% for intubated patients) and ipsilateral hyperresonance (26.7% vs 8.3%), perhaps due to compensatory mechanisms. In contrast, patients undergoing mechanical ventilation were markedly more likely to present with subcutaneous emphysema (30.9% vs 10.5% for independently breathing patients), hypotension (66.0% vs 16.3%), and cardiac arrest (28.9% vs 2.3%), likely due to the rapid escalation of intrapleural pressure. Accordingly, the diagnosis should be considered in any suddenly deteriorating patient on positive pressure ventilation.

The chest radiograph is traditionally "forbidden" in suspected tension pneumothoraces because of the associated delay in life-saving intervention while awaiting diagnostic confirmation. However, in an awake patient who has not yet developed hypoxia, hypotension, depressed respiratory rate (from fatigue), or altered mental status, a rapidly obtained confirmatory portable chest radiograph may be reasonable to avoid the risk of a potentially unnecessary thoracostomy. If available, POCUS may be used instead and can facilitate diagnosis with speed and accuracy.[245] The identification of "lung sliding,—the shimmering appearance generated on B-mode lung ultrasound as the visceral and parietal slide against one another with lung movement— serves to essentially rule out pneumothorax, with sensitivity of 86% to 98% across several studies.[276–280] A systematic review and meta-analysis including 1048 patients found a sensitivity of 90.9% (95% CI 86.5%–93.9%) and specificity of 98.2% (95% CI 97.0%–99.0%), far outperforming the 50.2% sensitivity of chest radiography.[281] It should be noted that absent lung sliding can only be seen over the pneumothorax itself, so the ultrasound probe must be positioned correctly to capture the area to which air will likely track (anteriorly for the supine patient, at the apex for the seated patient). Furthermore, the absence of lung sliding may be mimicked in other conditions, such as a COPD bleb, consolidated pneumonia or atelectasis, mainstem intubation, or scarring and interstitial lung disease.[245] Nevertheless, the findings of absent lung sliding in concert with a dilated inferior vena cava (IVC) or mediastinal shift should, in the appropriate clinical setting, raise clinical concern for the diagnosis of tension pneumothorax.[282] Altogether, ultrasound's improved test characteristics compared with chest radiography, its ease of use, and rapidity of diagnosis should make it the emergency physician's most desirable test for the unstable patient.

Lastly, improvement following needle decompression has often been considered a diagnostic test for tension pneumothorax, but it is well described in the literature as being imperfect, both diagnostically and therapeutically.[283] Although traditional Advanced Trauma Life Support guidelines encourage use of a 5-cm angiocatheter at the second intercostal space at the midclavicular line, a large meta-analysis showed failure rates as high as 38% with this approach, with better performance (13% failure rate) with catheter insertion at the fourth or fifth intercostal space and anterior axillary line.[284] Comparison of needle decompression in trauma patients using 5 cm versus 8 cm angiocatheters showed only 48% success rate with shorter catheters and improved to 83% with longer ones.[285] Although more data are needed, these results suggest that lack of a response to needle decompression should not prevent finger or tube thoracostomy in the appropriate clinical setting.

ESOPHAGEAL RUPTURE

First described in 1724 by Hermann Boerhaave in the case report of a Dutch admiral who died after vomiting,[286] full-thickness tears through the esophagus are relatively rare but carry a high morbidity and mortality, presumably due to delayed recognition of the ensuing mediastinitis and septic shock. In one case series of patients with atraumatic esophageal rupture, the median delay from admission to diagnosis was nearly 24 hours.[287] In another case series that included postendoscopic, traumatic, and erosive foreign body origins of esophageal ruptures, a shorter median time to diagnosis was reported, but time to diagnosis still ranged up to 96 hours.[288]

Data regarding patient presentation are limited to case series, but it seems that the classic "Mackler's triad" of esophageal rupture—chest pain, vomiting, and subcutaneous emphysema—occurs in the minority of cases.[287] Antecedent vomiting and sudden-onset chest pain or epigastric pain are the most commonly reported symptom in cases of spontaneous esophageal rupture,[286,287] although they may be absent in nearly a quarter[287] to half[289] of such cases, particularly if esophageal perforation is iatrogenic.[290] Other less commonly noted symptoms include dyspnea, fever, and dysphagia.[290] Patients may also demonstrate subcutaneous emphysema on physical examination. Other nonspecific signs include tachypnea and tachycardia, with 82% of patients meeting systemic inflammatory response syndrome criteria.[287]

Traumatic esophageal injury, although rare (overall prevalence of 0.02% of trauma patients), also carries significant morbidity and mortality. A review of data from the national trauma data bank showed an overall mortality rate of 12%,[291] whereas morbidity may be as high as 46%.[292] No signs or symptoms reliably diagnose traumatic esophageal injury,[292] so consideration of mechanism is paramount: approximately half of patients with traumatic esophageal injuries have a penetrating injury mechanism (gunshot or stab wound to the area) whereas 19% are injured in motor vehicle crashes.[291]

The upright chest radiograph is a useful screening tool for esophageal rupture, as 75% to 90% will be abnormal. Pneumomediastinum, mediastinal widening, hydropneumothoraces (usually left-sided because of the location of the distal esophagus), and pleural effusions are the most common findings. Confirmatory testing usually includes an esophagogram with water-soluble contrast agent. These agents are less likely to result in irritation and inflammation than barium if there is indeed a leak but also carry a false-negative rate of 10% to 25%. High-density barium adheres better to perforated sites and can diagnose 25% to 50% of esophageal perforations that were not diagnosed by previously performed water-soluble contrast studies.[293] Contrast CT is useful for assessing extraluminal manifestations of perforations,[294] such as air, fluid, or abscesses in the mediastinal, pleural, or pericardial regions. Finally, direct endoscopy most definitively assesses the site of leakage and length of tear.

Given the low prevalence of disease, unreliable history and examination findings, and high morbidity and mortality, a high index of suspicion must be maintained for esophageal rupture. In traumatic cases, early surgical consultation is crucial, as early surgical treatment is associated with improved survival.[291] Emergency physicians should have a low threshold for cross-sectional imaging, as it may aid in diagnosis and identify complications.

CARDIAC TAMPONADE

Cardiac tamponade is likely an underrecognized cause of death (particularly in intensive care patients[295]) and should be considered as a cause of unexplained shock in any critically ill patient.[296] Tamponade occurs when a pericardial effusion exerts enough pressure on the heart to blunt diastolic filling and thus impair cardiac output. Medical conditions at risk for pericardial effusions that can progress to tamponade include acute pericarditis, malignancy, AMI leading to wall rupture, proximal aortic dissection, uremia, congestive heart failure, collagen vascular disease, viral infection (including even the common influenza virus[297]), or bacterial infection (including tuberculosis[298,299]). Iatrogenic causes should also be considered in patients who have recently undergone cardiac surgery, PCI,[300] catheter ablation,[301] or wire insertion for pacemakers or implantable cardiac defibrillators.[302,303] Although overall mortality is high (in-hospital mortality of 16%–19%, 30-day mortality of 29%, and long-term mortality of 47%–48%), outcomes heavily depend on the cause of tamponade.[304,305] Iatrogenic tamponade and infectious/inflammatory causes of tamponade pose the lowest long-term mortality risk, whereas patients with post-MI or neoplastic disease have the poorest prognosis (80% and 68% 1-year mortality, respectively, in one study[304]).

The Rational Clinical Examination series in the *Journal of the American Medical Association* explored the utility of specific signs and symptoms for determining whether a patient with a known pericardial effusion has progressed to tamponade.[306] Conscious patients may report shortness of breath (pooled sensitivity 87%–88%) and chest pain (sensitivity 20%), in addition to other nonspecific symptoms, including fever, fullness, nausea, vomiting, or dysphagia. Tachycardia (pooled sensitivity of 77%), tachypnea (80%), and elevated jugular venous pressure (76%) are relatively sensitive signs for tamponade, whereas hypotension (26%) and diminished heart sounds (28%) are less reliable. Hypotension is a late finding and, in fact, some patients initially may even be *hypertensive* from increased adrenergic drive and resultant increased peripheral vascular resistance.[307,308] One physical examination finding, pulsus paradoxus (ie, a decrease in systolic blood pressure during inspiration of 10 mm Hg or greater[309]), has been shown to be correlated with the progression from effusion to tamponade. A pulsus of 10 mm Hg or greater is associated with a 3.3 LR for tamponade, and a pulsus greater than 12 mm Hg further increases the LR to 5.9. In contrast, a pulsus less than 10 mm Hg lowers the LR to 0.03. This finding, however, may also be seen in lung diseases such as COPD or massive PE or minimized by hypotension.[310]

Classically described ECG findings in tamponade are also insensitive. Low voltage is thought to be only 42% sensitive for the presence of cardiac tamponade, whereas electrical alternans is only 16% to 21% sensitive. The chest radiograph finding of cardiomegaly has a pooled sensitivity of 89%. Unfortunately, the often-described "globular" cardiac silhouette may require as much as 200 mL of fluid accumulation to be seen,[311] whereas much smaller yet rapidly accumulating effusions may just as readily cause tamponade physiology.

Although true hemodynamically significant tamponade is a clinical diagnosis, not an imaging one, several echocardiographic findings are suggestive. Subcostal views can identify as little as 15 mL of fluid, and an effusion's size can be roughly quantified by its maximal dimension in diastole.[311] Although it is not necessarily size but rather rate of accumulation generally that leads to tamponade physiology, larger effusions (>20 mm maximal thickness) and circumferential effusions are associated with more serious disease.[312] A distended inferior vena cava without normal respiratory variation is sensitive (97%) but not specific (40%) for tamponade.[313] Diastolic collapse of one or more heart chambers due to elevated pericardial pressure may also be diagnostic. Diastolic collapse of the right ventricle is specific for tamponade,[311,314] and right atrial collapse lasting more than one-third of the cardiac cycle is nearly 100% sensitive and specific.[315,316] Bulging of the interventricular septum into the LV may also be seen. Finally, Doppler echocardiography can be used to identify the pathophysiologic changes responsible for pulsus paradoxus: increased right-sided venous return with inspiration in the setting of a fixed high-pressure pericardial space will cause expansion of the RV and resultant compression of the LV, impairing left-sided filling. This results in the decreased systolic blood pressure seen with inspiration but can be measured directly with pulse wave Doppler assessments of mitral flow velocity. A reduction in flow velocity of 30% or more with inspiration is considered diagnostic.[317] Lastly, even if the emergency physician is uncomfortable or unable to perform some of these advanced echocardiographic assessments, the presence of a pericardial effusion and a distended IVC in the right clinical setting—that is, the hypotensive patient with any of the risk factors discussed earlier—should prompt expeditious therapeutic intervention, as the progression to cardiovascular collapse and PEA arrest may be precipitous.

SUMMARY

Patients with chest pain present one of the emergency medicine clinician's greatest challenges. Physicians must differentiate between the benign and life-threatening causes of chest pain, while also quickly identifying those patients who would benefit from immediate intervention. Complicating this already difficult task is the fact that therapy for one of these disease processes may be contraindicated for another (ie, anticoagulation in a patient presumed to have ACS when in fact they have an aortic dissection). Although *not* every case of missed ACS, TAD, or PE represents negligence or malpractice, it is critical for clinicians to realize the importance of clear documentation of risk factor assessment and thought processes. Reference to the various risk stratification tools and paradigms discussed here can provide a sound and evidence-based approach to doing so. When misses do occur, as they will for every emergency physician, it is imperative that documentation reflects careful, appropriate, and thoughtful management. Lastly, physicians should communicate clearly and frankly with their patients about the diagnoses being considered, the risks and benefits of diagnostic testing and treatment, and, when possible, should document shared decision-making regarding key management choices.

DISCLOSURE

Neither author has any disclosures to make.

REFERENCES

1. Tomaszewski CA, Nestler D, Shah KH, et al. Clinical policy: critical issues in the evaluation and management of emergency department patients with suspected non-ST-elevation acute coronary syndromes. Ann Emerg Med 2018;72(5): e65–106.

2. Riley RF, Miller CD, Russell GB, et al. Cost analysis of the history, ECG, age, risk factors, and initial troponin (HEART) pathway randomized control trial. Am J Emerg Med 2017;35(1):77–81.

3. Brown TW, McCarthy ML, Kelen GD, et al. An epidemiological study of closed emergency department malpractice claims in a national database of physician malpractice insurers. Acad Emerg Med 2010;17(5):553–60.

4. Dezman DZ, Mattu A, Body R. Utility of the history and physical examination in the detection of acute coronary syndromes in emergency department patients. West J Emerg Med 2017;18(4):752–60.

5. Heart disease facts, centers for disease control and prevention. Available at: https://www.cdc.gov/heartdiseasefacts.htm. Accessed July 1, 2019.

6. Go AS, Mozaffarian D, Roger VL, et al. Heart disease and stroke statistics—2014 update: a report from the American heart association. Circulation 2014; 129(3):e28–292.

7. Schor S, Behar S, Modan B, et al. Disposition of presumed coronary patients from an emergency room: a follow-up study. JAMA 1976;236(8):941–3.

8. Lee TH, Rouan GW, Weisberg MC, et al. Clinical characteristics and natural history of patients with acute myocardial infarction sent home from the emergency room. Am J Cardiol 1987;60:219–24.

9. McCarthy BD, Beshansky JR, D'Agostino RB, et al. Missed diagnoses of acute myocardial infarction in the emergency department: results from a multicenter study. Ann Emerg Med 1993;22:579–82.

10. Pope JH, Aufderheide TP, Ruthazer R, et al. Missed diagnosis of acute cardiac ischemia in the emergency department. N Engl J Med 2000;342:1163–70.

11. Schull MJ, Vermeulen MJ, Stukel TA. The risk of missed diagnosis of acute myocardial infarction associated with emergency department volume. Ann Emerg Med 2006;48(6):647–55.

12. Waxman DA, Kanzaria HK, Schriger DL. Unrecognized cardiovascular emergencies among medicare patients. JAMA Intern Med 2018;178(4):477–84.

13. Mehta RH, Eagle KA. Missed diagnoses of acute coronary syndromes in the emergency room—continuing challenges. N Engl J Med 2000;342(16):1207–10.

14. Pope JH, Selker HP. Acute coronary syndromes in the emergency department: diagnostic characteristics, tests, and challenges. Cardiol Clin 2005;23:423–51.

15. Katz DA, Williams GC, Brown RL, et al. Emergency physicians' fear of malpractice in evaluating patients with possible acute cardiac ischemia. Ann Emerg Med 2005;46(6):525–33.

16. Beckmann CH. How to avoid being swept away by the rising tide of malpractice litigation. Am J Cardiol 2003;91:585–6.

17. Weinstock MB, Weingart S, Orth F, et al. Risk for clinically relevant adverse cardiac events in patients with chest pain at hospital admission. JAMA Intern Med 2015;175(7):1207–12.

18. Laureano-Philips J, Robinson RD, Aryal S, et al. HEART score risk stratification of low-risk chest pain patients in the emergency department: a systematic review and meta-analysis. Ann Emerg Med 2019;74(2):187–203.

19. Kannel WB, Abbot RD. Incidence and prognosis of unrecognized myocardial infarction: an update of the Framingham Study. N Engl J Med 1984;311:1144–7.

20. Canto JG, Shlipak MG, Rogers WJ, et al. Prevalence, clinical characteristics, and mortality among patients with myocardial infarction presenting without chest pain. JAMA 2000;283:3223–9.

21. Dorsch MF, Lawrence RA, Sapsford RJ, et al. Poor prognosis of patients presenting with symptomatic myocardial infarction but without chest pain. Heart 2001;86:494–8.

22. Brieger D, Eagle KA, Goodman SG, et al. Acute coronary syndromes without chest pain, an underdiagnosed and undertreated high-risk group: insights from the Global Registry of Acute Coronary Events (GRACE). Chest 2004;126:461–9.

23. Coronado BE, Pope JH, Griffith JL, et al. Clinical features, triage, and outcome of patients presenting to the ED with suspected acute coronary syndromes but without pain: a multicenter study. Am J Emerg Med 2004;22:568–74.

24. Canto JG, Fincher C, Kiefe CI, et al. Atypical presentations among medicare beneficiaries with unstable angina pectoris. Am J Cardiol 2002;90:248–53.

25. Sederholm Lawesson S, Isaksson RM, Thylen I, et al. Gender differences in symptom presentation of ST-elevation myocardial infarction – an observational multicenter survey study. Int J Cardiol 2018;264:7–11.

26. Puymirat E, Aissaoui N, Bonello L, et al. Clinical outcomes according to symptom presentation in patients with acute myocardial infarction: results from the FAST-MI 2010 registry. Clin Cardiol 2017;40(12):1256–63.

27. Lee HO. Typical and atypical clinical signs and symptoms of myocardial infarction and delayed seeking of professional care among blacks. Am J Crit Care 1997;6(1):7–13.

28. Arslanian-Engoren C, Patel A, Fang J, et al. Symptoms of men and women presenting with acute coronary syndromes. Am J Cardiol 2006;98:1177–81.

29. Patel H, Rosengreen A, Ekman I. Symptoms in acute coronary syndromes: does sex make a difference? Am Heart J 2004;148:27–33.

30. Milner KA, Funk M, Richards S, et al. Gender differences in symptom presentation associated with coronary heart disease. Am J Cardiol 1999;84:396–9.

31. Kudenchuk PJ, Maynard C, Martin JS, et al. Comparison of presentation, treatment, and outcome of acute myocardial infarction in men versus women (the Myocardial Infarction Triage and Intervention Registry). Am J Cardiol 1996; 78:9–14.

32. Pilgrim T, Heg D, Tal K, et al. Age- and gender-related disparities in primary percutaneous coronary interventions for acute ST-segment elevation myocardial infarction. PLoS One 2015;10(9):e0137047.

33. Redfors B, Angeras O, Ramunddal T, et al. Trends in gender differences in cardiac care and outcome after acute myocardial infarction in western Sweden: a report from the Swedish web system for enhancement of evidence-based care in heart disease evaluated according to recommended therapies (SWEDE-HEART). J Am Heart Assoc 2015;4(7):e001995.

34. Johns PA, Lee TH, Cook F, et al. Effect of race on the presentation and management of patients with acute chest pain. Ann Intern Med 1993;118:593–601.

35. Lopez L, Wilper AP, Cervantes MC, et al. Racial and sex differences in emergency department triage assessment and test ordering for chest pain, 1997-2006. Acad Emerg Med 2010;17(8):801–8.

36. DeVon HA, Burke LA, Zerwic JJ, et al. Disparities in patients presenting to the emergency department with potential acute coronary syndrome: it matters if you are black or white. Heart Lung 2014;43(4):270–7.

37. Ferdinand KC, Yadav K, Nasser SA, et al. Disparities in hypertension and cardiovascular disease in blacks: the critical role of medication adherence. J Clin Hypertens (Greenwich) 2017;19(10):1015–24.

38. Alrwisan A, Eworuke E. Are discrepancies in waiting time for chest pain at emergency departments between African Americans and whites improving over time? J Emerg Med 2016;50(2):349–55.

39. Pezzin LE, Keyl PM, Green GB. Disparities in the emergency department evaluation of chest pain patients. Acad Emerg Med 2007;14:149–56.

40. Musey PL Jr, Kline JA. Do gender and race make a difference in acute coronary syndrome pretest probabilities in the emergency department? Acad Emerg Med 2017;24(2):142–51.

41. Egred M, Viswanathan G, Davis GK. Myocardial infarction in young adults. Postgrad Med J 2005;81:741–5.

42. Chen L, Chester M, Kaski JC. Clinical factors and angiographic features associated with premature coronary artery disease. Chest 1995;108(2):364–9.

43. Walker NJ, Sites FD, Shofer FS, et al. Characteristics and outcomes of young adults who present to the emergency department with chest pain. Acad Emerg Med 2001;8(7):703–8.
44. Goodacre S, Locker T, Campbell S. How useful are clinical features in the diagnosis of acute, undifferentiated chest pain? Acad Emerg Med 2002;9(3):203–8.
45. Chun AA, McGee SR. Bedside diagnosis of coronary artery disease: a systematic review. Am J Med 2004;117:334–43.
46. Swap CJ, Nagurney JT. Value and limitations of chest pain history in the evaluation of patients with suspected acute coronary syndromes. JAMA 2005;294(20):2623–9.
47. Solomon CG, Lee TH, Cook EF, et al. Comparison of clinical presentation of acute myocardial infarction in patients older than 65 years of age to younger patients: the multicenter chest pain study experience. Am J Cardiol 1989;63(12):772–6.
48. Hess EP, Brison RJ, Perry JJ, et al. Development of a clinical prediction rule for 30-day cardiac events in emergency department patients with chest pain and possible acute coronary syndrome. Ann Emerg Med 2012;59(2):115–25.e1.
49. Fanaroff AC, Rymer JA, Goldstein SA, et al. Does this patient with chest pain have acute coronary syndrome?: the rational clinical examination systematic review. JAMA 2015;314(18):1955–65.
50. Van der Meer MG, Backus BE, van der Graaf Y, et al. The diagnostic value of clinical symptoms in women and men presenting with chest pain at the emergency department, a prospective cohort study. PLoS One 2015;10(1):e0116431.
51. Panju AA, Hemmelgarn BR, Guyatt GH, et al. The rational clinical examination: is this patient having a myocardial infarction? JAMA 1998;280(14):1256–63.
52. Bruyninckx R, Aertgeerts B, Bruyninckx P, et al. Signs and symptoms in diagnosing acute myocardial infarction and acute coronary syndrome: a diagnostic meta-analysis. Br J Gen Pract 2008;58(547):105–11.
53. Body R, Carley S, Wibberley C, et al. The value of symptoms and signs in the emergent diagnosis of acute coronary syndromes. Resuscitation 2010;81(3):281–6.
54. Greenslade JH, Cullen L, Parsonage W, et al. Examining the signs and symptoms experienced by individuals with suspected acute coronary syndrome in the Asia-Pacific region: a prospective observational study. Ann Emerg Med 2012;60(6):777–85.e3.
55. Anderson JL, Adams CD, Antman EM, et al. ACC/AHA 2007 guidelines for the management of patients with unstable angina/non-ST-segment elevation myocardial infarction: a report of the American College of Cardiology/American Heart Association Task Force on Practice Guidelines (Writing committee to revise the 2002 guidelines for the management of patients with unstable angina/non-ST-elevation myocardial infarction): developed in collaboration with the American College of Emergency Physicians, American College of Physicians, Society for Academic Emergency Medicine, Society for Cardiovascular Angiography and Interventions, and Society for Thoracic Surgeons. J Am Coll Cardiol 2007;50:652–726.
56. Lee TH, Cook EF, Weisberg M, et al. Acute chest pain in the emergency room: identification and examination of low-risk patients. Arch Intern Med 1985;145:65–9.
57. Gordon T, Sorlie P, Kannel WB. Coronary heart disease, atherothrombotic brain infarction, intermittent claudication—a multivariate analysis of some factors

related to their incidence: Framingham Study, 16 year follow-up. Section 27, U.S. Govt. Print.Office; 1971.

58. Body R, McDowell G, Carley S, et al. Do risk factors for chronic coronary heart disease help diagnose acute myocardial infarction in the emergency department? Resuscitation 2008;79(1):41–5.

59. Jayes RL, Beshansky JR, D'Agostino RB, et al. Do patients' coronary risk factor reports predict acute cardiac ischemia in the emergency department? A multi-center study. J Clin Epidemiol 1992;45(6):621–6.

60. Wahrenberg A, Magnusson PK, Discacciati A, et al. Family history of coronary artery disease is associated with acute coronary syndrome in 28,188 chest pain patients. Eur Heart J Acute Cardiovasc Care 2019;24. 2048872619853521.

61. Han JH, Lindsell CJ, Storrow AB, et al. The role of cardiac risk factor burden in diagnosing acute coronary syndromes in the emergency department setting. Ann Emerg Med 2007;49(2):145–52, 152.e1.

62. Antman EM, Cohen M, Bernink PJL, et al. The TIMI risk score for unstable angina/non-ST elevation MI: a method for prognostication and therapeutic decision making. JAMA 2000;284(7):835–42.

63. Shry EA, Dacus J, Van De Graaff E, et al. Usefulness of the response to sublingual nitroglycerin as a predictor of ischemic chest pain in the emergency department. Am J Cardiol 2002;90(11):1264–6.

64. Henrikson CA, Howell EE, Bush DE, et al. Chest pain relief by nitroglycerin does not predict active coronary artery disease. Ann Intern Med 2003;139:979–86.

65. Diercks DB, Boghos E, Guzman H, et al. Changes in the numeric descriptive scale for pain after sublingual nitroglycerin do not predict cardiac etiology of chest pain. Ann Emerg Med 2005;45:581–5.

66. Servi RJ, Skiendzielewski JJ. Relief of myocardial ischemia pain with a gastrointestinal cocktail. Am J Emerg Med 1985;3(3):208–9.

67. Dickinson MW. The "GI cocktail" in the evaluation of chest pain in the emergency department. J Emerg Med 1996;14(2):245–6.

68. Chauhan A, Mullins PA, Taylor G, et al. Cardioesophageal reflex: a mechanism for "linked angina" in patients with angiographically proven coronary artery disease. J Am Coll Cardiol 1996;27(7):1621–8.

69. Dobrzycki S, Baniukiewicz A, Korecki J, et al. Does gastro-esophageal reflux provoke the myocardial ischemia in patients with CAD? Int J Cardiol 2005; 104:67–72.

70. Budzynski J, Klopocka M, Pulkowski G, et al. The effect of double dose of omeprazole on the course of angina pectoris and treadmill stress test in patients with coronary artery disease—a randomised, double-blind, placebo controlled, crossover trial. Int J Cardiol 2007;127:233–9.

71. Smith KS, Papp C. Episodic, postural, and "linked angina". Br Med J 1962; 2(5317):1425–30.

72. Chan S, Maurice AP, Davies SR, et al. The use of gastrointestinal cocktail for differentiating gastro-oesophageal reflux disease and acute coronary syndrome in the emergency setting: a systematic review. Heart Lung Circ 2014;23:913–23.

73. Fesmire FM, Percy RF, Bardoner JB, et al. Usefulness of automated serial 12-lead ECG monitoring during the initial emergency department evaluation of patients with chest pain. Ann Emerg Med 1998;31:3–11.

74. Fesmire FM, Decker WW, Diercks DB, et al. Clinical policy: critical issues in the evaluation and management of adult patients with non-ST-segment elevation acute coronary syndromes—from the American College of Physicians clinical polices subcommittee. Ann Emerg Med 2006;48:270–301.

75. Macias M, Peachey J, Mattu A, et al. The electrocardiogram in the ACS patient: high-risk electrocardiographic presentations lacking anatomically oriented ST-segment elevation. Am J Emerg Med 2016;34(3):611–7.

76. Miranda DF, Lobo AS, Walsh B, et al. New insights into the use of the 12-lead electrocardiogram for diagnosing acute myocardial infarction in the emergency department. Can J Cardiol 2018;34(2):132–45.

77. McCabe JM, Armstrong EJ, Ku I, et al. Physician accuracy in interpreting potential ST-segment elevation myocardial infarction electrocardiograms. J Am Heart Assoc 2013;2(5):e000268.

78. Masoudi FA, Magid DJ, Vinson DR, et al. Implications of the failure to identify high-risk electrocardiogram findings for the quality of care of patients with acute myocardial infarction—results of the Emergency Department Quality in Myocardial Infarction (EDQMI) Study. Circulation 2006;114:1565–71.

79. Brady WJ, Perron AD, Ullman E. Errors in emergency physician interpretation of ST-segment elevation in emergency department chest pain patients. Acad Emerg Med 2000;7:1256–60.

80. Brady WJ, Perron AD, Chan T. Electrocardiographic ST-segment elevation: correct identification of acute myocardial infarction (AMI) and non-AMI syndromes by emergency physicians. Acad Emerg Med 2001;8(4):349–60.

81. Erling BF, Perron AD, Brady WJ. Disagreement in the interpretation of electrocardiographic ST segment elevation: a source of error for emergency physicians? Am J Emerg Med 2004;22:65–70.

82. Snoey ER, Housset B, Guyon P, et al. Analysis of emergency department interpretation of electrocardiograms. J Accid Emerg Med 1994;11(3):149–53.

83. Todd KH, Hoffman JR, Morgan MT. Effect of cardiologist ECG review on emergency department practice. Ann Emerg Med 1996;27(1):16–21.

84. Balk EM, Ioannidis JPA, Salem D, et al. Accuracy of biomarkers to diagnose acute cardiac ischemia in the emergency department: a meta-analysis. Ann Emerg Med 2001;37:478–94.

85. Limkakeng A, Gibler WB, Pollack C, et al. Combination of Goldman risk and initial cardiac troponin I for emergency department chest pain patient risk stratification. Acad Emerg Med 2001;8:696–702.

86. Ebell MH, Flewelling D, Flynn CA. A systematic review of troponin T and I for diagnosing acute myocardial infarction. J Fam Pract 2000;49:550–6.

87. Smith SW, Tibbles CD, Apple FS, et al. Outcome of low-risk patients discharged home after a normal cardiac troponin I. J Emerg Med 2004;26(4):401–6.

88. Chapman AR, Lee KK, McAllister DA, et al. Association of high-sensitivity cardiac troponin I concentration with cardiac outcomes in patients with suspected acute coronary syndrome. JAMA 2017;318(19):1913–24.

89. Peacock WF, Baumann BM, Bruton D, et al. Efficacy of high-sensitivity troponin T in identifying very-low-risk patients with possible acute coronary syndrome. JAMA Cardiol 2018;3(2):104–11.

90. Ferencik M, Hoffman U, Bamberg F, et al. Highly sensitive troponin and coronary computed tomography angiography in the evaluation of suspected acute coronary syndrome in the emergency department. Eur Heart J 2016;37(30):2397–405.

91. Hollander JE. Managing troponin testing. Ann Emerg Med 2016;68(6):690–4.

92. Backus BE, Six AJ, Kelder JC, et al. A prospective validation of the HEART score for chest pain patients at the emergency department. Int J Cardiol 2013;168(3):2153–8.

93. MA OJ, Mateer JR, Blaivas M. Emergency ultrasound. 2nd edition. New York: McGraw-Hill; 2008.

94. Policy Statement, ACEP Board of Directors. Ultrasound guidelines: emergency, point-of-care and clinical ultrasound guidelines in medicine. Ann Emerg Med 2017;69(5):e27–54.

95. Croft PE, Strout TD, Kring RM, et al. WAMAMI: emergency physicians can accurately identify wall motion abnormalities in acute myocardial infarction. Am J Emerg Med 2019;37(12):2224–8.

96. Wohlgelernter D, Cleman M, Highman HA, et al. Regional myocardial dysfunction during coronary angioplasty: evaluation by two dimensional echocardiography and 13 lead electrocardiography. J Am Coll Cardiol 1986;7(6):1245–54.

97. Horowitz RS, Morganroth J, Parrotto C, et al. Immediate diagnosis of acute myocardial infarction by two-dimensional echocardiography. Circulation 1982; 65(2):323–9.

98. Sabia P, Afrookteh A, Touchstone DA, et al. Value of regional wall motion abnormality in the emergency room diagnosis of acute myocardial infarction. A prospective study using two-dimensional echocardiography. Circulation 1991; 84(3 Suppl):I85–92.

99. Kontos MC, Arrowood JA, Paulsen WH, et al. Early echocardiography can predict cardiac events in emergency department patients with chest pain. Ann Emerg Med 1998;31(5):550–7.

100. Frenkel O, Riguzzi C, Nagdev A. Identification of high-risk patients with acute coronary syndrome using point-of-care echocardiography in the ED. Am J Emerg Med 2014;32(6):670–2.

101. Pope JH, Ruthazer R, Beshansky JR, et al. Clinical features of emergency department patients presenting with symptoms suggestive of acute cardiac ischemia: a multicenter study. J Thromb Thrombolysis 1998;6:63–74.

102. Than M, Cullen L, Reid CM, et al. A 2-h diagnostic protocol to assess patients with chest pain symptoms in the Asia-Pacific region (ASPECT): a prospective observational validation study. Lancet 2011;377(9771):1077–84.

103. Than M, Cullen L, Aldous S, et al. 2-hour accelerated diagnostic protocol to assess patients with chest pain symptoms using contemporary troponins as the only biomarker: the ADAPT trial. J Am Coll Cardiol 2012;59(23):2091–8.

104. Zalenski RJ, McCarren M, Roberts R, et al. An evaluation of a chest pain diagnostic protocol to exclude acute cardiac ischemia in the emergency department. Arch Intern Med 1997;157:1085–91.

105. Polanczyk CA, Johnson PA, Hartley LH, et al. Clinical correlates and prognostic significance of early negative exercise tolerance test in patients with acute chest pain seen in the hospital emergency department. Am J Cardiol 1998;81:288–92.

106. Mikhail MG, Smith FA, Gray M, et al. Cost-effectiveness of mandatory stress testing in chest pain center patients. Ann Emerg Med 1997;29(1):88–98.

107. Amsterdam EA, Kirk JD, Diercks DB, et al. Immediate exercise testing to evaluate low-risk patients presenting to the emergency department with chest pain. J Am Coll Cardiol 2002;40:251–6.

108. Amsterdam EA, Wenger NK, Brindis RG, et al. 2014 AHA/ACC guideline for the management of patients with non-ST-elevation acute coronary syndromes: a report of the American college of cardiology/American heart association task force on practice guidelines. J Am Coll Cardiol 2014;64(24):e139–228.

109. Meyer MC, Mooney RP, Sekera AK. A critical pathway for patients with acute chest pain and low risk for short-term adverse cardiac events: role of outpatient stress testing. Ann Emerg Med 2006;47:427–35.

110. Lim SH, Anantharaman V, Sundram F, et al. Stress myocardial perfusion imaging for the evaluation and triage of chest pain in the emergency department: a randomized controlled trial. J Nucl Cardiol 2013;20(6):1002–12.

111. Frisoli TM, Nowak R, Evans KL, et al. Henry ford HEART score randomized trial: rapid discharge of patients evaluated for possible myocardial infarction. Circ Cardiovasc Qual Outcomes 2017;10(10):e003617.

112. Hermann LK, Newman DH, Pleasant WA, et al. Yield of routine provocative cardiac testing among patients in an emergency department-based chest pain unit. JAMA Intern Med 2013;173(12):1128–33.

113. Poldervaart JM, Six AJ, Backus BE, et al. The predictive value of the exercise ECG for major adverse cardiac events in patients who presented with chest pain in the emergency department. Clin Res Cardiol 2013;102(4):305–12.

114. Duseja R, Feldman JA. Missed acute cardiac ischemic in the ED: limitations of diagnostic testing. Am J Emerg Med 2004;22(3):219–25.

115. Smith SW, Jackson EA, Bart BA, et al. Incidence of myocardial infarction in emergency department chest pain patients with a recent negative stress imaging test [abstract]. Acad Emerg Med 2005;12(5 Suppl 1):51.

116. Walker J, Galuska M, Vega D. Coronary disease in emergency department chest pain patients with recent negative stress testing. West J Emerg Med 2010;11(4):384–8.

117. Raff GL, Gallagher MJ, O'Neill WW, et al. Diagnostic accuracy of noninvasive coronary angiography using 64-slice spiral computed tomography. J Am Coll Cardiol 2005;46:552–7.

118. Hoffmann U, Nagurney JT, Moselewski F, et al. Coronary multidetector computed tomography in the assessment of patietns with acute chest pain. Circulation 2006;114(21):2241–60.

119. Rubinshteim R, Halon DA, Gaspar T, et al. Usefulness of 64-slice cardiac computed tomographic angiography for diagnosing acute coronary syndromes and predicting clinical outcome in emergency department patients with chest pain of uncertain origin. Circulation 2007;115:1762–8.

120. Meijboom WB, Mollet NR, Mieghem CA, et al. 64-slice CT coronary angiography in patients with non-ST elevation acute coronary syndromes. Heart 2007;93: 1386–92.

121. Hollander JE, Chang AM, Shofer FS, et al. Coronary computed tomographic angiography for rapid discharge of low-risk patients with potential acute coronary syndromes. Ann Emerg Med 2009;53(3):295–304.

122. Hoffmann U, Bamberg F, Chae CU, et al. Coronary computed tomography angiography for early triage of patients with acute chest pain: the ROMICAT (rule out myocardial infarction using computer assisted tomography) trial. J Am Coll Cardiol 2009;53(18):1642–50.

123. Gallager MJ, Ross MA, Raff GL, et al. The diagnostic accuracy of 64-slice computed tomography coronary angiography compared with stress nuclear imaging in emergency department low-risk chest pain patients. Ann Emerg Med 2007;49:125–36.

124. Goldstein JA, Gallagher MJ, O'Neill WW, et al. A randomized controlled trial of multi-slice coronary computed tomography for evaluation of acute chest pain. J Am Coll Cardiol 2007;49:863–71.

125. Hoffmann U, Truong QA, Schoenfeld DA, et al. Coronary CT angiography versus standard evaluation in acute chest pain. N Engl J Med 2012;367(4):299–308.

126. Litt HI, Gatsonis C, Snyder B, et al. CT angiography for safe discharge of patients with possible acute coronary syndromes. N Engl J Med 2012;366(15):1393–403.

127. Barnett K, Feldman JA. Noninvasive imaging techniques to aid in the triage of patients with suspected acute coronary syndrome: a review. Emerg Med Clin North Am 2005;23:977–98.

128. Truong QA, Schulman-Marcus J, Zakroysky P, et al. Coronary CT angiography versus standard emergency department evaluation for acute chest pain and diabetic patients: is there benefit with early coronary CT angiography? Results of the randomized comparative effectives ROMICAT II trial. J Am Heart Assoc 2016;5(3):e003137.

129. Poon M, Cortegiano M, Abramowicz AJ, et al. Associations between routine coronary computed tomographic angiography and reduced unnecessary hospital admissions, length of stay, recidivism rates, and invasive coronary angiography in the emergency department triage of chest pain. J Am Coll Cardiol 2013;62(6):543–52.

130. Braunwald E, Brown J, Brown L, et al. Unstable angina: diagnosis and management. Clinical practice guideline number 10. Rockville (MD): Agency for Health Care Policy and Research, US Public Health Service, US Department of Health and Human Services; 1994.

131. Selker HP, Griffith JL, D'Agostino RB. A tool for judging coronary care unit admission appropriateness, valid for both real-time and retrospective use: a time-insensitive predictive instrument (TIPI) for acute cardiac ischemia: a multicenter study. Med Care 1991;29(7):610–27.

132. Six AJ, Backus BE, Kelder JC. Chest pain in the emergency room: value of the HEART score. Neth Heart J 2008;16(6):191–6.

133. Sun BC, Laurie A, Fu R, et al. Comparison of the HEART and TIMI risk scores for suspected acute coronary syndrome in the emergency department. Crit Pathw Cardiol 2016;15(1):1–5.

134. Poldervaart JM, Reitsma JB, Backus BE, et al. Effect of using the HEART score in patients with chest pain in the emergency department: a stepped-wedge, cluster randomized trial. Ann Intern Med 2017;166(10):689–97.

135. Van Den Berg P, Body R. The HEART score for early rule out of acute coronary syndromes in the emergency department: a systematic review and meta-analysis. Eur Heart J Acute Cardiovasc Care 2018;7(2):111–9.

136. Mahler SA, Miller CD, Hollander JE, et al. Identifying patients for early discharge: performance of decision rules among patients with acute chest pain. Int J Cardiol 2013;168(2):795–802.

137. Mahler SA, Riley RF, Hiestand BC, et al. The HEART pathway randomized trial: identifying emergency department patients with acute chest pain for early discharge. Circ Cardiovasc Qual Outcomes 2015;8(2):195–203.

138. Pollack CV, Sites FD, Shofer FS, et al. Application of the TIMI risk score for unstable angina and non-ST elevation acute coronary syndrome to an unselected emergency department chest pain population. Acad Emerg Med 2006;13(1):13–8.

139. Chase M, Robey JL, Zogby KE, et al. Prospective validation of the Thrombolysis in Myocardial Infarction Risk score in the emergency department chest pain population. Ann Emerg Med 2006;48(3):252–9.

140. Jaffery Z, Hudson MP, Jacobsen G, et al. Modified thrombolysis in myocardial infarction (TIMI) risk score to risk stratify patients in the emergency department

with possible acute coronary syndrome. J Thromb Thrombolysis 2007;24: 137–44.

141. Ramsay G, Podogrodzka M, McClure, et al. Risk prediction in patients presenting with suspected cardiac pain: the GRACE and TIMI risk scores. QJM 2007; 100(1):11–8.

142. Than M, Flaws D, Sanders S, et al. Development and validation of the emergency department assessment of chest pain score and 2 h accelerated diagnostic protocol. Emerg Med Australas 2014;26(1):34–44.

143. Stopyra JP, Miller CD, Hiestand BC, et al. Performance of the EDACS-accelerated diagnostic pathway in a cohort of US patients with acute chest pain. Crit Pathw Cardiol 2015;14(4):134–8.

144. Rusnak RA, Stair TO, Hansen K, et al. Litigation against the emergency physician: common features in cases of missed myocardial infarction. Ann Emerg Med 1989;18:1029–34.

145. Acute myocardial infarction study. Rockville (MD): Physician Insurers Association of America; 1996.

146. Croskerry P. Achilles heels of the ED: delayed or missed diagnoses. ED Legal Letter 2003;109–20.

147. Freas GC. Medicolegal aspects of acute myocardial infarction. Emerg Med Clin North Am 2001;19(2):511–21.

148. Wu KH, Yen YL, Wu CH, et al. Learning from an analysis of closed malpractice litigation involving myocardial infarction. J Forensic Leg Med 2017;48:41–5.

149. Kachalia A, Gandhi TK, Puopolo AL, et al. Missed and delayed diagnoses in the emergency department: a study of closed malpractice claims from 4 liability insurers. Ann Emerg Med 2007;49(2):196–205.

150. Brooker JA, Hastings JW, Major-Monfried H, et al. The association between medicolegal and professional concerns and chest pain admission rates. Acad Emerg Med 2015;22(7):883–6.

151. Hess EP, Hollander JE, Schaffer JT, et al. Shared decision making in patients with low risk chest pain: prospective randomized pragmatic trial. BMJ 2016; 355:i6165.

152. Ferguson B, Geralds J, Patrey J, et al. Malpractice in emergency medicine – a review of risk and mitigation practices for the emergency medicine provider. J Emerg Med 2018;55(5):659–65.

153. Vukmir RB. Medical malpractice: managing the risk. Med Law 2004;23(3): 495–513.

154. Klompas M. Does this patient have an acute aortic dissection? JAMA 2002; 287(17):2262–72.

155. Mussa FF, Horton JD, Moridzadeh R, et al. Acute aortic dissection and intramural hematoma: a systematic review. JAMA 2016;316(7):754–63.

156. Nienaber CA, Clough RE. Management of acute aortic dissection. Lancet 2015; 385(9970):800–11.

157. Chen K, Varon J, Wenker O, et al. Acute thoracic aortic dissection: the basics. J Emerg Med 1997;15(6):859–67.

158. Strayer RJ. Thoracic aortic syndromes. Emerg Med Clin North Am 2017;34(4): 713–25.

159. Meszaros I, Morocz J, Szlavi J, et al. Epidemiology and clinicopathology of aortic dissection. Chest 2000;117(5):1271–8.

160. Kouchokis N, Dougenis D. Surgery of the thoracic aorta. N Engl J Med 1997; 336(26):1876–88.

161. Hagan PG, Nienaber CA, Isselbaher EM, et al. The international registry of acute aortic dissection (IRAD). JAMA 2000;283(7):897–903.

162. Slater E, DeSanctis RW. The clinical recognition of dissecting aortic aneurysm. Am J Med 1976;60:625–33.

163. Massumi A, Mathur VS. Clinical recognition of aortic dissection. Tex Heart Inst J 1990;17:254–6.

164. Bossone E, Pyeritz RE, O'Gara P, et al. Acute aortic dissection in blacks: insights from the International Registry of Acute Aortic Dissection. Am J Med 2013; 126(10):909–15.

165. Westover AN, Nakonezny PA. Aortic dissection in young adult who abuse amphetamines. Am Heart J 2010;160(2):315–21.

166. Crawford ES. The diagnosis and management of aortic dissection. JAMA 1990; 264:2537–41.

167. Bordeleau L, Cwinn A, Turek M, et al. Aortic dissection and Turner's syndrome: case report and review of the literature. J Emerg Med 1998;16:593–6.

168. Smith K, Gros B. Pregnancy-related acute aortic dissection in Marfan syndrome: a review of the literature. Congenit Heart Dis 2017;12(3):251–60.

169. Silaschi M, Byrne J, Wendler O. Aortid dissection: medical, interventional and surgical management. Heart 2017;103(1):78–87.

170. Sullivan PR, Wolfson AB, Leckey RD, et al. Diagnosis of acute thoracic aortic dissection in the emergency department. Am J Emerg Med 2000;18:46–50.

171. Rosman HS, Patel S, Bzorak S, et al. Quality of history taking in patients with aortic dissection. Chest 1998;114:793–5.

172. Alter SM, Eskin B, Allegra JR. Diagnosis of aortic dissection in emergency department patients is rare. West J Emerg Med 2015;16(5):629–31.

173. Pesola GR, Pesola HR, Lin M, et al. The normal difference in bilateral indirect blood pressure recordings in hypertensive individuals. Acad Emerg Med 2002;9:342–5.

174. Singer AJ, Hollander JE. Blood pressure: assessment of interarm differences. Arch Intern Med 1996;156:2005–8.

175. Fan KL, Leung LP. Clinical profile of patients of acute aortic dissection presenting to the ED without chest pain. Am J Emerg Med 2017;35(4):599–601.

176. Imamura H, Sekiguchi Y, Iwashita T, et al. Painless acute aortic dissection. – Diagnostic, prognostic, and clinical implications. Circ J 2011;75(1):59–66.

177. Harris KM, Strauss CE, Eagle KA, et al. Correlates of delayed recognition and treatment of acute type A aortic dissection: the international registry of acute aortic dissection (IRAD). Circulation 2011;124(18):1911–8.

178. Kurabayashi M, Miwa N, Ueshima D, et al. Factors leading to failure to diagnose acute aortic dissection in the emergency room. J Cardiol 2011;58(3):287–93.

179. Hirata K, Kyushima M, Asato H. Electrocardiographic abnormalities in patients with acute aortic dissection. Am J Cardiol 1995;76:1207–12.

180. Pourafkari L, Tajil A, Ghaffari S, et al. Electrocardiography changes in acute aortic dissection – association with troponin leak, coronary anatomy, and prognosis. Am J Emerg Med 2016;34(8):1431–6.

181. Ohtani H, Kiyokawa K, Asada H, et al. StanfordtypeAacutedissectiondeveloping acute myocardial infarction. Jpn J Thorac Cardiovasc Surg 2000;48:69–72.

182. Gregorio MC, Baumgartner FJ, Omari BO. The presenting chest roentgenogram in acute type A aortic dissection: a multidisciplinary study. Am Surg 2002; 68(1):6–10.

183. Sommer T, Fehske W, Holzknecht N, et al. Aortic dissection: A comparative study of diagnosis with spiral CT, multiplanar transesophageal echocardiography, and MR imaging. Radiology 1996;199:347–52.

184. Baliga RR, Nienaber CA, Bossone E, et al. The role of imaging in aortic dissection and related syndromes. JACC Cardiovasc Imaging 2014;7(4):406–24.

185. Moore AG, Eagle KA, Bruckman D, et al. Choice of computed tomography, transesophageal echocardiography, magnetic resonance imaging and aortography in acute aortic dissection: International registry of acute aortic dissection (IRAD). Am J Cardiol 2002;89:1235–7.

186. Diercks DB, Promes SB, Schuur JD, et al. Clinical policy: critical issues in the evaluation and management of adult patients with suspected acute nontraumatic thoracic aortic dissection. Ann Emerg Med 2015;65(1):32–42.e12.

187. Silvey SV, Stoughton TL, Pearl W, et al. Rupture of the outer partition of aortic dissection during transesophageal echocardiography. Am J Cardiol 1991; 68(2):286–7.

188. Hayter RG, Rhea JT, Small A, et al. Suspected aortic dissection and other aortic disorders: Multi-detector CT in 373 cases in the emergency setting. Radiology 2006;238(3):841–52.

189. Wen D, Zhou XL, Li JJ, et al. Biomarkers in aortic dissection. Clin Chim Acta 2011;412(9–10):688–95.

190. Suzuki T, Katoh H, Tsuchio, et al. Diagnostic implications of elevated levels of smooth-muscle myosin heavy-chain protein in acute aortic dissection. Ann Intern Med 2000;133(7):537–41.

191. Ranasinghe AM, Bonser RS. Biomarkers in acute aortic dissection and other aortic syndromes. J Am Coll Cardiol 2010;56(19):1535–41.

192. Weber T, Hogler S, Auer J, et al. D-dimer in acute aortic dissection. Chest 2003; 123:1375–8.

193. Perez A, Abbet P, Drescher MJ. D-dimers in the emergency department evaluation of aortic dissection. Acad Emerg Med 2004;11:397–400.

194. Eggebrecht H, Naber CK, Bruch C, et al. Value of plasma fibrin D-dimers for detection of acute aortic dissection. J Am Coll Cardiol 2004;44:804–9.

195. Sodeck G, Domanovits H, Schillinger M, et al. D-dimer in ruling out acute aortic dissection: A systematic review and prospective cohort study. Eur Heart J 2007; 28:3067–75.

196. Hazui H, Nishimoto M, Hoshiga M, et al. Young adult patients with short dissection length and thrombosed false lumen without ulcer-like projections are liable to have false-negative results of D-dimer testing for acute aortic dissection based on a study of 113 cases. Circ J 2006;70(12):1598–601.

197. Januzzi JL, Isselbacher EM, Fatorri R, et al. Characterizing the young patient with aortic dissection: results from the international registry of aortic dissection (IRAD) [abstract 1081–154]. J Am Coll Cardiol 2003;41(6):235A.

198. Hansen MS, Nogareda GJ, Hutchison SJ. Frequency of and inappropriate treatment of misdiagnosis of acute aortic dissection. Am J Cardiol 2007;99:852–6.

199. Spittell PC, Spittell JA, Joyce JW, et al. Clinical features and differential diagnosis of aortic dissection: Experience with 236 cases (1980 through 1990). Mayo Clin Proc 1993;68:642–51.

200. Cohen S, Littman D. Painless dissecting aneurysm of the aorta. N Engl J Med 1964;271:143–5.

201. Alsous F, Silam A, Ezeldin A, et al. Potential pitfalls in the diagnosis of aortic dissection. Conn Med 2003;67(3):131–4.

202. Nallamothu BK, Eagle KA. When zebras run with the horses: The diagnostic dilemma of acute aortic dissection complicated by myocardial infarction. J Interv Cardiol 2002;15:297–300.

203. Piney SP, Wasserman HS. Anterior myocardial infarction, acute aortic dissection and anomalous coronary artery. J Interv Cardiol 2002;15:293–6.

204. Elefteriades JA, Barrett PW, Kopf GS. Litigation in nontraumatic aortic diseases—a tempest in the malpractice maelstrom. Cardiology 2008;109:263–72.

205. Hiratzka LF, Bakris GL, Beckman JA, et al. 2010 ACCF/AHA/AATS/ACR/ASA/SCA/SCAI/SIR/STS/SVM guidelines for the diagnosis and management of patients with thoracic aortic disease: a report of the American college of cardiology foundation/American heart association task force on practice guidelines, American association for thoracic surgery, American college of radiology, America stroke association, society of cardiovascular anesthesiologists, society for cardiovascular angiography and interventions, society of interventional radiology, society of thoracic surgeons, and society for vascular medicine. Circulation 2010;121(13):e266–369.

206. Rogers AM, Hermann LK, Booher AM, et al. Sensitivity of the aortic dissection detection risk score, a novel guideline-based tool for identification of acute aortic dissection at initial presentation: results from the international registry of acute aortic dissection. Circulation 2011;123(20):2213–8.

207. Nazerian P, Giachino F, Vanni S, et al. Diagnostic performance of the aortic dissection detection risk score in patients with suspected acute aortic dissection. Eur Heart J Acute Cardiovasc Care 2014;3(4):373–81.

208. Heit JA, O'Fallon WM, Petterson TM, et al. Relative impact of risk factors for deep vein thrombosis and pulmonary embolism. Arch Intern Med 2002;162:1245–8.

209. Wolf SJ, Hahn SA, Nentwich LM, et al. Clinical policy: critical issues in the evaluation and management of adult patients presenting to the emergency department with suspected acute venous thromboembolic disease. Ann Emerg Med 2018;71(5):e59–109.

210. Spencer FA, Emery C, Lessard D, et al. The Worcester Thromboembolism Study. A population-based study of the clinical epidemiology of venous thromboembolism. J Gen Intern Med 2006;21:722–7.

211. Konstantinides S, Geibel A, Olschewski M, et al. Association between thrombolytic treatment and the prognosis of hemodynamically stable patients with major pulmonary embolism: results of a multicenter registry. Circulation 1997;96(3):882–8.

212. Goldhaber SZ, Visani L, DeRosa M. Acute pulmonary embolism: clinical outcomes in the International Cooperative Pulmonary Embolism Registry (ICOPER). Lancet 1999;353:1386–9.

213. Carson JL, Kelle MA, Duff A, et al. The clinical course of pulmonary embolism. N Engl J Med 1992;326(19):1240–5.

214. Becattini C, Agnelli G. Acute pulmonary embolism: risk stratification in the emergency department. Intern Emerg Med 2007;2:119–29.

215. Smith SB, Geske JB, Maguire JM, et al. Early anticoagulation is associated with reduced mortality for acute pulmonary embolism. Chest 2010;137(6):1382–90.

216. Torbicki A, van Beek EJR, Charbonnier B, et al. Guidelines on diagnosis and management of acute pulmonary embolism. Eur Heart J 2000;21:1301–36.

217. Stein PD, Beemath A, Matta F, et al. Clinical characteristics of patients with acute pulmonary embolism: data from PIOPED II. Am J Med 2007;120:871–9.

218. Stein PD, Henry JW. Clinical characteristics of patients with acute pulmonary embolism stratified according to their presenting syndromes. Chest 1997;112: 974–9.
219. Elliot CG, Goldhaber SZ, Visani L, et al. Chest radiographs in acute pulmonary embolism. Chest 2000;118:33–8.
220. Stein PD, Hull RD, Patel KC, et al. D-dimer for the exclusion of acute venous thrombosis and pulmonary embolism: a systematic review. Ann Intern Med 2004;140(8):589–602.
221. Brown MD, Rowe BH, Reeves MJ, et al. The accuracy of the enzyme-linked immunosorbent assay D-dimer test in the diagnosis of pulmonary embolism: a meta-analysis. Ann Emerg Med 2002;40(2):133–44.
222. Brown MD, Lau J, Nelson RD, et al. Turbidimetric D-dimer test in the diagnosis of pulmonary embolism: a metaanalysis. Clin Chem 2003;49(11):1846–53.
223. Di Nisio M, Squizzato A, Rutjes AW, et al. Diagnostic accuracy of D-dimer test for exclusion of venous thromboembolism: a systematic review. J Thromb Haemost 2007;5(2):296–304.
224. Fesmire FM, Brown MD, Espinosa JA, et al. Critical issues in the evaluation and management of adult patients presenting to the emergency department with suspected pulmonary embolism. Ann Emerg Med 2011;57(6):628–52.e75.
225. Qaseem A, Snow V, Barry P, et al. Current diagnosis of venous thromboembolism in primary care: a clinical practice guideline from the American academy of family physicians and the American college of physicians. Ann Intern Med 2007;146(6):454–8.
226. Brown MD, Vance SJ, Kline JA. An emergency department guideline for the diagnosis of pulmonary embolism: an outcome study. Acad Emerg Med 2005; 12(1):20–5.
227. Righini M, Goehring C, Bounameaux H, et al. Effects of age on the performance of common diagnostic tests for pulmonary embolism. Am J Med 2000;109: 357–61.
228. Hogg K, Dawson D, Mackway-Jones K. The emergency department utility of Simplify D-dimer to exclude pulmonary embolism in patients with pleuritic chest pain. Ann Emerg Med 2005;46(4):305–10.
229. Kutinsky I, Blakely S, Roche V, et al. Normal D-dimer levels in patients with pulmonary embolism. Arch Intern Med 1999;159:1569–72.
230. Kabrhel C. Outcomes of high pretest probability patients undergoing D-dimer testing for pulmonary embolism: a pilot study. J Emerg Med 2008;35(4):373–7.
231. Chabloz P, Reber G, Boehlen F, et al. TAFI antigen and D-dimer levels during normal pregnancy and at delivery. Br J Haematol 2001;115:150–2.
232. Kline JA, Williams GW, Hernandez-Nino J. D-dimer concentrations in normal pregnancy: new diagnostic thresholds are needed. Clin Chem 2005;51(5): 825–9.
233. ten Wolde M, Kraaijenhagen RA, Prins MH, et al. The clinical usefulness of D-dimer testing in cancer patients with suspected deep venous thrombosis. Arch Intern Med 2002;162:1880–4.
234. Righini M, Van Es J, Den Exter PL, et al. Age-adjusted D-dimer cutoff levels to rule out pulmonary embolism: the ADJUST-PE study. JAMA 2014;311(11): 1117–24.
235. Van Es N, van der Hulle T, van Es J, et al. Wells rule and d-dimer testing to rule out pulmonary embolism: a systematic review and individual-patient data meta-analysis. Ann Intern Med 2016;165(4):253–61.

236. Flores J, Garcia de Tena J, Galipienzo J, et al. Clinical usefulness and safety of an age-adjusted D-dimer cutoff levels to exclude pulmonary embolism: a retrospective analysis. Intern Emerg Med 2016;11(1):69–75.

237. Moores LK, Jackson WL Jr, Shorr AF, et al. Meta-analysis: outcomes in patients with suspected pulmonary embolism managed with computed tomographic pulmonary angiography. Ann Intern Med 2004;141(11):866–74.

238. Quiroz R, Kucher N, Zou KH, et al. Clinical validity of a negative computed tomography scan in patients with suspected pulmonary embolism. JAMA 2005; 293:2012–7.

239. Van Belle A, Buller HR, Huisman MV, et al. Effectiveness of managing suspected pulmonary embolism using an algorithm combining clinical probability, d-dimer testing, and computed tomography. JAMA 2006;295(2):172–9.

240. Perrier A, Roy PM, Sanchez O, et al. Multidetector-row computed tomography in suspected pulmonary embolism. N Engl J Med 2005;352(17):1760–8.

241. Righini M, Le Gal G, Aujesky D, et al. Diagnosis of pulmonary embolism by multidetector CT alone or combined with venous ultrasonography of the leg: a randomized non-inferiority trial. Lancet 2008;371(9621):1343–52.

242. Musset D, Parent F, Meyer G, et al. Diagnostic strategy for patients with suspected pulmonary embolism: a prospective multicentre outcome study. Lancet 2002;360(9349):1914–20.

243. Stein PD, Fowler SE, Goodman LR, et al. Multidetector computed tomography for acute pulmonary embolism. N Engl J Med 2006;354:2317–27.

244. Madan A, Schwartz C. Echocardiographic visualization of acute pulmonary embolus and thrombolysis in the ED. Am J Emerg Med 2004;22(4):294–300.

245. Perera P, Mailhot T, Riley D, et al. The RUSH exam: rapid ultrasound in shock in the evaluation of the critically ill. Emerg Med Clin North Am 2010;28(1):29–56.

246. Grifoni S, Olivotto I, Cecchini P, et al. Utility of an integrated clinical, echocardiographic, and venous ultrasonographic approach for triage of patients with suspected pulmonary embolism. Am J Cardiol 1998;82(10):1230–5.

247. Miniati M, Monti S, Pratali L, et al. Value of transthoracic echocardiography in the diagnosis of pulmonary embolism: results of a prospective study in unselected patients. Am J Med 2001;110(7):528–35.

248. Elfwen L, Hildebrand K, Schierbeck S, et al. Focused cardiac ultrasound after return of spontaneous circulation in cardiac-arrest patients. Resuscitation 2019;142:16–22.

249. Wicki J, Pereger T, Junod A, et al. Assessing clinical probability of pulmonary embolism in the emergency ward: a simple score. Arch Intern Med 2001; 161:92–7.

250. Wells PS, Ginsberg JS, Anderson DR, et al. Use of a clinical model for safe management of patients with suspected pulmonary embolism. Ann Intern Med 1998; 129:997–1005.

251. Kline JA, Mitchell AM, Kabrhel C, et al. Clinical criteria to prevent unnecessary diagnostic testing in emergency department patients with suspected pulmonary embolism. J Thromb Haemost 2004;2(8):1247–55.

252. Le Gal G, Righini M, Roy PM, et al. Prediction of pulmonary embolism in the emergency department: the revised Geneva score. Ann Intern Med 2006; 144(3):165–71.

253. Klok FA, Kruisman E, Spaan J, et al. Comparison of the revised Geneva score with the Wells rule for assessing clinical probability of pulmonary embolism. J Thromb Haemost 2008;6(1):40–4.

254. Klok FA, Mos IC, Nijkeuter M, et al. Simplification of the revised Geneva score for assessing clinical probability of pulmonary embolism. Arch Intern Med 2008; 168(19):2131–6.

255. Wells PS, Anderson DR, Rodger M, et al. Derivation of a simple clinical model to categorize patients probability of pulmonary embolism: increasing the models utility with the simpleRED d-dimer. Thromb Haemost 2000;83(3):416–20.

256. Wells PS, Anderson DR, Rodger M, et al. Excluding pulmonary embolism at the bedside without diagnostic imaging: management of patients with suspected pulmonary embolism presenting to the emergency department by using a simple clinical model and d-dimer. Ann Intern Med 2001;135(2):98–107.

257. Kline JA, Courtney DM, Kabrhel C, et al. Prospective multicenter evaluation of the pulmonary embolism rule-out criteria. J Thromb Haemost 2008;6(5):772–80.

258. Penaloza A, Verschuren F, Dambrine S, et al. Performance of the pulmonary embolism rule-out criteria (the PERC rule) combined with low clinical probability in high prevalence population. Thromb Res 2012;129(5):e189–93.

259. Wolf SJ, McCubbin TR, Nordenholz KE, et al. Assessment of the pulmonary embolism rule-out criteria rule for evaluation of suspected pulmonary embolism in the emergency department. Am J Emerg Med 2008;26(2):181–5.

260. Singh B, Parsaik AK, Agarwal D, et al. Diagnostic accuracy of pulmonary embolism rule-out criteria: a systematic review and meta-analysis. Ann Emerg Med 2012;59(6):517–20.e1-4.

261. Hugli O, Righini M, Le Gal G, et al. The pulmonary embolism rule-out criteria (PERC) rule does not safely exclude pulmonary embolism. J Thromb Haemost 2011;9(2):300–4.

262. Chagnon I, Bounameaux H, Aujesky D, et al. Comparison of two clinical prediction rules and implicit assessment among patients with suspected pulmonary embolism. Am J Med 2002;133(4):269–75.

263. Kabrhel C, Mark Courtney D, Camargo CA Jr, et al. Potential impact of adjusting the threshold of the quantitative D-dimer based on pretest probability of acute pulmonary embolism. Acad Emerg Med 2009;16(4):325–32.

264. Runyon MS, Webb WB, Jones AE, et al. Comparison of the unstructured clinician estimate of pretest probability for pulmonary embolism to the Canadian score and the Charlotte rule: a prospective observational study. Acad Emerg Med 2005;12(7):587–93.

265. Stone SE, Morris TA. Pulmonary embolism during and after pregnancy. Crit Care Med 2005;33(10):S294–300.

266. Chunilal SD, Wikelboom JW, Attia J, et al. Does this patient have pulmonary embolism? JAMA 2003;290(21):2849–58.

267. Timmons S, Kingston M, Hussain M, et al. Pulmonary embolism: differences in presentation between older and younger patients. Age Ageing 2003;32:601–5.

268. The PIOPED Investigators. Value of the ventilation/perfusion scan in acute pulmonary embolism: results of the Prospective Investigation of Pulmonary Embolism Diagnosis (PIOPED). JAMA 1990;263:1753–9.

269. Boie ET. Initial evaluation of chest pain. Emerg Med Clin North Am 2005;23: 937–57.

270. Stein PD, Sostman HD, Bounameaux H, et al. Challenges in the diagnosis of acute pulmonary embolism. Am J Med 2008;121(7):565–71.

271. Currie GP, Alluri R, Christie GL, et al. Pneumothorax: an update. Postgrad Med J 2007;83:461–5.

272. Holloway VJ, Harris JK. Spontaneous pneumothorax: is it under tension? J Accid Emerg Med 2000;17:222–3.

273. Weissberg D, Refaely Y. Pneumothorax: experience with 1,199 patients. Chest 2005;117(5):1279–85.

274. Leigh-Smith S, Harris T. Tension pneumothorax—time for a rethink? Emerg Med J 2005;22:8–16.

275. Roberts DJ, Leigh-Smith S, Faris PD, et al. Clinical presentation of patients with tension pneumothorax: a systematic review. Ann Surg 2015;261(6):1068–78.

276. Lichtenstein DA, Menu Y. A bedside ultrasound sign ruling out pneumothorax in the critically ill. Lung sliding. Chest 1995;108(5):1245–8.

277. Knudtson JL, Dort JM, Helmer SD, et al. Surgeon-performed ultrasound for pneumothorax in the trauma suite. J Trauma 2004;56(3):527–30.

278. Blaivas M, Lyon M, Duggal S. A prospective comparison of supine chest radiography and bedside ultrasound for the diagnosis of traumatic pneumothorax. Acad Emerg Med 2005;12(9):844–9.

279. Soldati G, Testa A, Sher S, et al. Occult traumatic pneumothorax: diagnostic accuracy of lung ultrasound in the emergency department. Chest 2008;133(1): 204–11.

280. Zhang M, Lui ZH, Yan JX, et al. Rapid detection of pneumothorax by ultrasonography in patients with multiple trauma. Crit Care 2006;10(4):R112.

281. Alrajhi K, Woo MY, Vaillancourt C. Test characteristics of ultrasonography for the detection of pneumothorax, a systematic review and meta-analysis. Chest 2012; 141(3):703–8.

282. Inocencio M, Childs J, Chilstrom ML, et al. Ultrasound findings in tension pneumothorax: a case report. J Emerg Med 2017;52(6):e217–20.

283. Jones R, Hollingsworth J. Tension pneumothorax not responding to needle thoracentesis. Emerg Med J 2002;19:176–7.

284. Laan DV, Vu TD, Thiels CA, et al. Chest wall thickness and decompression failure: a systematic review and meta-analysis comparing anatomic locations in needle thoracostomy. Injury 2016;47(4):797–804.

285. Aho JM, Thiels CA, El Khatib MM, et al. Needle thoracostomy: clinical effectiveness is improved using a longer angiocatheter. J TraumaAcuteCare Surg 2016; 80(2):272–7.

286. Velasco Hernandez DN, Horiuchi HR, Rivaletto LA, et al. Boerhaave's syndrome with late presentation. Experience in an Argentine single center: case series. Ann Med Surg (London) 2019;45:59–61.

287. Griffin SM, Lamb PJ, Shenfine J, et al. Spontaneous rupture of the oesophagus. Br J Surg 2008;95:1115–20.

288. Eroglu A, Kurkcuoglu IC, Karaoglanoglu N, et al. Esophageal perforation: the importance of early diagnosis and primary repair. Dis Esophagus 2004;17:91–4.

289. Blencowe NS, Strong S, Hollowood AD. Spontaneous oesophageal rupture. BMJ 2013;346:f3095.

290. Lemke T, Jagminas L. Spontaneous esophageal rupture: a frequently missed diagnosis. Am Surg 1999;65:449–52.

291. Vidarsdottir H, Blondal S, Alfredsson H, et al. Oesophageal perforations in Iceland: a whole population study on incidence, aetiology and surgical outcome. Thorac Cardiovasc Surg 2010;58(8):476–80.

292. Aiolfi A, Inaba K, Recinos G, et al. Non-iatrogenic esophageal injury: a retrospective analysis from the national trauma data bank. World J Emerg Surg 2017;12:19.

293. Petrone P, Kassimi K, Jimenez-Gomez M, et al. Management of esophageal injuries secondary to trauma. Injury 2017;48(8):1735–42.

294. Rubesin SE, Levin MS. Radiologic diagnosis of gastrointestinal perforation. Radiol Clin North Am 2003;41:1095–115.
295. White CS, Templeton PA, Attar S. Esophageal perforation: CT findings. AJR Am J Roentgenol 1993;160:767–70.
296. Nadrous HF, Afess B, Pfeifer EA, et al. The role of autopsy in the intensive care unit. Mayo Clin Proc 2003;78:947–50.
297. Wacker DA, Winters ME. Shock. Emerg Med Clin North Am 2014;32(4):747–58.
298. Mamas MA, Nair S, Fraser D. Cardiac tamponade and heart failure as a presentation of influenza. Exp Clin Cardiol 2007;12(4):214–6.
299. Gladych E, Goland S, Attali M, et al. Cardiac tamponade as a manifestation of tuberculosis. Southampt Med J 2001;94(5):525–8.
300. Goldberger ZD, Loge AS. Three's company: an unusual clue. Am J Med 2008; 121(9):774–6.
301. Fejka M, Dixon SR, Safian RD, et al. Diagnosis, management, and clinical outcome of cardiac tamponade complicating percutaneous coronary intervention. Am J Cardiol 2002;90:1183–6.
302. Yetter E, Brazg J, Del Valle D, et al. Delayed cardiac tamponade: a rare but life-threatening complication of catheter ablation. Am J Emerg Med 2017;35(5): 803.e1-3.
303. Gerson T, Kuruppu J, Olshaker J. Delayed cardiac tamponade after pacemaker insertion. J Emerg Med 2000;18(3):355–9.
304. Moazzami K, Dolmatova E, Kothari N, et al. Trends in cardiac tamponade among recipients of permanent pacemakers in the United States: from 2008 to 2012. JACC Clin Electrophysiol 2017;3(1):41–6.
305. Orbach A, Schliamser JE, Glugelman MY, et al. Contemporary evaluation of the causes of cardiac tamponade: acute and long-term outcomes. Cardiol J 2016; 23(1):57–63.
306. Sanchez-Enrique C, Nunez-Gil IJ, Viana-Tejedor A, et al. Cause and long-term outcome of cardiac tamponade. Am J Cardiol 2016;117(4):664–9.
307. Roy CL, Minor MA, Brookhart MA, et al. Does this patient with a pericardial effusion have a cardiac tamponade? JAMA 2007;297(16):1810–8.
308. Brown J, MacKinnon D, King A, et al. Elevated arterial blood pressure in cardiac tamponade. N Engl J Med 1992;327(7):463–6.
309. Hoit BD. Pericardial disease and pericardial tamponade. Crit Care Med 2007; 35(8 Suppl):S355–64.
310. Adler Y, Charron P, Imazio M, et al. 2015 ESC guidelines for the diagnosis and management of pericardial diseases: the task force for the diagnosis and management of pericardial diseases of the European society of cardiology (ESC) endorsed by: the European association for cardio-thoracic surgery (EACTS). Eur Heart J 2015;36(42):2921–64.
311. Curtiss EI, Reddy PS, Uretsky BF, et al. Pulsus paradoxus: definition and relation to the severity of cardiac tamponade. Am Heart J 1988;115(2):385–90.
312. Kearns MJ, Walley KR. Tamponade: hemodynamic and echocardiographic diagnosis. Chest 2018;153(5):1266–75.
313. Maisch B, Seferovic PM, Ristic AD, et al. Guideliens on the diagnosis and management of pericardial diseases executive summary; the task force on the diagnosis and management of pericardial diseases of the European society of cardiology. Eur Heart J 2004;25(7):587–610.
314. Guntheroth WG. Sensitivity and specificity of echocardiographic evidence of tamponade: implications for ventricular interdependence and pulsus paradoxus. Pediatr Cardiol 2007;28:358–62.

315. Singh S, Wann LS, Schuchard GH, et al. Right ventricular and right atrial collapse in patients with cardiac tamponade – a combined echocardiographic and hemodynamic study. Circulation 1984;70(6):966–71.
316. Kronzon I, Cohen ML, Winer HE. Diastolic atrial compression: a sensitive echocardiographic sign of cardiac tamponade. J Am Coll Cardiol 1983;2(4):770–5.
317. Klein AL, Abbara S, Agler DA, et al. American society of echocardiography clinical recommendations for multimodality cardiovascular imaging of patients with pericardial disease: endorsed by the society for cardiovascular magnetic resonance and society of cardiovascular computed tomography. J Am Soc Echocardiogr 2013;26(9):965–1012.e15.

High-Risk Chief Complaints
III: Abdomen and Extremities

Sharon Bord, MD*, Christopher El Khuri, MD

KEYWORDS

- Abdominal complaints • Extremity complaints • Risk management
- Orthopedic injuries • Soft tissue injuries

KEY POINTS

- Patients who present to the emergency department with abdominal pain should always have a thorough history and physical examination completed to minimize missed diagnoses.
- Imaging of both patients with abdominal pain and patients with extremity injuries should be carefully considered, weighing risks and benefits.
- Extremity injuries can be high risk for litigation, particularly in patients who work in jobs that require manual labor.

INTRODUCTION

Abdominal and extremity complaints are commonly noted in the emergency department (ED) and clinical vigilance is vital in order not to miss the timely diagnosis of occult or delayed emergencies. If not timely managed, such emergencies are sources of significant patient morbidity and mortality, and may expose ED physicians to possible litigation. Each patient complaint yields to a nuanced approach in diagnostics and therapeutics that can lead the physician toward the ruling in or out of the correct high-risk diagnosis. This article provides an overview of the approach and risk management of this high-risk subset of abdominal and extremity diagnoses in both adult and pediatric populations.

The abdominal diseases covered include appendicitis, abdominal aortic aneurysm (AAA), mesenteric ischemia, and bowel obstruction. For the extremity diseases, the article discusses foreign bodies, hand and finger lacerations, and compartment syndrome. For each complaint, the article highlights the limitations of the history, physical examination, and diagnostic findings; touches on the treatment of these diagnoses; and ends with a summary regarding the risk management of these diseases based on the most recent evidence.

Department of Emergency Medicine, Johns Hopkins University School of Medicine, 1830 E Monument Street, Balitmore, MD 21287, USA
* Corresponding author.
E-mail address: Sbord1@jh.edu

Emerg Med Clin N Am 38 (2020) 499–522
https://doi.org/10.1016/j.emc.2020.02.005
0733-8627/20/© 2020 Elsevier Inc. All rights reserved.
emed.theclinics.com

APPENDICITIS
Epidemiology

Appendicitis is one of the most common abdominal emergencies worldwide, with a lifetime risk ranging from 6% to 9%, a 4 to 1 male to female ratio across all age groups, and a peak incidence between the ages of 10 and 30 years.[1] The cause is poorly understood, and the preoperative diagnosis may be difficult because it must be considered in any patients presenting with acute abdominal pain.[2] Failure to diagnose these patients early (in 1 retrospective study, >36 hours' delay) can lead to increased incidence of appendiceal rupture and unwanted morbidity and mortality.[3] Misdiagnosis is common, with less than 50% of patients presenting with the common signs and symptoms of appendicitis and atypical presentations permeating the populations of the elderly, women, and children.[4] Despite its limitations, clinical examination remains the standard by which emergency physicians determine the probability of appendicitis and further the patients' management in the ED (level B recommendation, American College of Emergency Physicians [ACEP] clinical policies, 2010).[5]

History and Physical Examination

Individually, history and physical examination elements are poor at distinguishing appendicitis from other abdominal disorders. In 1 retrospective study comparing simple versus complicated appendicitis, the top predictive findings of complicated appendicitis were:[6]

- Generalized tenderness (odds ratio [OR], 5.36)
- Symptom duration greater than 12 hours (OR, 3.29)
- Body temperature greater than 38°C or 100.4°F (OR, 2.38)

The findings are congruent with what is seen clinically and support the need to make the diagnosis early. Atypical presentations occur because of anatomic differences and in special populations:

- The anatomy of the appendix can lead to atypical presentations such as right flank pain and right testicular pain (retrocecal), suprapubic pain, and urinary frequency (subcecal), and even left-sided abdominal pain.[7]
- In pregnancy, right lower quadrant (RLQ) abdominal pain and tenderness continues to be the most common symptom and sign, but 20% of patients had right upper quadrant pain, and nonspecific symptoms such as nausea, vomiting, and anorexia were also common among the studied population.[8]
- In children, appendicitis can occur in all age groups but mainly occurs in school children (5–12 years of age). Again, RLQ pain was the most common symptom, but clinicians should also have a high degree of suspicion when children have difficulty with walking or jumping; pain with percussion; and generalized malaise, nausea, or vomiting.[9]
- Elderly have increased morbidity and mortality with perforation of the appendix. RLQ pain and tenderness are most often seen (84%), but the diagnosis should be considered in patients without the classic finding and associated nausea, vomiting, and anorexia.[10]

A commonly referred to symptom of pain while traveling over speed bumps was studied as well and was found to have a modest negative likelihood ratio (LR) 0.1 but poor positive LR 1.4.[11] Overall, history and examination findings alone cannot make the diagnosis but push clinicians' pretest probability toward the best next step in management. In an attempt to objectify the findings, clinical scores based on history, physical examination, and laboratory findings have been developed, such as Alvarado[12] and Appendicitis Inflammatory Response (AIR) score.[2] In a systematic review, the Alvarado score had good sensitivity, poor specificity, but in the end was not any better than a physician's clinical judgment.[12] In recent years, the AIR score has been externally validated in 941 patients, for ages 2 to 96 years, and was found to outperform the Alvarado score with a sensitivity of 93% and a specificity of 85%.[13,14] Although not currently in official guidelines, these scores can be used to further the physician's gestalt and consideration for laboratory tests, imaging, and therapy (**Table 1**).

Laboratory Testing

Several tests, including complete blood count, urinalysis, pregnancy test, and inflammatory markers, are often used in the initial evaluation of appendicitis. A meta-analysis on blood tests in pediatric and adult patients (excluding pregnant patients) with suspected appendicitis noted that, when both tests (white blood cell count [WBC] $\geq$ 10,000 cells/μL and C-reactive protein $\geq$8 mg/dL) were positive, they had a positive LR greater than 23, and, if both were less than this range, there was a negative LR of 0.03.[15] Viewed in isolation, these are neither sensitive nor specific for the diagnosis.

During pregnancy, laboratory tests are even less reliable because of physiologic changes and an inherit mild leukocytosis in this population.[8] Total bilirubin level

Table 1		
Comparison between the Alvarado and Appendicitis Inflammatory Response scores		
Alvarado Score	**AIR Score**	
Ages 4–80 y	Ages 2–96 y	
Nausea or vomiting[1]	Vomiting[1]	
RLQ abdominal pain[1]	Right iliac fossa pain[1]	
Rebound tenderness[1]	Rebound tenderness	Light[1] Medium[2] Severe[3]
Increased temperature (37.3°C or 99.1°F)[1]	Temp $\geq$ 38.5°C (101.3°F)[1]	
Leukocyte left shift >75% neutrophils[1]	Polymorphonuclear leukocytes (%)	<70[1] 70–84[2] $\geq$85
Leukocytosis (>10,000/mm³)[2]	White blood cell count (× 10⁹/L)	<10[1] 10–14.9[2] >15[3]
Migration of pain to the right lower quadrant[1] and/or anorexia[1]	CRP level (mg/L)	<10[1] 10–49[2] $\geq$50[3]
0–3, unlikely appendicitis	0–4, outpatient management	
4–6, CT scan recommended	5–8, indeterminate	
7–9, surgical consultation	9–12, surgical exploration	

Abbreviations: CRP, C-reactive protein; CT, computed tomography.
Adapted from Bhangu A, Soreide K, Di Saverio S, Assarsson JH, Drake FT. Acute appendicitis: Modern understanding of pathogenesis, diagnosis, and management. *Lancet.* 2015;386(10000):1278-1287. Doi: S0140-6736(15)00275-5 [pii].

greater than 1 mg/dL has been shown to have a modest predictive value for a perforated appendix in adults, with 70% sensitivity 86% specificity as well.[16] Procalcitonin, amyloid, and calprotectin have been investigated but none of them were found to be robust enough in ruling in or out the diagnosis.[17,18] Urinalysis is essential in the diagnosing of other causes of lower abdominal pain, but up to 40% of patients with appendicitis can have urinalysis abnormalities, including pyuria, hematuria, or bacteriuria.[19]

Radiologic Evaluation

Various imaging techniques are available to clinicians when the diagnosis of acute appendicitis is being entertained, including ultrasonography (US), computed tomography (CT), and MRI. The choice of imaging modality depends on several patient-specific factors, reader proficiency, and technology limitations.

CT is the most common modality used in the United States in adolescents and adults with suspected appendicitis and is currently recommended for confirmation before surgery by the ACEP (level B evidence).[2,5] The use of low versus standard radiation dosing, contrast versus noncontrast imaging, and focused scanning have been debated in the literature:

- Low-radiation-dose versus standard-radiation-dose CT scan, with or without contrast, was found to have a 96% sensitivity and 93% specificity according to a recent systematic review.[20]
- CT with or without contrast had similar sensitivity and specificity in detecting appendicitis based on multiple studies.[21,22] ACEP (level B) advocates that intravenous (IV) versus oral contrast may increase sensitivity, but this continues to be debated with the recent literature that has been released.[5] The use of oral or IV contrast may be useful in patients with low body mass index (BMI) because it is difficult to appreciate fat stranding in this population or diagnose other disorders, such as inflammatory disease and diverticulitis.

Because of the inherent risks and radiation exposure associated with CT scans, US has been added in lieu of or in addition to other imaging modalities for making the diagnosis of appendicitis, particularly in children and pregnant patients. In 1 recent systematic review, pooled sensitivity and specificity of 69% and 81% make US poor at ruling out, but possibly helpful at ruling in, the diagnosis across all populations.[23] Subgroup analysis in another systematic review showed that the younger the patient (<19 years of age), the more sensitive the US,[24] likely because of thinner wall musculature, less abdominal fat, and trained pediatric US operators because of the need of avoiding radiation in this population. The use of US for the confirmation of appendicitis in children, but not for excluding it, is endorsed by ACEP (level B) and encouraged as the initial imaging modality (level C).[5] US may also be useful in pregnant patients or women because it can also be used to evaluate for other pelvic emergencies.

The final modality to consider is MRI, whose utility in being specific and sensitive in ruling out appendicitis must be balanced by its cost burden, time constraints, and limited availability to emergency physicians.[25] At present, MRI use should be limited to nondiagnostic US in pregnant patients and children, with the caveat of avoiding gadolinium in first-trimester pregnancies.[25]

Treatment

Per the American College of Surgeons, the current gold standard intervention for uncomplicated appendicitis in all age groups is appendectomy.[26] The role of emergency physicians is to make the patient comfortable, decrease complications, and ensure a timely and safe transport to the operating room:

- Patients should be treated with appropriate analgesics in the setting of appendicitis. Although a Cochrane Review showed a nonsignificant pain reduction with morphine, it did not mask examination findings or impair diagnosis.[27]
- Narrow-spectrum antibiotics (cefotetan, cefoxitin, or cefazolin plus metronidazole) more than 60 minutes before surgery for uncomplicated appendicitis is recommended to cover gram-negative aerobes and anaerobes and decrease postoperative infection rates.[28,29] Antibiotics should be escalated if there is any risk of perforation or other signs of complicated appendicitis. These antibiotics include carbapenems and combination antibiotics for broader coverage.[28]
- Although still being studied, antibiotics can treat uncomplicated appendicitis in some patients without surgery but the recurrence rate is 5% to 15% within 1 year without differences in major or minor complications.[30]
- These recommendations hold for pregnant patients as well as pediatrics, although their nuanced approaches would be best discussed with the consulting surgeon.

Risk Management Strategy

A high index of suspicion is required for all comers to the ED with abdominal pain, especially in the elderly, children, and pregnant populations. Effectively, emergency physicians need to risk manage 2 unique diagnostic dilemmas: those patients with low pretest probability of the disease versus those with a moderate to high pretest probability and negative imaging findings but a continued concerning clinical picture. At present, the best approach to determine the pretest probability involves a thorough history and physical examination and, although not incorporated into national guidelines, physicians can use scores such as the AIR score for adult patients to more objectively analyze a patient's risk. There is limited use for these in pregnant and elderly patients.

- For low-risk patients, a patient-centered shared decision-making conversation should be conducted with strict return precautions well delineated, verbally communicated, and clearly written on the discharge instructions. Patients should be able to gauge the risk of the diagnostic modalities and risks of surgery versus observation in the ED versus observation at home. For those staying in the ED, documentation of serial abdominal examinations and discussion with consultants and primary care physicians is vital.
- For moderate-risk to high-risk patients with negative CT scans and a persistent clinical suspicion, physicians should not hesitate to keep these patients in the ED for observation or admit them for serial abdominal examinations. Their discharge process should be as nuanced as for those that are low risk.

ABDOMINAL AORTIC ANEURYSM
Epidemiology

An AAA is a high-risk diagnosis in patients presenting to the ED because of the high mortality associated with aneurysmal rupture. Although current literature is inconsistent on its epidemiology, roughly 15,000 deaths in the United States are attributed to ruptured AAAs, with incidences ranging from less than 1% to 12% in the United Statespopulation.[31] Globally, the incidence of AAA has decreased over the past

2 decades and most diagnoses are found incidentally in asymptomatic patients.[32] Astute emergency physicians should always keep this diagnosis on the differential, and fine tune pretest probability based on high-risk features on the history and physical examination.[33]

History and Physical Examination

In patients in whom the diagnosis of AAA is being considered, a thorough review of the patient's risk factors is the most important part of the history. Risk factors for AAA include male sex, untreated hyperlipidemia, smoking (especially in those >40 years of age), hypertension (blood pressure >160/100 mm Hg), family history of AAA, history of large vessel aneurysms, and increasing age (>65 years of age) per epidemiologic studies.[34] Recently, fluoroquinolone use within 60 days has also been implicated, with a hazard ratio of 1.9 in adults more than 50 years of age.[35] Factors associated with decreased risk of AAA include black race, Hispanic ethnicity, and diabetes.[36]

AAA clinically presents in 3 ways: asymptomatic, symptomatic nonruptured, and symptomatic ruptured.

- The most common presentation is asymptomatic, which poses a diagnostic conundrum for ED physicians. These patients may be managed without ever being formally diagnosed with AAA or found to have an incidental AAA on radiographic imaging obtained for another purpose. Specialist consultation in the ED versus outpatient follow-up should dictated by the size of the AAA.[32]
- In patients with symptomatic nonruptured AAA, symptoms are vague and may include indolent abdominal discomfort, lower back pain, or flank pain.[37]
- In 1 retrospective study of 66 patients with symptomatic ruptured AAA, 25% did not present with pain, 45% presented with abdominal pain, and 17% presented with flank pain.[38] From 25% to 50% of patients present with the classic triad of abdominal pain, hypotension, and pulsatile abdominal mass.[32] Despite these percentages, abdominal pain and/or back pain coupled with hypotension should bring the diagnosis of ruptured AAA immediately to mind.

Because of the vague clinical presentations of AAA, a good physical examination is critical.[32] A pulsatile abdominal mass is the most common physical examination finding in AAA. In 1 study, abdominal palpation had a sensitivity of 91% if the patient's abdominal girth was less than 102 cm (40 inches) but decreased to 82% if the girth was any larger. The physical examination's diagnostic performance expectantly improves with enlargement of the AAA and decrease in abdominal circumference.[33] Ecchymosis around the flanks (Grey Turner), periumbilical (Cullen), scrotum (Bryant), and proximal thigh (Fox) are nonspecific for the diagnosis.[39] A lower extremity examination to assess for distal limb ischemia is strongly recommended by the Society of Vascular Surgeons in patients suspected of having AAA.[40]

Laboratory Work

No current laboratory tests can significantly sway physicians to image for AAA. Biomarkers of coagulation and specifically D dimer have been studied with mixed results. D dimer level has been shown to increase sequentially with increasing AAA size but no real cutoff has been suggested because of poor sensitivity and specificity.[41] Further research is warranted, and the utility of laboratory work is to assess for other diagnoses or sequelae of AAA, such as severe blood loss, infected aneurysm, and preoperative testing.

Radiologic Evaluation

Although CT scan continues to be most used test for most abdominal disorders, US remains the gold standard for the diagnosis and monitoring of patients with AAA.[42] The United States Preventive Services Task Force (USPSTF) has been using US for the monitoring of asymptomatic AAA larger than 3 cm for more than a decade in male patients more than 65 years of age with a history of smoking, with excellent sensitivity and specificity.[42] In addition, based on a systematic review, bedside US in the ED had a sensitivity and specificity of 99% in symptomatic patients.[43] These findings were across different patient populations and ultrasonographers, but increased BMI, nonfasting state, and ileus are all associated with poorer-quality images.[43]

Especially in the setting of symptomatic AAA, CT is necessary for a definitive diagnosis because it is more reproducible, more reliable, and allows better visualization of the aneurysm and its tributaries.[40] Although contrast is not required for ruptured aneurysms, it is highly desired for those patients being considered for endovascular therapy and should be the go-to modality in the ED.[40] CT can also better stratify patients' US readings that are equivocal, because AAAs of less than 5-cm diameter are underestimated by 0.5 mm by US.[44] Furthermore, CT can also differentiate AAA from other common causes of abdominal pain that masquerade as flank pain and lower back pain (eg, nephrolithiasis, appendicitis).

The use of MRI is limited in AAA considering its emergent quality as a diagnosis. One possible use is in patients who are allergic to iodinated contrast and require definitive abdominal imaging.[32]

Treatment

Initial management in the ED for symptomatic nonruptured AAA and ruptured AAA can be summarized by the following 4 items:

- Emergent consultation to vascular surgery, because the definitive treatment is open versus endovascular repair.
- Preparation of blood products and appropriate preoperative laboratory testing. There should be no delay in transfusion, and the emergency physician should transfuse uncrossmatched blood products as necessary in patients with symptomatic ruptured AAA and/or hemodynamically unstable patients.
- Based on trauma literature and observational studies on AAA, permissive hypotension of systolic blood pressure of 80 to 100 mm Hg may prevent further aortic wall tearing.[45] The use of antihypertensives, such as esmolol, to achieve this is still under debate.
- Control pain, which can contribute to increase in blood pressure.

Risk Management Strategy

ED physicians should consider this diagnosis in patients more than 50 years of age, presenting with abdominal pain, hypotension, or any associated symptoms of poor perfusion (eg, light headedness, syncope, decreased lower extremity pulses, mottled lower extremity skin). Patients with risk factors or with vague symptoms such as lower back pain or flank pain should also raise suspicion of the diagnosis and prompt a good abdominal examination with palpation for an enlarged abdominal aorta. Be wary of the first diagnosis of renal colic in these groups of patients, and remember that, despite its utility, the abdominal examination is only 82% sensitive for AAA in patients with increased abdominal girth.[33] Stable, symptomatic, unruptured patients should undergo bedside US, followed by CT scan with IV contrast.

Emergency physicians should consider obtaining urgent vascular consultation depending on pretest probability and the findings on the bedside US. Unstable ruptured patients should undergo basic emergency resuscitation and emergent vascular consultation, with the bedside US being critical in the early recognition of these patients.[40]

MESENTERIC ISCHEMIA
Epidemiology

Mesenteric ischemia is reported to account for about 1% of all acute abdomens presenting to the ED, increasing to about 10% in patients more than 70 years of age, and has high mortality across all age groups.[46] Mesenteric ischemia occurs when blood supply to the intestines fails to meet metabolic demand. The 4 major mechanisms behind this disease are arterial embolism (40%–50%); arterial thrombosis/atherosclerosis (25%–30%); nonocclusive ischemia, seen usually in low-flow states such as hemodialysis or extracorporeal membrane oxygenation (ECMO) (20%); and mesenteric venous thrombosis (10%–25%).[47] The rare incidence as well as the different causes make the diagnosis of mesenteric ischemia challenging in ED patients with acute abdominal pain.

History and Physical Examination

Based on cross-sectional studies, mesenteric ischemia tends to occur more in older adults more than 60 years of age and those with typical cardiovascular risk factors such as nicotine use, diabetes, hypertension, and dyslipidemia.[48,49] A large number of patients with mesenteric ischemia caused by an arterial embolism or thrombosis were found to have atrial fibrillation or other cardiovascular risk factors.[50] As mentioned, nonocclusive mesenteric ischemia occurred more in long-term dialysis and cardiac surgery patients requiring ECMO.[47] Expectantly, those with mesenteric venous thrombosis were more likely to have thrombophilias and diseases that cause an acquired hypercoagulable state.[46]

A careful history is necessary to tease out patients with this diagnosis because of the different causes and risk factors. Of note, one-third of patients with arterial embolic mesenteric ischemia have had a similar episode in the past. A personal or family history of pulmonary embolism or deep vein thrombosis is noted in almost one-half of patients diagnosed with mesenteric venous thrombosis.[51] It is best to approach the history and physical examination from a causal standpoint as well:

- Classically, patients with acute occlusive arterial disease present with abdominal cramping for a few hours followed by a pain-free interval, followed by peritonitis. They may or may not have gastrointestinal bleeding and other systemic complaints.[48]
- Arterial thrombotic disease presents more subacutely because of the production of collaterals, delaying an acute presentation by days to weeks.[46]
- For nonocclusive disease, progressively worsening abdominal pain is expected in the right clinical context.[47]
- Mesenteric venous thrombosis presents abruptly and can be difficult to differentiate from acute occlusive arterial disease without a detailed history and past medical history.[46]

The classic physical examination finding is pain out of proportion to examination because there is minimal abdominal tenderness preceding the progression to transmural bowel ischemia and subsequent peritonitis. This finding is neither specific nor sensitive. Occult blood may be found during the examination as well.[46] In short, the history and physical examination can provide clues for the clinician as to the cause and possibly the stage of ischemia but is far from being a definitive tool for the diagnosis of mesenteric ischemia.

Laboratory Work

Laboratory work is used to rule out other causes of acute abdomen with no laboratory finding that can definitively rule out the diagnosis. Clinicians should keep mesenteric ischemia higher on the differential with abdominal pain and concurrent metabolic acidosis or uptrending lactate as a subtle indicator of possible intra-abdominal ischemia. Although D dimer has been studied in ruling out mesenteric ischemia, there continue to be limited data on its use.[52]

Radiologic Evaluation

Historically, the gold standard for diagnosing mesenteric ischemia was arteriography, but that has since been supplanted by more practical imaging modalities in the ED, such as CT angiography (CTA) and magnetic resonance angiography (MRA):

- CTA is considered the gold standard for the diagnosis in the ED, with sensitivity and specificity approaching 100% for arterial occlusive and thrombotic disease.[38,53] CTA continues to be diagnostic in most patients with venous occlusive disease and nonocclusive disease.[53] Typical use of CTA is with IV contrast only.
- MRA can be considered in those in whom radiation needs to be limited but time constraints and issues with resolution in the distal branches of intestinal arteries limit its utility.[38]

Treatment

For most patients, surgical intervention is the definitive therapy. In the ED, clinicians should focus on basic resuscitation, attempting to restore intestinal blood flow and pain control, and avoid worsening the underlying problem. Per the American Cardiology Conference/American Heart Association (ACC/AHA), the most important step is reversal of shock with IV fluids and monitoring of urine output hourly, in addition to other markers of systemic perfusion such as serum lactate.[38] Attempt to avoid vasopressors and vasoconstrictive medications. If advanced blood pressure therapy is required, dobutamine, low-dose dopamine, or milrinone can be considered.[38] Timely administration of heparin, regardless of suspected cause, and antibiotics (second-generation cephalosporins or levofloxacin plus metronidazole) are important steps in the resuscitation of these patients.[38,47] Consider keeping patients nil by mouth so as not to exacerbate the underlying ischemia.[46]

Risk Management

In a recent systematic review, the pooled mortality of acute mesenteric ischemia was 47%. All emergency physicians should keep this diagnosis high on the differential for patients presenting with abdominal pain, especially in the elderly with a concerning past medical history and history of presenting illness.[54] Based on laboratory findings of metabolic acidosis, increased WBC counts, and a concerning story, surgical consultation should be called early and CTA ordered. However, at this time there are no validated scores or well-studied laboratory tests to rule the diagnosis in or out, and clinicians must base their pretest probability on the evidence available. In patients in whom mesenteric ischemia is diagnosed, initiation of therapy expeditiously and prompt discussion of management with the surgery team is essential. For those with negative CTA but a heightened clinical suspicion, observation in the ED or hospital is reasonable. It is also essential to documented serial abdominal examination and progressively improving pain scores during the patient's clinical course.

SMALL BOWEL OBSTRUCTION
Epidemiology

Small bowel obstruction (SBO) is a common diagnosis in the ED, accounting for 12% to 16% of all surgical admissions to the hospital.[55] In addition, a recent systematic review noted an incidence of 9% from any cause after abdominal surgery.[56] The most common cause of SBO is postsurgical adhesions, accounting for more than two-thirds of all cases, followed by malignancy and hernias.[56] Although the clinical course of SBO tends toward self-resolution despite the grade of obstruction, it carries a significant risk of bowel necrosis, perforation, and subsequent peritonitis, making it a required part of the ED physician's differential for acute abdominal pain.[55]

History and Physical Examination

Risk factors for SBO are directly related to the most common cause for the disease. Physicians must ask for previous surgical history, abdominal hernias, intestinal inflammation, history of malignancies, and any history of abdominal radiation.[55] Classically, adhesions caused by previous surgeries are the main cause for this disease, but 3% to 9% of patients with SBO caused by adhesions have no previous history of surgery.[57] A history of previous partial obstructions also increases the risk of subsequent episodes.[55]

In terms of history, a recent systematic review suggested that historical elements could significantly increase the likelihood of the disease without any 1 element sufficient to rule it out.[58] In a population of 2500 with 4% having SBO, the following 3 elements were most predictive:

- History of constipation (90%–95% specific)
- History of previous abdominal surgery (74%–78% specific)
- Relief with vomiting (93%–94% specific)

The same systematic review showed that no examination finding can exclude the diagnosis of SBO, but abdominal distention was most predictive, with 89% to 96% specificity. The literature describes auscultation of tinkling bowel sounds representing increased intestinal peristalsis followed by decrease in abdominal sounds with prolonged obstruction. The utility of this finding is questionable in terms of distinguishing power because the systematic review showed increased, decreased, and abnormal bowel sounds having similar predictive value in making the diagnosis. ED physicians should also observe for any signs of dehydration with prolonged obstruction and vital sign changes that could signal perforation, peritonitis, or infection.[58] Of note, the diagnosis of SBO can exist without abdominal pain or abdominal tenderness on examination.

Laboratory Work

Blood tests are geared toward the sequelae of SBO, such as vomiting and bowel ischemia, and not for making the diagnosis. Although not specifically studied, complete blood count and a chemistry panel can be considered in the assessment and triage of these patients and can assist with ruling out other medical illness, including electrolyte abnormalities. Serum lactate has been investigated and can be 90% sensitive with a negative predictive value of 96% in ruling out intestinal ischemia.[59]

Imaging

As with all previously described abdominal disorders, multiple imaging modalities have been studied in SBO, and CT with IV contrast and without oral contrast is currently the gold standard and initial choice per The Eastern Association for the Surgery of Trauma (EAST) guidelines.[55] The current recommendations for CT scan are:

- Oral contrast is contraindicated, because of side effects and delay in diagnosis.[55]
- If IV contrast is contraindicated, CT without contrast has comparable diagnostic power.[55]
- Although it is considered the first-line imaging modality, CT scan with IV contrast has 87% sensitivity and 81% specificity for the diagnosis.[58]

Abdominal radiographs are another consideration but their diagnostic power is poor in diagnosing SBO (75% sensitivity, 65% specificity).[58] US is gaining increasing traction in the diagnosis of SBO, especially point-of-care US (POCUS) in the ED. A recent study comparing POCUS with CT showed comparable sensitivity of around 88% when ED physicians looked for intraperitoneal fluid, abnormal peristalsis, small bowel edema, and small bowel dilatation to greater than 25 mm.[60] Formal and emergency US were also studied in a systematic review and found to have acceptable sensitivity and specificity of greater than 90%, but the review was limited by heterogeneity.[58] US continues to have the limitation of poor image quality in obese patients and is operator dependent.

In addition, MRI can be considered for pregnant patients, children, and young patients with a history of multiple CT scans.[55] MRI with and without contrast has been shown to have comparable diagnostic value compared with CT.[58]

Treatment

Not all patients diagnosed with SBO require surgery. Up to 80% of patients with adhesive SBO can be treated nonoperatively.[61] For those treated nonoperatively, a small portion (3%–6%) go on to have bowel ischemia and other complications.[62] Indications for surgery include clinical findings that suggest peritonitis, perforation, or bowel ischemia. These findings include fever, tachycardia, continuous pain, and laboratory findings of ischemia.[55] Surgical consultation should be obtained for disposition planning and clinical input.

Aside from basic resuscitation with IV fluids, implementing bowel rest in the setting of multiple episodes of nausea and vomiting, and adequate pain control, treatment may include the insertion of a nasogastric (NG) tube for bowel decompression. Copious 2% lidocaine jelly application or 4 mL of 10% nebulized lidocaine should be used for comfort.[63] NG tube use has not been studied in the setting of SBO. A risk/benefit consideration may be wise, because a meta-analysis regarding NG tube placement postlaparotomy improved nausea, vomiting, and abdominal distention but did increase the risk of fever, atelectasis, and pneumonia.[64]

Risk Management

Although most SBO cases are treated nonoperatively, those that do require surgery and have high-grade obstructions can reach high levels of mortality.[55] In addition, over 5 years, patients admitted for SBO can have up to a 19% readmission rate, based on 1 study.[65] A good past medical and surgical history can provide clues for the clinician to the diagnosis and sway the pretest probability toward imaging. During the history and physical examination, history of constipation, relief with vomiting, and abdominal distention on examination had the most predictive power for the diagnosis.

However, it is important to remember that SBO can occur without abdominal pain or tenderness on examination. Laboratory tests may help with assessing for surgical need and guide resuscitation, but do not assist in making the diagnosis. CT with IV contrast and without oral contrast is the recommended imaging modality. US is slowly gaining traction in this realm. In the management of these patients, as with all abdominal emergencies, serial abdominal examinations and solid documentation are essential. Physicians should always be ready to escalate diagnostics in patients who are not obviously improving in terms of oral intake, pain, or serial laboratory work during their ED course. The choice to go for surgery versus observation should be made in conjunction with the consultant.

RETAINED FOREIGN BODY IN ACUTE WOUNDS
Epidemiology

Patients presenting with lacerations to the ED made up approximately 5% of visits, or 7 million patients.[66] Of these patients who present to the ED with a laceration or open wound, only a small percentage are complicated by a retained foreign body (FB). Despite being unusual, they have been found to be often missed, with 1 study revealing that 75 of 200 FBs in the hand were missed.[67] Wounds complicated by FBs are most common during warmer weather because of increased exposure of bare skin and outdoor activities.[68] Wounds that are at highest risk of retained FBs include puncture wounds and wounds that were caused by shattering glass. Among patients with injuries from shattered glass, 15% were found to have retained glass.[69] The most common FBs include wood (eg, splinters), metal (eg, BB pellets), and glass/ceramic.[70] Unrecognized retained FBs may lead to infection and persistent pain, which may in turn result in malpractice claims.

History and Physical Examination

The focus of the history should be on the mechanism of injury. In a study of 490 patients with ICD-9 (International Classification of Diseases, Ninth Revision) diagnosis of wound with FB, approximately two-thirds were caused by either stepping on something or sustaining a wound from a foreign material.[70] This study also found that most patients present in the first 48 hours following the trauma.[70] A patient reporting an FB sensation to the provider has a positive predictive value of 31%.[69] It is also important to ascertain the patient's past medical history to assess for risk factors for wound infections, such as diabetes or immunosuppressive therapy.

The focus in the physical examination should consist of assessing the wound, carefully examining the wound for FBs, and examining the skin for palpable FBs under the surface. FBs may also damage nerves or blood vessels, making it imperative to perform a thorough neurovascular examination of the injured area.[68] It is important to remember that even small wounds can harbor retained FBs.[67]

Imaging

Determining which imaging study to obtain in a case of suspected retained FB can be challenging. The pearls and pitfalls of plain film radiograph, US, and CT scan re discussed here to assist in determining the presence or absence of an FB. Some clinicians argue that, in the case of visualized FB, no additional imaging is necessary, but, in wounds that primarily had glass FBs, there is usually more than 1 FB present.[70]

Plain Film Radiograph

Radiography is most helpful when looking for a radio-opaque FB, most commonly glass or metal but also including bone, teeth, gravel/rock, and some fish spines.[68]

In 1 study of 490 cases of FB, in which half the patients had radiographs performed, the sensitivity of radiography was 75% for glass, 98% for metal, and 7% for wood.[70]

- Radiography remains the criterion standard for diagnosis of FBs, with a sensitivity of 83% to 99% when looking for glass.[71]
- Based on current evidence, radiography has a 0.6% to 4.3% rate of retained FB after adequate wound exploration.[71]

Computed Tomography Scan

CT scan can be used to detect both radio-opaque and radiolucent FBs, but has a greater sensitivity for radio-opaque ones such as glass or metal.

- CT scan to detect radiolucent FBs performed better than plain radiography, but still is notable for having intermediate sensitivity.
- CT scans are associated with higher levels of ionized radiation and increased patient cost, but may be of benefit if an FB is strongly suspected but not visualized on other imaging modalities.
- CT may be useful in the setting of possible abscess or infection because it can also help detect inflammation or damage to deeper tissues.[72]

Ultrasonography

Performance of bedside US in the ED is extraordinarily common and easily accessible. US can look for both radio-opaque and radiolucent FBs, both of which are hyperechoic on imaging and produce posterior shadowing.

- US can be most helpful when looking for a radiolucent FB such as wood or plastic. FBs made of these substances are not reliably visualized on plain radiography.[73]
- The sensitivity of US to detect FB has been found to range between 43% to 98% with a specificity of 59% to 98%.[72] One study found that US performed by emergency medicine physicians had a sensitivity of 96.7%, identifying 29 of 30 FBs.[74] A systematic review found extensive heterogeneity and potential bias among studies, but concluded that US has high specificity and moderate sensitivity for detection of FBs.[75]
- US may be limited by air in the soft tissue, in which case, CT scan may be more beneficial.[72]

Treatment

Treatment of a wound FB depends on the material of the FB as well as how accessible it is for removal. FBs that are superficial can likely easily be removed in the ED. FBs that are deeper and have a low potential for infection can often remain in place; however, consideration should be made for relationship to critical surrounding structures, such as nerves and blood vessels.[67] Patients with persistent FB sensation, those at high risk for infection such as organic matter, and those with FB with close proximity to a critical structure should be referred to a surgical service for further management.

Risk Management Discussion

Patients with a retained FB are at risk for infection, chronic pain, or damage to soft tissue or surrounding structures if not recognized in a timely fashion. Wound management that includes FB retention has been consistently found to be one of the top causes of litigation, representing 10.7% of malpractice claims.[76] The diagnosis of FB should be suspected based on the patient's history and physical examination. A concerning history should prompt further exploration for FB. Decision for imaging modality should be made based on composition of the FB, with plain radiographs used in locating a radio-opaque FB such as glass or metal. CT and US may be helpful in determining the presence of organic matter or radio-opaque FBs. If a wound FB is located, the ED provider should consider ease of removal of the FB and engage the patient in discussion regarding risks and benefits of removal. If a patient has a wound with high risk for FB or a persistent FB sensation but no FB is found during the ED evaluation, the patient should be informed of the risk for missed FB and be provided with strict return precautions. At times, surgical consultants may need to be involved in more complicated cases that require removal.[67]

HAND AND FINGER LACERATIONS
Epidemiology

Simple hand lacerations are a common reason for ED visits. A 2007 study found that 1.8 million presentations were for hand laceration, with 1.6 million of those individuals requiring laceration repair. Hand injury is also associated with up to 8% of trauma-related visits.[77] An important risk management discussion related to this topic is wound infection, but the data regarding infection following simple hand laceration are antiquated and disparate, ranging from less than 1% to 12%,[78] and it remains unclear what places patients in a higher risk group for infection. In addition, hand injuries with possible tendon, nerve, or vascular damage can lead to diminished functional status following the injury, mandating extreme care be taken when managing these injuries.[79]

History and Physical Examination

Obtaining a careful medical history can aid with identification of patients at increased risk of wound infection. It is important to ask patients the mechanism of the injury and to ascertain whether there was any bite-related injury or risk for FB, because these may increase infection risk.[77] Although there are no clearly defined risks for patients with simple hand lacerations, a study of 23,000 surgical incisions found that patients with diabetes mellitus, obesity, malnutrition, advanced age, and steroid use were at increased risk.[80] Tetanus vaccination history should be obtained.

Examination of the wound must take place with optimal lighting and visualization of the affected area. A thorough neurovascular examination should be performed to assess for circulation and pulses distal to the wound as well as limitations in strength and changes in sensation. Examination, particularly the sensory examination, should take place before anesthetizing the area. The wound must also be assessed for bleeding and surrounding tissue damage.[77] Thorough documentation of both the wound as well as the neurovascular examination and tendon function is of utmost importance in patients with hand injuries.

Treatment

The current standard of care for management of hand wounds includes irrigation of the wound, debridement, and removal of FBs as indicated, followed by repair of the wound.[79] Repair of hand lacerations is generally accomplished using simple interrupted sutures, because these sutures provide a high-tensile strength, which is needed because of extensive movement of hands. Local anesthetics used either directly at the wound or via regional anesthesia or digital block remain the mainstay for analgesia when repairing hand lacerations.[77] There are several controversies that exist within management of lacerations:

- Irrigation procedure: normal saline or tap water can be used to irrigate the laceration. There have been several studies that have examined infection rates in patients whose lacerations were irrigated with sterile normal saline versus tap water and repeatedly infection rates have been found to be similar in both groups.[81,82] Pressurized irrigation has been found to lead to decreased bacterial contamination in wounds; however, the optimal pressure has been debated. The goal of pressurized irrigation is to clean the wound, but too much pressure can cause damage to surrounding tissues.[77]
- Prophylactic antibiotics: based on current literature, it is unclear which patients with hand lacerations are at risk of infection. A multicenter study sought to determine risk factors for infection following traumatic laceration, not limited to just the hand. They examined 2663 patients and found that a history of diabetes, wound contamination, and wounds greater than 5 cm in length put patients in a higher-risk category with wound infections of greater than 5%. Interestingly, no association was found between wound infection and timing between injury and repair.[83] In 1 randomized controlled trial in which patients with hand lacerations were given cephalexin, clindamycin, or placebo, the infection rate was 1% in all groups. This study had a small enrollment of 78 patients and the investigators concluded that larger studies need to be completed before conclusions can be made on this topic.[79] A systematic review of 3 articles was completed and there was no statistical difference in infection rates in patients who received either antibiotics or placebo.[84] Individuals with lacerations related to bites should receive prophylactic antibiotics because of infection risk.

Risk Management Considerations

Hand lacerations and wounds are common causes for litigation. Tendon injuries and wound complications have been cited as a high-risk area.[76] One study from France found them to represent 10% of all emergency medicine–related personal injury claims in 2013. The most common injury sites that triggered a claim were the thumb and the index finger. Claims were filed because of inadequate wound exploration, stiffness of the involved area, and dysesthesias. The most common missed lesions were damage to a tendon or a nerve.[85] In patients with hand lacerations, ED physicians can minimize risk by performing a thorough physical examination with focus on circulation, sensation, and motor distal to the injury. Patients should be provided with appropriate wound care instructions and strict return precautions to include signs or symptoms of infection. In addition, patients should be referred to hand surgery for follow-up in cases of persistent pain or suspected tendon or nerve injury.

COMPARTMENT SYNDROME
Epidemiology

Acute compartment syndrome is caused by increased pressure within a closed compartment, which in turn leads to decreased perfusion of the soft tissue. This condition is generally caused by either an increase in the contents of an enclosed space, such as occurs with bleeding or swelling, or a decrease in the volume of an enclosed space caused by a tight cast or ace wrap.[86] It requires early recognition and acute surgical intervention and has an high morbidity and mortality associated with missed diagnosis.

- Acute compartment syndrome is most common among individuals less than 35 years old because of increased muscle bulk, stronger fascial tissue, and higher-risk injuries. Men are affected 10 times more than women.[87]

- Among studies from 2 large trauma centers, patients with trauma had a rate of acute compartment syndrome of approximately 1%, which is in contrast with prior studies that found a rate of 0.7 per 100,000 among women but as high as 7.3 per 100,000 among male patients. Mechanisms of injury that were most commonly associated with development of acute compartment syndrome include motorcycle accident, pedestrians being struck, gunshot wounds, and stab wounds.[88,89]
- The most common cause of compartment syndrome is fractures, with tibial fractures being the most commonly associated fracture, representing 2% to 9% of acute compartment syndromes.[87] However, there are many other causes of compartment syndrome, which include blunt injury, acute ischemia with reperfusion, deep venous thrombosis, overexertion, drug use, and iatrogenic causes such as contrast dye extravasation.[87,88]
- The most common location for compartment syndrome is the anterior tibial compartment, but it can also occur in the hand, forearm, foot, thigh, and buttocks.[90]

History and Physical Examination

Initially the provider should take a thorough history to determine the mechanism of injury. It is important to perform a full trauma survey in the appropriate clinical situation. Special concern for compartment syndrome should be maintained for patients with altered mental status, intoxication, or loss of consciousness, because they may not be able to communicate regarding pain in the extremity.[87]

The history and physical examination should focus on the 5 Ps (pain, paresthesia, paralysis, pallor and pulselessness) although overall these signs and symptoms have low sensitivity but high specificity for diagnosing acute compartment syndrome.[87] Pain is the earliest sign of compartment syndrome and is often noted to be out of proportion to what was expected from the original injury.[91] However, measuring pain is subjective, making its use in diagnosis more challenging.[87] Pulselessness is a late sign that often indicates a poor outcome for the patient.[92] Inspecting and palpating the compartment may reveal firmness or swelling, but again this finding alone is unreliable.[87] It is possible to increase the sensitivity by combining multiple findings. Pain with passive stretch and paresthesias and pain with rest increase sensitivity to 93%, and adding in paresis increases sensitivity to 98%.[87] Serial examinations should be performed, ideally by the same clinician.

Diagnosis

A high level of suspicion is the first step in diagnosing acute compartment syndrome because many of the signs, symptoms, and testing can be nonspecific or inconclusive. Emergency consultation with either orthopedic or plastic/hand surgery should be obtained for all patients in whom the diagnosis of compartment syndrome is suspected. Diagnostic testing for compartment syndrome includes measurement of creatine kinase (CK), renal function, and urinalysis to assess for myoglobinuria. CK levels continue to increase as compartment syndrome progresses, making it less useful for early diagnosis.[87,92] Imaging studies should be obtained to evaluate for fracture if not performed earlier in the patient's evaluation.

Intracompartmental pressure measurement can confirm the diagnosis of compartment syndrome in patients in whom there is not a clear diagnosis based on clinical signs and symptoms. Pressures can be measured by the ED team or by the consulting surgical service depending on availability of equipment, familiarity with the procedure, and available resources at the institution. Compartment pressure is measured using a variety of devices that can detect what the pressure is within the compartment. The pressure should be measured approximately 5 cm from the fracture level, if present. Normal compartment pressure is generally less than 10 to 12 mm Hg in adult patients. The pressure that supports the diagnosis of compartment syndrome remains controversial. Some studies have found that a pressure of greater than 45 mm Hg was concerning, whereas others prefer to use a lower threshold of greater than 30 mm Hg as a cutoff. In addition, a difference between diastolic blood pressure and intracompartmental pressure of less than 30 mm Hg has been shown to support the diagnosis of acute compartment syndrome.[86,87,91] If there is persistent concern despite normal measurements, serial pressures should be measured and testing of adjacent compartments may be indicated.[87] There are some newer technologies that show promise in the diagnosis of compartment syndrome. Near-infrared spectroscopy can evaluate for a decrease in tissue oxygenation noninvasively,[93] and US may reveal changes in arterial waveform in patients with acute compartment syndrome.[94]

Treatment

Immediate management of acute compartment syndrome should consist of removal of constrictive dressing and emergent surgical consultation with an orthopedic or plastic surgeon. A cast that is in place can be bivalved, which has been shown to reduce pressure by 55%, whereas complete cast removal, if it is an option, can further reduce pressure by up to 85%.[87,91] Patients who are at high risk for development of compartment syndrome should be considered for observation or admission and have serial examinations performed with possible repeat compartment pressure measurements. The patient's pain should be adequately treated, but regional anesthesia should be avoided because it may complicate future examinations.[87]

Once the diagnosis has been established based on signs, symptoms, and compartment pressure measurements, fasciotomy should be performed. It is important to remember that surgeons may have different thresholds for operative management of compartment syndrome. The generally accepted indications for fasciotomy include an intracompartmental pressure of greater than 30 mm Hg, a delta pressure of less than 30 mm Hg, clinical signs or symptoms highly suspicious for acute compartment syndrome, or interrupted arterial circulation of greater than 4 hours. Special consideration should be given to performing fasciotomy at lower compartment pressure measurements (<20 mm Hg) in hypotensive patients.[87,90,91] The fasciotomy procedure involves making incisions in the soft tissue to aid in decreasing pressure in the compartments.

Risk Management

Acute compartment syndrome is a common cause for litigation. In patients with compartment syndrome, expedient diagnosis and management can have a significant effect on reducing negative patient outcomes, which include contractures, chronic pain, and limb function. One study examined 19 cases of litigation associated with acute compartment syndrome and found that approximately 50% of these claims were awarded to the patients.[95] Another study of 66 claims found that 48 of those were in favor of the patient.[96] In most of these cases, one of the classic presenting symptoms(5 Ps) was present. Many of these cases were caused by a delay in treatment or misdiagnosis. Rulings were more likely to be in favor of the defendant if the cases were in women or children.[97]

The earlier that acute compartment syndrome is recognized and definitive treatment given, the better the patient outcomes. Up to one-third of patients had necrosis, which can occur as early as 3 hours after injury.[87] Another study found that fasciotomy performed within 4 hours always resulted in restoration of nerve function, whereas, after 12 hours, nerve conduction was never restored.[87] Clinician inexperience, patient sedation, polytrauma, soft tissue injury, and reliance on clinical signs and symptoms alone are associated with missed diagnosis.[87] The main way to reduce risk with the diagnosis of acute compartment syndrome is to maintain a high suspicion for this diagnosis in patients with extremity trauma or prolonged immobilization, with special consideration given to patients who are unable to cooperate with the examination or communicate about pain levels.

REFERENCES

1. Addiss DG, Shaffer N, Fowler BS, et al. The epidemiology of appendicitis and appendectomy in the united states. Am J Epidemiol 1990;132(5):910–25.
2. Bhangu A, Soreide K, Di Saverio S, et al. Acute appendicitis: modern understanding of pathogenesis, diagnosis, and management. Lancet 2015; 386(10000):1278–87.
3. Bickell NA, Aufses AH, Rojas M, et al. How time affects the risk of rupture in appendicitis. J Am Coll Surg 2006;202(3):401–6.
4. Flum DR. Clinical practice. Acute appendicitis–appendectomy or the "antibiotics first" strategy. N Engl J Med 2015;372(20):1937–43.
5. Howell JM, Eddy OL, Lukens TW, et al. Clinical policy: critical issues in the evaluation and management of emergency department patients with suspected appendicitis. Ann Emerg Med 2010;55(1):71–116. Accessed June 8, 2019.
6. Mahattanobon S, Samphao S, Pruekprasert P. Clinical features of complicated acute appendicitis. J Med Assoc Thai 2014;97(8):835–40. Accessed June 6, 2019.
7. Schwartz JH, Manco LG. Left-sided appendicitis. J Am Coll Surg 2008;206(3): 590. Accessed June 6, 2019.
8. Mahmoodian S. Appendicitis complicating pregnancy. South Med J 1992;85(1): 19–24. Accessed June 6, 2019.
9. Colvin JM, Bachur R, Kharbanda A. The presentation of appendicitis in preadolescent children. Pediatr Emerg Care 2007;23(12):849–55. Accessed June 6, 2019.
10. Omari AH, Khammash MR, Qasaimeh GR, et al. Acute appendicitis in the elderly: Risk factors for perforation. World J Emerg Surg 2014;9(1):6. Accessed June 6, 2019.
11. Ashdown HF, D'Souza N, Karim D, et al. Pain over speed bumps in diagnosis of acute appendicitis: Diagnostic accuracy study. BMJ 2012;345:e8012. Accessed June 6, 2019.
12. Ohle R, O'Reilly F, O'Brien KK, et al. The Alvarado score for predicting acute appendicitis: A systematic review. BMC Med 2011;9:139. Accessed Jun 6, 2019.
13. Kollár D, McCartan DP, Bourke M, et al. Predicting acute appendicitis? A comparison of the Alvarado score, the appendicitis inflammatory response score and clinical assessment. World J Surg 2015;39(1):104–9. Accessed June 6, 2019.
14. de Castro SMM, Ünlü C, Steller EP, et al. Evaluation of the appendicitis inflammatory response score for patients with acute appendicitis. World J Surg 2012; 36(7):1540–5. Accessed June 6, 2019.
15. Andersson REB. Meta-analysis of the clinical and laboratory diagnosis of appendicitis. Br J Surg 2004;91(1):28–37. Accessed June 8, 2019.

16. Estrada JJ, Petrosyan M, Barnhart J, et al. Hyperbilirubinemia in appendicitis: a new predictor of perforation. J Gastrointest Surg 2007;11(6):714–8. Accessed June 8, 2019.
17. Schellekens DH, Hulsewé KWE, van Acker, et al. Evaluation of the diagnostic accuracy of plasma markers for early diagnosis in patients suspected for acute appendicitis. Acad Emerg Med 2013;20(7):703–10. Accessed June 8, 2019.
18. Yu C-, Juan L-, Wu M-, et al. Systematic review and meta-analysis of the diagnostic accuracy of procalcitonin, C-reactive protein and white blood cell count for suspected acute appendicitis. Br J Surg 2013;100(3):322–9. Accessed June 8, 2019.
19. Petroianu A. Diagnosis of acute appendicitis. Int J Surg 2012;10(3):115–9. Accessed June 8, 2019.
20. Yun SJ, Ryu C, Choi NY, et al. Comparison of low- and standard-dose CT for the diagnosis of acute appendicitis: A meta-analysis. AJR Am J Roentgenol 2017;208(6):W198–207. Accessed June 8, 2019.
21. Neumayer L, Kennedy A. Imaging in appendicitis: A review with special emphasis on the treatment of women. Obstet Gynecol 2003;102(6):1404–9. Accessed Jun 8, 2019.
22. Anderson SW, Soto JA, Lucey BC, et al. Abdominal 64-MDCT for suspected appendicitis: The use of oral and IV contrast material versus IV contrast material only. AJR Am J Roentgenol 2009;193(5):1282–8. Accessed Jun 8, 2019.
23. Giljaca V, Nadarevic T, Poropat G, et al. Diagnostic accuracy of abdominal ultrasound for diagnosis of acute appendicitis: Systematic review and meta-analysis. World J Surg 2017;41(3):693–700. Accessed June 17, 2019.
24. Yu SH, Kim CB, Park JW, et al. Ultrasonography in the diagnosis of appendicitis: evaluation by meta-analysis. Korean J Radiol 2005;6(4):267–77. Accessed June 17, 2019.
25. Duke E, Kalb B, Arif-Tiwari H, et al. A systematic review and meta-analysis of diagnostic performance of MRI for evaluation of acute appendicitis. AJR Am J Roentgenol 2016;206(3):508–17. Accessed June 17, 2019.
26. Schuster KM, Holena DN, Salim A, et al. American association for the surgery of trauma emergency general surgery guideline summaries 2018: Acute appendicitis, acute cholecystitis, acute diverticulitis, acute pancreatitis and small bowel obstruction. Trauma Surg Acute Care Open 2019;4:e000281. Accessed June 17, 2019.
27. Manterola C, Vial M, Moraga J, et al. Analgesia in patients with acute abdominal pain. Cochrane Database Syst Rev 2011;(1):CD005660. Accessed June 17, 2019.
28. Solomkin JS, Mazuski JE, Bradley JS, et al. Diagnosis and management of complicated intra-abdominal infection in adults and children: Guidelines by the surgical infection society and the infectious diseases society of America. Clin Infect Dis 2010;50(2):133–64. Accessed June 17, 2019.
29. Bratzler DW, Dellinger EP, Olsen KM, et al. Clinical practice guidelines for antimicrobial prophylaxis in surgery. Am J Health Syst Pharm 2013;70(3):195–283. Accessed June 17, 2019.
30. Findlay JM, Kafsi JE, Hammer C, et al. Nonoperative management of appendicitis in adults: A systematic review and meta-analysis of randomized controlled trials. J Am Coll Surg 2016;223(6):814–24.e2. Accessed June 17, 2019.
31. Stather PW, Sidloff DA, Rhema IA, et al. A review of current reporting of abdominal aortic aneurysm mortality and prevalence in the literature. Eur J Vasc Endovasc Surg 2014;47(3):240–2. Accessed June 21, 2019.

32. Sakalihasan N, Michel J, Katsargyris A, et al. Abdominal aortic aneurysms. Nat Rev Dis Primers 2018;4(1):34. Accessed June 21, 2019.

33. Fink HA, Lederle FA, Roth CS, et al. The accuracy of physical examination to detect abdominal aortic aneurysm. Arch Intern Med 2000;160(6):833–6.

34. Törnwall ME, Virtamo J, Haukka JK, et al. Life-style factors and risk for abdominal aortic aneurysm in a cohort of finnish male smokers. Epidemiology 2001;12(1): 94–100. Accessed June 21, 2019.

35. Pasternak B, Inghammar M, Svanström H. Fluoroquinolone use and risk of aortic aneurysm and dissection: Nationwide cohort study. BMJ 2018;360:k678. Accessed June 21, 2019.

36. Keisler B, Carter C. Abdominal aortic aneurysm. Am Fam Physician 2015;91(8): 538–43. Accessed June 21, 2019.

37. Hirsch AT, Haskal ZJ, Hertzer NR, et al. ACC/AHA 2005 practice guidelines for the management of patients with peripheral arterial disease (lower extremity, renal, mesenteric, and abdominal aortic): a collaborative report from the American association for vascular surgery/society for vascular surgery, society for cardiovascular angiography and interventions, society for vascular medicine and biology, society of interventional radiology, and the ACC/AHA task force on practice guidelines (writing committee to develop guidelines for the management of patients with peripheral arterial disease): Endorsed by the American association of cardiovascular and pulmonary rehabilitation; national heart, lung, and blood institute; society for vascular nursing; TransAtlantic inter-society consensus; and vascular disease foundation. Circulation 2006;113(11):463. Accessed June 21, 2019.

38. Rinckenbach S, Albertini J, Thaveau F, et al. Prehospital treatment of infrarenal ruptured abdominal aortic aneurysms: A multicentric analysis. Ann Vasc Surg 2010;24(3):308–14. Available at: http://www.sciencedirect.com.proxy1.library. jhu.edu/science/article/pii/S0890509609002556.

39. David M, Pelberg J, Kuntz C. Grey Turner's sign. QJM 2013;106(5):481–2.

40. Chaikof EL, Dalman RL, Eskandari MK, et al. The society for vascular surgery practice guidelines on the care of patients with an abdominal aortic aneurysm. J Vasc Surg 2018;67(1):2–77.e2. Accessed June 21, 2019.

41. Golledge J, Muller R, Clancy P, et al. Evaluation of the diagnostic and prognostic value of plasma D-dimer for abdominal aortic aneurysm. Eur Heart J 2011;32(3): 354–64. Accessed June 22, 2019.

42. Erbel R, Aboyans V, Boileau C, et al. 2014 ESC guidelines on the diagnosis and treatment of aortic diseases: Document covering acute and chronic aortic diseases of the thoracic and abdominal aorta of the adult. The task force for the diagnosis and treatment of aortic diseases of the European society of cardiology (ESC). Eur Heart J 2014;35(41):2873–926. Accessed June 22, 2019.

43. Rubano E, Mehta N, Caputo W, et al. Systematic review: emergency department bedside ultrasonography for diagnosing suspected abdominal aortic aneurysm. Acad Emerg Med 2013;20(2):128–38. Accessed June 22, 2019.

44. Vidakovic R, Feringa HHH, Kuiper RJ, et al. Comparison with computed tomography of two ultrasound devices for diagnosis of abdominal aortic aneurysm. Am J Cardiol 2007;100(12):1786–91. Accessed June 22, 2019.

45. Hamilton H, Constantinou J, Ivancey K, et al. The role of permissive hypotension in the management of ruptured abdominal aortic aneurysms. J Cardiovasc Surg (Torino) 2014;55(2):151–9. Accessed June 22, 2019.

46. Wyers MC. Acute mesenteric ischemia: diagnostic approach and surgical treatment. Semin Vasc Surg 2010;23(1):9–20. Accessed June 30, 2019.

47. Clair DG, Beach JM. Mesenteric ischemia. N Engl J Med 2016;374(10):959–68. Accessed June 30, 2019.
48. Hawkins BM, Khan Z, Abu-Fadel MS, et al. Endovascular treatment of mesenteric ischemia. Catheter Cardiovasc Interv 2011;78(6):948–52. Accessed June 30, 2019.
49. van den Heijkant, Teun C, Aerts BAC, et al. Challenges in diagnosing mesenteric ischemia. World J Gastroenterol 2013;19(9):1338–41. Accessed June 30, 2019.
50. Acosta S, Björck M. Acute thrombo-embolic occlusion of the superior mesenteric artery: a prospective study in a well defined population. Eur J Vasc Endovasc Surg 2003;26(2):179–83. Accessed June 30, 2019.
51. Harward TR, Green D, Bergan JJ, et al. Mesenteric venous thrombosis. J Vasc Surg 1989;9(2):328–33. Accessed June 30, 2019.
52. Chiu Y, Huang M, How C, et al. D-dimer in patients with suspected acute mesenteric ischemia. Am J Emerg Med 2009;27(8):975–9. Accessed June 30, 2019.
53. Furukawa A, Kanasaki S, Kono N, et al. CT diagnosis of acute mesenteric ischemia from various causes. AJR Am J Roentgenol 2009;192(2):408–16. Accessed June 30, 2019.
54. Cudnik MT, Darbha S, Jones J, et al. The diagnosis of acute mesenteric ischemia: A systematic review and meta-analysis. Acad Emerg Med 2013;20(11): 1087–100. Accessed June 30, 2019.
55. Maung AA, Johnson DC, Piper GL, et al. Evaluation and management of small-bowel obstruction: An eastern association for the surgery of trauma practice management guideline. J Trauma Acute Care Surg 2012;73(5 Suppl 4):362. Accessed June 30, 2019.
56. ten Broek, Richard PG, Issa Y, et al. Burden of adhesions in abdominal and pelvic surgery: systematic review and met-analysis. BMJ 2013;347:f5588. Accessed June 30, 2019.
57. Butt MU, Velmahos GC, Zacharias N, et al. Adhesional small bowel obstruction in the absence of previous operations: management and outcomes. World J Surg 2009;33(11):2368–71. Accessed June 30, 2019.
58. Taylor MR, Lalani N. Adult small bowel obstruction. Acad Emerg Med 2013;20(6): 528–44. Accessed June 30, 2019.
59. Murray MJ, Gonze MD, Nowak LR, et al. Serum D(-)-lactate levels as an aid to diagnosing acute intestinal ischemia. Am J Surg 1994;167(6):575–8. Accessed July 1, 2019.
60. Becker BA, Lahham S, Gonzales MA, et al. A prospective, multicenter evaluation of point-of-care ultrasound for small-bowel obstruction in the emergency department. Acad Emerg Med 2019. https://doi.org/10.1111/acem.13713. Accessed July 1, 2019.
61. Cox MR, Gunn IF, Eastman MC, et al. The safety and duration of non-operative treatment for adhesive small bowel obstruction. Aust N Z J Surg 1993;63(5): 367–71. Accessed July 3, 2019.
62. Fevang BT, Jensen D, Svanes K, et al. Early operation or conservative management of patients with small bowel obstruction? Eur J Surg 2002;168(8–9):475–81. Accessed July 3, 2019.
63. Wolfe TR, Fosnocht DE, Linscott MS. Atomized lidocaine as topical anesthesia for nasogastric tube placement: a randomized, double-blind, placebo-controlled trial. Ann Emerg Med 2000;35(5):421–5. Accessed July 3, 2019.
64. Cheatham ML, Chapman WC, Key SP, et al. A meta-analysis of selective versus routine nasogastric decompression after elective laparotomy. Ann Surg 1995; 221:469–76 [discussion: 476–8].

65. Foster NM, McGory ML, Zingmond DS, et al. Small bowel obstruction: a population-based appraisal. J Am Coll Surg 2006;203(2):170–6. Accessed July 3, 2019.

66. Mankowitz SL. Laceration management. J Emerg Med 2017;53(3):369–82. Available at: http://www.sciencedirect.com.proxy1.library.jhu.edu/science/article/pii/S0736467917304729 https://doi-org.proxy1.library.jhu.edu/10.1016/j.jemermed.2017.05.026.

67. Anderson MA, Newmeyer WL, Kilgore ES. Diagnosis and treatment of retained foreign bodies in the hand. Am J Surg 1982;144(1):63–7. https://www.sciencedirect.com/science/article/pii/0002961082906031.

68. Halaas GW. Management of foreign bodies in the skin. Am Fam Physician 2007; 76(5):683. Available at: https://www.ncbi.nlm.nih.gov/pubmed/17894138.

69. Steele MT, Tran LV, Watson WA, et al. Retained glass foreign bodies in wounds: Predictive value of wound characteristics, patient perception, and wound exploration. Am J Emerg Med 1998;16(7):627–30. Available at: https://www.sciencedirect.com/science/article/pii/S0735675798901619.

70. Levine MR, Gorman SM, Young CF, et al. Clinical characteristics and management of wound foreign bodies in the ED. Am J Emerg Med 2008;26(8):918–22. Available at: http://www.sciencedirect.com/science/article/pii/S0735675707007851.

71. Weinberger LN, Chen EH, Mills AM. Is screening radiography necessary to detect retained foreign bodies in adequately explored superficial glass-caused wounds? Ann Emerg Med 2008;51(5):666–7. Available at: http://www.sciencedirect.com/science/article/pii/S0196064407006099.

72. Blankenship RB, Baker T. Imaging modalities in wounds and superficial skin infections. Emerg Med Clin North Am 2007;25(1):223–34. Available at: http://www.sciencedirect.com.proxy1.library.jhu.edu/science/article/pii/S0733862707000120 https://doi-org.proxy1.library.jhu.edu/10.1016/j.emc.2007.01.011.

73. Horton LK, Jacobson JA, Powell A, et al. Sonography and radiography of soft-tissue foreign bodies. AJR Am J Roentgenol 2001;176(5):1155–9. Available at: https://www.ncbi.nlm.nih.gov/pubmed/11312171.

74. Nienaber A, Harvey M, Cave G. Accuracy of bedside ultrasound for the detection of soft tissue foreign bodies by emergency doctors. Emerg Med Australas 2010; 22(1):30–4. Available at: https://onlinelibrary.wiley.com/doi/abs/10.1111/j.1742-6723.2009.01255.x.

75. Davis J, Czerniski B, Au A, et al. Diagnostic accuracy of ultrasonography in retained soft tissue foreign bodies: A systematic review and meta-analysis. Acad Emerg Med 2015;22(7):777–87.

76. Ferguson B, Geralds J, Petrey J, et al. Malpractice in emergency Medicine—A review of risk and mitigation practices for the emergency medicine provider. J Emerg Med 2018;55(5):659–65. Available at: http://www.sciencedirect.com.proxy1.library.jhu.edu/science/article/pii/S0736467918306486 https://doi-org.proxy1.library.jhu.edu/10.1016/j.jemermed.2018.06.035.

77. Hollander JE, Singer AJ. Laceration management. Ann Emerg Med 1999;34(3): 356–67. Available at: https://www.sciencedirect.com/science/article/pii/S0196064499701319.

78. Zehtabchi S, Yadav K, Brothers E, et al. Prophylactic antibiotics for simple hand lacerations: Time for a clinical trial? Injury 2012;43(9):1497–501. Available at: http://www.sciencedirect.com.proxy1.library.jhu.edu/science/article/pii/S002013831100811 https://doi-org.proxy1.library.jhu.edu/10.1016/j.injury.2011.05.001.

79. Berwald N, Khan F, Zehtabchi S. Antibiotic prophylaxis for ED patients with simple hand lacerations: A feasibility randomized controlled trial. Am J Emerg

Med 2014;32(7):768–71. Available at: http://www.sciencedirect.com.proxy1.library.jhu.edu/science/article/pii/S0735675714002319 https://doi-org.proxy1.library.jhu.edu/10.1016/j.ajem.2014.03.043.

80. Cruse PJE, Foord R. A five-year prospective study of 23,649 surgical wounds. Arch Surg 1973;107(2):206–10.

81. Bansal BC, Wiebe RA, Perkins SD, et al. Tap water for irrigation of lacerations. Am J Emerg Med 2002;20(5):469–72. Available at: http://www.sciencedirect.com.proxy1.library.jhu.edu/science/article/pii/S0735675702000426 https://doi-org.proxy1.library.jhu.edu/10.1053/ajem.2002.35501.

82. Moscati RM, Mayrose J, Reardon RF, et al. A multicenter comparison of tap water versus sterile saline for wound irrigation. Acad Emerg Med 2007;14(5):404–9. Available at: https://doi-org.proxy1.library.jhu.edu/10.1111/j.1553-2712.2007.tb01798.x.

83. Quinn JV, Polevoi SK, Kohn MA. Traumatic lacerations: What are the risks for infection and has the 'golden period' of laceration care disappeared? Emerg Med J 2014;31(2):96–100.

84. Zehtabchi S. The role of antibiotic prophylaxis for prevention of infection in patients with simple hand lacerations. Ann Emerg Med 2007;49(5):682–9.e1. Available at: http://www.sciencedirect.com.proxy1.library.jhu.edu/science/article/pii/S0196064406026837 https://doi-org.proxy1.library.jhu.edu/10.1016/j.annemergmed.2006.12.014.

85. Mouton J, Houdre H, Beccari R, et al. Surgical exploration of hand wounds in the emergency room: Preliminary study of 80 personal injury claims. Orthop Traumatol Surg Res 2016;102(8):1009–12. Available at: http://www.sciencedirect.com.proxy1.library.jhu.edu/science/article/pii/S1877056816301645 https://doi-org.proxy1.library.jhu.edu/10.1016/j.otsr.2016.09.018.

86. Taylor R, Sullivan M, Mehta S. Acute compartment syndrome: Obtaining diagnosis, providing treatment, and minimizing medicolegal risk. Curr Rev Musculoskelet Med 2012;5(3):206–13. Available at: https://www.ncbi.nlm.nih.gov/pubmed/22644598.

87. Long B, Koyfman A, Gottlieb M. Evaluation and management of acute compartment syndrome in the emergency department. J Emerg Med 2019;56(4):386–97. Available at: http://www.sciencedirect.com.proxy1.library.jhu.edu/science/article/pii/S0736467918312137 https://doi-org.proxy1.library.jhu.edu/10.1016/j.jemermed.2018.12.021.

88. Schellenberg M, Chong V, Cone J, et al. Extremity compartment syndrome. Curr Probl Surg 2018;55(7):256–73. Available at: http://www.sciencedirect.com.proxy1.library.jhu.edu/science/article/pii/S0011384018301126 https://doi-org.proxy1.library.jhu.edu/10.1067/j.cpsurg.2018.08.002.

89. Zuchelli D, Divaris N, McCormack JE, et al. Extremity compartment syndrome following blunt trauma: A level I trauma center's 5-year experience. J Surg Res 2017;217:131–6. Available at: http://www.sciencedirect.com.proxy1.library.jhu.edu/science/article/pii/S0022480417302664 https://doi-org.proxy1.library.jhu.edu/10.1016/j.jss.2017.05.012.

90. Mabee JR. Compartment syndrome: a complication of acute extremity trauma. J Emerg Med 1994;12(5):651–6.

91. Gourgiotis S, Villias C, Germanos S, et al. Acute limb compartment syndrome: a review. J Surg Educ 2007;64(3):178–86. Available at: http://www.sciencedirect.com.proxy1.library.jhu.edu/science/article/pii/S1931720407001079 https://doi-org.proxy1.library.jhu.edu/10.1016/j.jsurg.2007.03.006.

92. Raza H, Mahapatra A. Acute compartment syndrome in orthopedics: Causes, diagnosis, and management. Adv Orthop 2015;2015:543412–8.
93. Gentilello L, Sanzone A, Wang L, et al. Near-infrared spectroscopy versus compartment pressure for the diagnosis of lower extremity compartmental syndrome using electromyography-determined measurements of neuromuscular function. J Trauma 2001;51(1):1–9. Available at: http://ovidsp.ovid.com/ovid web.cgi?T=JS&NEWS=n&CSC=Y&PAGE=fulltext&D=ovft &AN=00005373-200107000-00001.
94. Lynch JE, Lynch JK, Cole SL, et al. Noninvasive monitoring of elevated intramuscular pressure in a model compartment syndrome via quantitative fascial motion. J Orthop Res 2009;27(4):489–94. Available at: https://onlinelibrary.wiley.com/doi/abs/10.1002/jor.20778.
95. Bhattacharyya T, Vrahas M. Medical legal aspects of compartment syndrome. J Bone Joint Surg Am 2004;86(4):864–8.
96. Marchesi M, Marchesi A, Calori GM, et al. A sneaky surgical emergency: Acute compartment syndrome. retrospective analysis of 66 closed claims, medicolegal pitfalls and damages evaluation. Injury 2014;45:S16–20. Available at: https://www.clinicalkey.es/playcontent/1-s2.0-S0020138314005026.
97. DePasse JM, Sargent R, Fantry AJ, Bokshan SL. Assessment of malpractice claims associated with acute compartment syndrome. J Am Acad Orthop Surg 2017;25(6):e109–13.

High-Risk Chief Complaints
III: Neurologic Emergencies

Danielle E. Smith, MS4[a], Matthew S. Siket, MD, MS[b],*

KEYWORDS

- Stroke • Subarachnoid hemorrhage • Status epilepticus • Cauda equina
- Diagnostic error

KEY POINTS

- Patients presenting with headache should be screened for red-flag criteria that suggest a dangerous secondary cause warranting imaging and further diagnostic workup.
- Dizziness is a vague complaint, and focusing on timing, triggers, and examination findings can help reduce diagnostic error.
- Most patients presenting with back pain do not require emergent imaging, but those with new neurologic deficits or signs/symptoms concerning for acute infection or cord compression warrant MRI.
- Treatment of seizures should be swift and algorithm driven.

INTRODUCTION

The assessment, diagnosis, and management of acute neurologic dysfunction in the Emergency Department (ED) can be challenging, even for the most seasoned clinician. Patients may present with vague, subtle, seemingly benign, or even transient symptoms and be harboring devastating neurologic disability if not promptly and correctly diagnosed. Misdiagnoses of the neurologic emergencies are common, particularly among ED chief complaints, such as headache, dizziness, back pain, and weakness. Uncovering the high-risk "subtle yet dangerous" presentation in a chaotic work environment is a challenge unique to emergency medicine.[1] Tools to aid the frontline provider in accurate diagnosis of the neurologic emergencies and tips to improve timely treatment decisions are the focus of this article in hopes of reducing diagnostic error and medicolegal risk and optimizing care delivery for patients.

Headache

Headache is a common chief complaint seen in the ED, representing 2% of all patient visits.[2] Of patients with neurologic problems, headache is the presenting chief

[a] Robert Larner College of Medicine of the University of Vermont, 89 Beaumont Avenue, Burlington, VT 05405, USA; [b] Surgery, Larner College of Medicine at the University of Vermont, 111 Colchester Avenue, EC 2, Burlington, VT 05401, USA
* Corresponding author.
E-mail address: matthew.siket@uvmhealth.org

Emerg Med Clin N Am 38 (2020) 523–537
https://doi.org/10.1016/j.emc.2020.02.006
0733-8627/20/© 2020 Elsevier Inc. All rights reserved.
emed.theclinics.com

complaint in 13% to 20% of patients.[3,4] Primary headache disorders are experienced by 46% of the world's population,[5] making it one of the most common disease pathologic conditions of human existence. Although most headaches are benign, there are dangerous causes that represent high-risk neurologic emergencies that convey significant morbidity and mortality risk for the patient. Many of these high-risk causes, including subarachnoid hemorrhage (SAH), cerebral venous sinus thrombosis (CVST), cervical arterial dissections (CAD), and pituitary apoplexy, may present with severe, rapid-onset headache, otherwise known as thunderclap headache (TCH), where maximum pain intensity is reached within 1 minute of onset.[6] Despite its severe presentation, the incidence of TCH is only 43 per 100,000 people,[7] and 80% of patients presenting with TCH eventually become diagnosed with a primary headache disorder.[8] Headaches that signify high-risk intracranial pathologic conditions are rare and present a diagnostic challenge for emergency physicians (EP). Physicians must choose between the benefits of increased diagnostic accuracy and potential for reduced morbidity and mortality in a small number of patients with high-risk pathologic conditions against the risks associated with evaluating for the disease (increased radiation exposure, resource utilization, higher costs to patients) or missed diagnosis of these headache emergencies.[8-10]

In order to avoid missing the proverbial "needle-in-the-haystack" dangerous headache diagnosis, the ED evaluation requires a thorough history and physical examination with particular attention paid to exposing "red flags." Some of the dangerous secondary causes of headache are listed in **Table 1**. In a study of 55 fatal headache cases with headache as the initial presenting symptom, new onset headache in the patient over age of 50 (55%), collapse or loss of consciousness (53%), thunderclap (51%), worst headache ever experienced (46%), altered mental status (33%), progressive visual or neurologic symptoms (33%), nausea/vomiting (31%), and focal neurologic deficits (22%) were the most common red-flag symptoms associated with fatality.[11] Other red flags include fever, weight loss, significant hypertension, pregnancy, onset triggered by exertion, and postural headaches.[12] However, the EP must be mindful that history and physical examination findings are heterogenous in patients with headache emergencies, and no single historical factor can predict likelihood of intracranial pathologic condition.[10] For example, the presenting headache in SAH is most commonly localized to the occipital region, but it is by no means specific for this. In fact, it is also a common site for headache in vertebral artery dissection.[13] Conversely, presence of neck stiffness on examination has a strongly positive likelihood ratio of 6.59 in association with SAH.[10] Collectively, this suggests that individual

Table 1	
Dangerous secondary causes of headache	
Hemorrhagic	Subarachnoid, subdural, epidural, intracerebral hemorrhage
Infectious	Meningitis, encephalitis, abscess
Vascular	Dissection, sinus thrombosis, posterior reversible encephalopathy syndrome, reversible cerebral vasoconstriction syndrome
Intracranial pressure related	Idiopathic intracranial hypotension, intracranial hypotension, colloid cyst of the third ventricle
Endocrine	Pituitary apoplexy, pheochromocytoma, diabetic ketoacidosis
Toxicologic	Carbon monoxide, solvents, vapors
Oncologic	Tumor
Ophthalmologic	Giant cell arteritis, angle closure glaucoma

physical examination findings or historical factors may predict distinct causes of headache emergencies, but no 1 finding is sufficient to predict general intracranial pathologic condition.

Timely diagnosis of headache emergencies in the ED is imperative to avoid poor outcomes. Although not all patients presenting to the ED with a headache warrant neuroimaging, patients exhibiting any red-flag signs/symptoms should typically undergo an expeditious workup that includes a noncontrast head computed tomographic (CT) scan (NCHCT).[8] NCHCT is likely to be diagnostic in most patients with mass lesions causing headache (brain tumor, abscess, and so forth) and intracranial bleeding. In addition, the sensitivity and specificity of NCHCT for CVST are 85% and 87%, respectively, making this the preferred first diagnostic test for CVST.[14] Other causes of headache emergencies presenting with TCH, including CAD, reversible cerebral vasoconstriction syndrome, and posterior reversible encephalopathy syndrome, may require more advanced neuroimaging before a diagnosis will be achieved.[8]

Advances in CT technology over the past decade have increased the sensitivity of NCHCT for intracranial bleeding to nearing 100%.[15,16] If performed within the first 6 hours following headache onset, the sensitivity of NCHCT for SAH is 98.7%.[16] Historically, diagnosis of SAH involved NCHCT followed by lumbar puncture (LP) with evidence of red blood cells and xanthochromia in the cerebral spinal fluid. However, recent literature has sparked controversy regarding the need for LP following an NCHCT within 6 hours of headache onset given the near perfect sensitivity of CT in this timeframe.[9,17,18] LP can cause complications for patients, including subdural hematoma, introduction of infection into the cerebrospinal fluid (CSF), and postspinal headache, which has prompted many investigations into its utility in the diagnosis of SAH.[18] LP in SAH is also limited by the possibility of traumatic taps and the introduction of observer bias in interpretation of xanthochromia.[10] Despite its limitations, LP is known to establish a differing diagnosis (meningitis, idiopathic intracranial hypertension, spontaneous intracranial hypotension) from SAH in approximately 3% of patients.[19] Many EPs are changing their practice to minimize administration of LPs following the recent trend in literature. However, this area of clinical decision making in the management of headache is still controversial.

The medicolegal implications of missed diagnoses of neurologic emergencies presenting with headache are significant and far-reaching. Neurologic emergencies can be challenging to recognize and diagnose and often do not present with the "classic symptoms" that students, trainees, and providers are taught.[20,21] Many factors contribute to missed diagnoses, including EP knowledge gaps, cognitive errors, and systems-based errors.[22] In those neurologic emergencies that present with headaches, atypical presentations, failure to follow an algorithmic workup, and the misinterpretation of neuroimaging represent the most common sources for missed diagnosis.[20,22]

Of the available literature regarding litigation and the medicolegal consequences of missed diagnoses in headache, most pertain to missed SAH. Mortality after SAH was found to be 20% at 3 days and 36% at 7 days in 1 study,[23] and these figures do not consider those cases of SAH that involved a delayed or missed diagnosis. Of patients presenting with SAH, 5.4% have an initial missed diagnosis.[24] In another study, 19% of patients with SAH who presented with normal mental status were initially misdiagnosed, most commonly with migraine and tension-type headaches.[25] The most common reason for misdiagnosis in SAH is failure to obtain an NCHCT.[8,25] Misdiagnosis is associated with poorer outcomes and increased mortality and can lead to litigation involving EPs and residents.[26] EPs were the primary defendants in 20% of malpractice claims from 1985 to 2007.[27] In this timeframe, the court ruled in favor of the physician in 70% of cases. Despite the likelihood of favorable outcomes for physicians, malpractice claims secondary to missed diagnoses continue to represent a significant financial burden placed on individual physicians and hospital groups.

Dizziness

Dizziness is a commonly reported symptom in the ED, particularly among elderly patients,[28] and is a notoriously imprecise symptom, because it means different things to different people. More than half of ED patients report having experienced the symptom of dizziness within the past 7 days, and differentiating the dangerous from benign causes can be particularly challenging. Most causes have an underlying medical (cardiovascular, toxic, metabolic, infectious, and so forth) or benign vestibular cause, but approximately 15% have a dangerous underlying cause (cardiovascular, cerebrovascular, medical) for which accurate and timely diagnosis is paramount.

The classic diagnostic paradigm of dichotomizing dizziness into symptoms of "lightheadedness" or "vertigo" is a common cause of diagnostic error and should be avoided. In 1 study, ED patients were asked to choose 1 of 6 symptom descriptors that best characterized their presenting complaint (spinning/vertigo, about to faint, unsteady on my feet, dizzy, lightheaded, or disoriented/confused), and then they were asked the same question again 6 minutes later by research staff. The study found a concordance rate of less than 50%.[29] Rather, focusing the diagnostic approach on timing and triggers can more accurately individualize the differential diagnosis and determine ED test utilization.[30] The mnemonic ATTEST (Associated symptoms, Timing, Triggers, Exam Signs, and Testing) has been proposed to encourage EPs to think broadly and reduce diagnostic error when approaching the undifferentiated dizzy patient.[31] By focusing on timing and triggers, rather than symptoms quality, the EP can distinguish different "vestibular syndromes," namely acute vestibular syndrome (AVS), triggered episodic vestibular syndrome (t-EVS), and spontaneous episodic vestibular syndrome (s-EVS), each with a unique list of differential diagnoses informing subsequent testing and resource utilization.

Patients presenting with AVS have acute-onset, persistent, and continuous dizziness usually associated with nausea and/or vomiting. These patients warrant a targeted physical examination to differentiate peripheral causes, such as vestibular neuronitis, and labyrinthitis from central causes, namely posterior circulation stroke. Testing for focal neurologic deficits in the brainstem (cranial nerves, concerning nystagmus) and cerebellum (dysmetria, dysdiadochokinesia, ataxia) is generally indicated. The HINTS examination (Head Impulse, Nystagmus, and Test of Skew) is a battery of 3 tests developed to aid in the differentiation of central from peripheral causes of AVS and has been shown to outperform early MRI in the diagnosis of stroke in appropriately selected dizzy patients.[32]

Ischemic stroke accounts for an estimated 4% to 5% (120,000–200,000) of dizziness presentations annually, of which 35% are missed initially.[33,34] Strokes in the posterior fossa (ie, cerebellum and brainstem) are the most likely to be misdiagnosed, because symptoms may be atypical, minimal, or even go undetected using the gold-standard acute stroke assessment tool, the National Institutes of Health Stroke Scale (NIHSS), which is preferentially weighted toward the anterior circulation. **Table 2** lists several components of the neurologic examination that may be useful to perform and document in patients presenting with dizziness. Younger patients, those with milder symptoms (such as isolated dizziness), and those with stroke caused by a vertebral artery dissection are more likely to be missed initially.[35–37] As

Table 2 Components of the neurologic examination in dizzy patients	
Eyes	Pupillary response, extraocular movements, presence and type of nystagmus, visual fields, vertical refixation on alternating cover test, vestibuloocular reflex, papilledema, afferent pupillary defect
Face	Cranial nerves, facial symmetry
Speech	Articulation, fluency, aphasia
Extremities	Strength, sensation
Coordination	Rapid-alternating movements, dysmetria, cerebellar rebound, truncal and gait ataxia

a general rule, dizzy patients with AVS and focal neurologic deficits should be evaluated for stroke, and neurology consultation is warranted.

Patients with s-EVS or t-EVS typically present with episodes of dizziness that are separated by periods of complete resolution of symptoms. If there is a clear precipitating trigger (such as head turning or standing upright), then t-EVS is suspected. Common causes include benign paroxysmal position vertigo (BPPV), for which provocative maneuvers can be performed for both diagnostic confirmation and therapeutic resolution, as well as orthostatic hypotension. A common pitfall in the misdiagnosis of dizzy patients occurs when providers are falsely reassured when patients with acute and persistent dizziness note worsening of symptoms with provocative maneuvers. These maneuvers to test for BPPV should be reserved for patients with t-EVS and generally not applied to patients with AVS.

If episodes of dizziness are spontaneous and without a clear precipitating trigger, then s-EVS is suspected. The differential diagnosis of s-EVS is broad, and typically these patients warrant a thorough and thoughtful history and examination, despite typically being asymptomatic at the time of evaluation. Causes of s-EVS include transient ischemic attack (TIA), vestibular migraine, paroxysmal cardiac arrhythmia, and Meniere disease, among others. If TIA is suspected, then particular caution should be used in patients with stuttering symptoms, additional focal neurologic dysfunction, known cardioembolic causes, and those with significant risk factors for stroke. These patients represent a high-risk population and generally warrant cerebrocephalic vascular imaging when feasible.

Posttraumatic dizziness caused by minor head injury, concussion, perilymphatic fistula, or barotrauma can also be challenging for both providers and patients. Although less common, they may have medicolegal implications related to the traumatic event (such as a motor vehicle accident). Although numerous potentially debilitating causes exist, some patients may be presenting with a source of secondary gain. Generally, this is beyond the scope of the EP, and referral to a vestibular specialist is warranted in these cases.[38]

Although most patients with dizziness are not experiencing a neurologic emergency, the EP should be thoughtful about excluding the dangerous causes before providing reassurance. Ask yourself: "Does this patient have AVS, s-EVS, or t-EVS?" Distinguish likely causes based on the ATTEST mnemonic and cater your targeted physical examination and diagnostic test utilization to the individualized list of suspect causes. If focal neurologic deficits are present, a concerning HINTS examination is noted in patients with AVS, or the underlying presentation seems suggestive of a TIA with high-risk features, then an underlying central neurologic cause should be suspected. Although not all misdiagnosis in dizziness is preventable, standardizing the approach will likely help improve diagnostic accuracy and subvert medicolegal risk.

Back Pain

Back pain is one of the 5 most common chief complaints seen in EDs nationally and represents approximately 5% of all patient evaluations.[39,40] Back pain and its sequelae affect more than 100 million individuals in the United States and cost upwards of 200 million dollars annually.[41] The differential diagnosis of back pain is expansive and includes musculoskeletal, cardiovascular, gastrointestinal, renal, infectious, and malignant causes. Most patients with back pain have a benign, nonemergent cause for their pain and will improve without major medical intervention. Back pain emergencies, however, require expeditious intervention to prevent significant morbidity and/or mortality for the patient. Neurologic emergencies presenting with back pain include, but are not limited to, cauda equina syndrome (CES), spinal epidural abscess (SEA), spinal epidural hematoma, and severe nucleus pulposus herniation.[20] Unfortunately, these emergencies are often missed or misdiagnosed because of the heterogeneity of clinical presentation, rarity of incidence, and failure to obtain further imaging and laboratory studies.[27,42] Failure to recognize these neurologic emergencies may demonstrate future medicolegal implications for EPs.

A thorough history and physical examination are warranted for any patient presenting to the ED with back pain. In 1 study, 42% of malpractice claims involving EPs involved failure to perform an adequate history or physical examination.[43] The history and physical examination should focus on elucidating the presence of "red flags" concerning for emergent causes. Red flags associated with back pain include age greater than 50, fever, bowel or bladder incontinence, urinary retention, saddle anesthesia, history of cancer, unexplained weight loss, intravenous drug use, alcoholism, diabetes, immunosuppression, and previous spinal surgery.[40,44] The presence of red flags should alert the EP to the potential for a serious cause, and further laboratory and imaging studies are usually required for diagnosis.

Benign causes of acute onset low back pain most often do not require imaging, and plain film radiographs are indicated only in the context of trauma or if pathologic fracture is suspected.[40,45] Despite this fact, 30% of patients with low back pain have plain films obtained in the ED.[45] Failure of physicians to follow an algorithmic approach often causes increased resource utilization and radiation exposure to patients. When red flags are present, gadolinium-enhanced MRI is the gold standard for advanced neuroimaging of the spine given its better resolution and visualization of soft tissue structures, although an unenhanced MRI is often sufficient to assess for spinal cord compression.[46] The ability of EPs to obtain emergent MRI poses a significant barrier to the timely diagnosis and subsequent management of these neurologic emergencies.[20] Establishing institutional protocols for emergent MRI utilization and interfacility transfer is 1 possible solution to avoid adverse outcomes because of logistical delays.

CES presents a diagnostic challenge for EPs. The classic clinical features of CES include low back pain, bilateral sciatica, motor dysfunction, saddle anesthesia, and sphincter dysfunction. In 1 study, only 19% of patients presented with the classic symptoms.[47] CES is a surgical emergency and requires rapid decompression. Studies suggest that neurosurgical intervention within 48 hours produces improved patient outcomes, including return of function, length of hospital stay, and costs incurred by the patient.[48–50] CES is often initially misdiagnosed because of lack of inclusion into the EP's differential, failure to obtain advanced imaging, and inappropriate referral.[47] Delay in diagnosis of CES causing surgical intervention to be initiated after 48 hours of symptom onset represents a significant proportion of medical malpractice claims associated with CES whereby the court ruled in favor of the patient.[51]

A large proportion of the back pain–related medicolegal literature is focused on missed SEA. Less than 15% of patients with SEA present with the classic triad of spinal pain, fever, and focal neurologic deficits.[52,53] SEAs are also rare, with an incidence of 0.2 to 2.8 cases/10,000 admissions annually.[54] In 1 study evaluating the effectiveness of implementing clinical decision guidelines, 83% of patients with SEA were initially misdiagnosed before guideline implementation. Following the adoption of clinical decision rules, the rate of misdiagnosis dropped significantly.[55,56] Unfortunately, the rate of misdiagnosis remains high. In malpractice claims involving EPs, the plaintiff (patient) was more likely to win if a delay in diagnosis or treatment occurred or the patient became paraplegic or quadriplegic as a result of the SEA.[51,55]

Hematomas can occur as a result of trauma or iatrogenic injury (such as following an LP) or can occur spontaneously. The incidence is less than 1:100,000 and typically presents with axial spine pain with progressive neurologic dysfunction.[57] Early diagnosis is the key to preventing neurologic sequelae, and EP suspicion should be high in patients with a history of invasive spinal procedures, injections, or underlying coagulopathy or antithrombotic use.

Neurologic emergencies presenting with back pain cause diagnostic dilemmas for EPs who are required to balance utilization of resources and radiation exposure with the probability of an emergent cause of back pain. Providers should consider the presence of red flags and risk factors in their diagnostic evaluation of back pain.

Weakness

The chief complaint of "weakness" represents one of the most challenging diagnostic ventures undertaken by the EP on a daily basis. Patients present with this nonspecific complaint commonly, and the differential diagnosis is extremely broad. Weakness can be caused by nearly every system in the body, which necessitates an exhaustive workup associated with procurement of extensive laboratory tests, diagnostic imaging, procedures, and specialty services. In 1 study, the most common underlying cause of weakness in the ED was infections (32%), closely followed by metabolic dysfunction (18%) and malignancies (10%).[57] Although neurologic emergencies do not signify the largest contingent of disorders presenting with weakness, they are potentially fatal, often cause significant morbidity, and may require immediate intervention on the part of the EP.[20,58] To place in perspective, stroke remains the fourth leading cause of death, causes an estimated loss of 72 million disability-adjusted life years worldwide, and costs the US health care system an estimated 70 billion dollars annually.[59] When evaluating a patient with weakness, the EP must remain vigilant and keep a high clinical suspicion for neurologic causes to avoid a missed diagnosis with potential medicolegal implications.

One of the most important aspects of the initial evaluation of weakness is delineating whether the patient has perceived weakness, otherwise known as fatigue or malaise, or true neuromuscular weakness.[60] The history and physical examination are key components in this distinction and should be detailed and thorough. True neuromuscular weakness, as evidenced by weakness on the neurologic examination, can be generalized or localized, with each category possessing its own distinct differential and diagnostic challenges. Neurologic causes of generalized weakness include Guillain-Barre syndrome (GBS), myasthenia gravis (MG), Lambert-Eaton myasthenic syndrome, transverse myelitis, and more rare disorders, including botulism, hypokalemic periodic paralysis, and tick paralysis.[20,60] All of these possess the potential for rapid deterioration or mortality and often present atypically, making recognition critically important.[61,62]

GBS is the most common cause of acute paralysis seen in the ED with a reported incidence of 0.4 to 4 per 100,000 people annually.[63] Mortality in patients with GBS ranges from 3% to 10% and was 3.9% 12 months after diagnosis in 1 study.[64] GBS progresses to respiratory failure in 20% to 30% of patients.[62] The constellation of progressive bilateral symmetric limb paralysis and areflexia, usually with sensory involvement and 1 to 2 weeks following an immune stimulation, should raise concern for the diagnosis of GBS. Prompt and accurate diagnosis of GBS improves patient outcomes by decreasing time to immunologic treatment (intravenous immunoglobulin and plasma exchange), thereby preventing progression to respiratory compromise. Unfortunately, most patients with GBS are initially misdiagnosed and present to health care on at least 2 occasions on average before establishing the correct diagnosis.[63] Traditionally, GBS has been associated with elevated CSF protein levels. Despite this classic teaching, 50% of patients will have normal protein in their CSF 1 week after symptom onset.[65] This atypical presentation further complicates the accurate diagnosis of GBS.

MG can present as isolated weakness or a fulminant myasthenic crisis leading to respiratory collapse. Diagnosis can be challenging in the acute setting, but progressive muscle fatigue that improves with rest should raise concern. Ocular myasthenia is a variant that may present with ocular disturbance, ptosis, and ophthalmoplegia. Rapid sequence intubation in patients with undiagnosed MG can be complicated by the succinylcholine resistance and increased sensitivity to nondepolarizing agents seen in this disease pathologic condition.[66] Early diagnosis can aid EPs in avoiding the high-stress intubation of a complicated airway. Once the diagnosis of MG is entertained, neurology consultation is recommended as well as confirmation with the Tensilon test.

Transverse myelitis is very rare with an annual incidence of 1.3 to 8 cases per million people.[67,68] Its presentation tends to involve bilateral weakness. However, unilateral and asymmetric weakness as well as hyporeflexia has been reported.[67] This overlap in symptoms creates diagnostic uncertainty for the EP and can lead to misdiagnosis. Botulism, hypokalemic periodic paralysis, and tick paralysis are extremely rare diagnoses that are usually initially misdiagnosed because of lack of inclusion in the differential diagnosis by infectious disease and EPs.[69–71] A careful history should be obtained to identify possible underlying triggers for neuromuscular disease.

Most patients presenting with true focal neuromuscular weakness are suffering from some type of cerebrovascular event.[4] In 1 study, 76% of patients with focal weakness had either TIA, ischemic stroke, or intracranial hemorrhage.[57] Anterior circulation strokes more often present with the classic findings of facial droop, speech impairment, and lateralizing motor weakness compared with posterior circulation strokes. The rate of missed diagnosis for acute stroke in the ED varies from as low as 2% to as high as 20% in recent studies.[20,35,72,73] Missed diagnosis rates tend to be higher at nonteaching hospitals[72] and can be as high as 30% in the prehospital setting.[74] Factors associated with missed diagnosis of stroke include young age and presentation with atypical symptoms, including headache, dizziness, generalized weakness, ataxia, and altered mental status.[73–75] Many clinical decision tools have been developed to aid emergency medical services (EMS), registered nurses (RNs), and EPs in the accurate and rapid diagnosis of acute stroke. In the prehospital setting, the FAST scale (Face Arm Speech Test) used by EMS has a sensitivity of 81% and a specificity of 39% for acute stroke.[76] In the ED, both the NIHSS and the Recognition of Stroke in the Emergency Room (ROSIER) scale are currently used as screening tools. In 1 study, RNss using the ROSIER tool were able to diagnose stroke with a sensitivity of 98% and a positive predictive value of 83%, which was similar in comparison to physicians using the standard neurologic assessment.[77] Although both the NIHSS and the ROSIER tool aid in diagnosis, both possess limitations and can be negative even in patients with stroke.[20,76] The diagnostic accuracy of an NCHCT for intracranial hemorrhage approaches 100%.[16] Unfortunately, NCHCT does not adequately capture large proportions of acute ischemic strokes, especially small territory infarcts. Conversely, CT perfusion studies, often ordered by EPs to increase diagnostic accuracy of ischemic strokes, have a pooled sensitivity of 55.7% and a specificity of 92% for acute ischemic stroke.[78] Young patients and those with atypical symptoms may benefit from early MRI scanning.[75]

The medicolegal literature regarding patients with weakness focuses almost exclusively on the administration or the failure to administer tissue plasminogen activator (tPA) for acute ischemic stroke. Treatment of stroke with tPA has been a topic of significant debate since the 1990s. Although current clinical guidelines, including the American College of Emergency Physicians and American Heart Association/American Stroke Association (AHA/ASA), support its administration up to 4.5 hours of last known well (LKW) in patients meeting inclusion criteria and without contraindications, treatment is associated with an increased risk of intracranial bleeding, leading many providers, patients, and family members to be reluctant to make a treatment decision.[79] The administration of tPA represents a double-edged sword for the EP. Although substantial evidence exists for its benefit in specific patient populations, those patients who do have a complication from tPA tend to have severe complications with poor outcomes.[80] From a medicolegal standpoint, most malpractice claims associated with tPA and stoke are those whereby tPA was not given in an eligible patient.[79,81] In 1 review, 70% of malpractice claims involved failure to treat with tPA, and only 5% involved a complication from receiving tPA.[81] In another study, 88% of malpractice claims involved failure to give tPA, and EP were the most common defendants in these litigations.[82]

Regardless of medicolegal risk, ED providers are encouraged to make individual reperfusion decisions based on clinical judgment as well as the best interests and wishes of each patient. Providers are encouraged to make these decisions in consultation with neurologists when feasible and to use shared decision making with patients and family members after a brief discussion of risks and benefits of treatment. Visual aids can assist in this discussion, and institutions are encouraged to have management algorithm that can help streamline decision making, expedite treatment times, and maximize the likelihood of a good outcome.

In recent years, endovascular therapy with mechanical thrombectomy for large vessel occlusion (LVO) has become an additional time-dependent treatment option in certain acute ischemic strokes and led to an evolution in standard of care. Current AHA/ASA guidelines strongly support endovascular intervention in confirmed LVO when treatment can be initiated within 6 hours of onset.[83] Treatment has also been shown to be efficacious up to 24 hours from when the patient was LKW when favorable imaging criteria are present. For these reasons, EPs are encouraged to screen for LVO in patients with suspected acute stroke and significant neurologic deficits. Systems of care should be designed to streamline prehospital and early hospital stroke detection with expedited access to reperfusion therapies, including endovascular intervention.[84]

An often unrecognized and underappreciated cerebrovascular emergency is the TIA. Patients with transient neurologic dysfunction pose many challenges to the EP, because they are neurologically at baseline by definition at the time of their evaluation. However, it is estimated that stroke is preceded by TIA in 12% to 20% of patients, and the risk of stroke is highest in the first 24 hours.[85,86] In order to reduce the short-term stroke risk and optimize individual secondary stroke prevention strategies, it is generally recommended that patients with suspected TIA undergo a front-loaded diagnostic evaluation at the time of their initial contact with a health care provider. Cerebrocephalic vascular imaging (such as CT or magnetic resonance angiography or carotid duplex ultrasonography) in addition to brain imaging (diffusion-weighted MRI preferred to CT when feasible) is generally recommended.[87] Although clinical risk stratification tools are somewhat useful in predicting short-term stroke risk following TIA, they are imperfect, and their routine use to guide disposition decisions is generally discouraged.[87] Front-loading the diagnostic workup in the ED or observation unit and initiation of secondary prevention strategies (such as a daily aspirin and intensive stating therapy for most patients in addition to optimizing treatment of medical comorbidities) in all suspected TIA patients is 1 strategy to reduce stroke events following discharge.

Seizure

The clinical presentation of generalized convulsive status epilepticus is rarely subtle and is usually recognized swiftly in the ED unlike partial seizures or nonconvulsive status epilepticus, which may be easily missed. Failure of or delay to diagnosis and initiation of definitive management may lead to adverse outcomes and medicolegal implications.

The patient presenting with a first-time seizure poses many challenges for the EP. First, a reasonable attempt should be made to differentiate the provoked from unprovoked seizure. Provoked seizures have an underlying trigger, such as a metabolic or toxicologic cause, stroke, tumor, trauma, or infection.[88] A reasonable attempt should be made to exclude common precipitating triggers of a first-time seizure, such as obtaining serum glucose, electrolytes, and a pregnancy test in women of childbearing age. Whenever feasible, neuroimaging (most commonly CT scan of the head) should be obtained.

Patients with continuous seizure activity for greater than 5 minutes' duration or who have intermittent seizures without regaining consciousness between events are considered to be in status epilepticus. These patients have the potential for high morbidity and mortality, especially if diagnosis and treatment are delayed. Management should follow typical resuscitation algorithms, including a primary and secondary survey and initial assessment of ABCs (airway, breathing, and circulation). The next top priority is to terminate seizure activity as quickly as possible. Generally, benzodiazepines are considered the first-line treatment of choice, followed by antiepileptic agents, such as levetiracetam, phenytoin, fosphenytoin, and valproic acid.[89] Treatment algorithms are recommended to improve outcomes and have been shown to lead to faster seizure control and decreased hospital length of stay.[90–92]

The issue of driving restrictions following a first-time seizure is a frequent topic of ethical and medicolegal debate. Although patient autonomy should be preserved as much as possible, physicians have a legal and ethical obligation to comply with the law. Each state has its own process of self-reporting, and state laws vary on requirements for physician reporting.[82] The Epilepsy Foundation's State Driving Laws Database (https://www.epilepsy.com/driving-laws) is a resource to aid providers in how to best counsel patients in their region. As a general rule, it is reasonable for ED providers to counsel patients who are being discharged after a first-time seizure to refrain from driving until they have been seen in follow-up.[93]

SUMMARY

Neurologic emergencies are heterogenous in their presentation to the ED, ranging from seemingly benign to life-threatening critical illness. Subtle presentations of dangerous conditions, such as posterior stroke presenting as isolated dizziness or aneurysmal SAH mimicking a benign headache syndrome, are among the most commonly misdiagnosed and pose medicolegal risk to the ED provider. A thoughtful history, focused neurologic examination, and knowledge of red-flag signs and symptoms of the "cannot miss" diagnoses are the best protections against these unfortunate outcomes. Efficient diagnosis of time-critical neurologic emergencies, such as acute ischemic stroke, status epilepticus, and acute spinal cord injury, may allow for more rapid treatment and improved outcomes for patients. ED providers should be supported with institutional and multidisciplinary clinical pathways that aid in timely decision making and mitigate unnecessary risk.

REFERENCES

1. Newman-Toker DE, Perry JJ. Acute diagnostic neurology: challenges and opportunities. Acad Emerg Med 2015;22(3):357–61.
2. Goldstein JN, Camargo CA Jr, Pelletier AJ, et al. Headache in United States emergency departments: demographics, work-up and frequency of pathological diagnoses. Cephalalgia 2006;26(6):684–90.
3. Royl G, Ploner CJ, Möckel M, et al. Neurological chief complaints in an emergency room. Nervenarzt 2010;81(10):1226–30 [in German].
4. Rizos T, Jüttler E, Sykora M, et al. Common disorders in the neurological emergency room–experience at a tertiary care hospital. Eur J Neurol 2011;18(3): 430–5.
5. Stovner LJ, Hagen K, Jensen R, et al. The global burden of headache: a documentation of headache prevalence and disability worldwide. Cephalalgia 2007; 27(3):193–210 [Review].
6. Ducros A, Bousser MG. Thunderclap headache. BMJ 2013;346:e8557.
7. Landtblom AM, Fridriksson S, Boivie J, et al. Sudden onset headache: a prospective study of features, incidence and causes. Cephalalgia 2002;22(5):354–60.
8. Edlow JA. Managing patients with nontraumatic, severe, rapid-onset headache. Ann Emerg Med 2018;71(3):400–8 [Review].
9. Montemayor ET, Long B, Pfaff JA, et al. Patient with a subarachnoid headache. Clin Pract Cases Emerg Med 2018;2(3):193–6.
10. Carpenter CR, Hussain AM, Ward MJ, et al. Spontaneous subarachnoid hemorrhage: a systematic review and meta-analysis describing the diagnostic accuracy of history, physical examination, imaging, and lumbar puncture with an exploration of test thresholds. Acad Emerg Med 2016;23(9):963–1003 [Review].
11. Lynch KM, Brett F. Headaches that kill: a retrospective study of incidence, etiology and clinical features in cases of sudden death. Cephalalgia 2012;32(13): 972–8.
12. Cady R, Garas SY, Patel K, et al. Symptomatic overlap and therapeutic opportunities in primary headache. J Pharm Pract 2015;28(4):413–8 [Review].
13. Mortimer AM, Bradley MD, Stoodley NG, et al. Thunderclap headache: diagnostic considerations and neuroimaging features. Clin Radiol 2013;68(3): e101–13 [Review].
14. Avsenik J, Oblak JP, Popovic KS. Non-contrast computed tomography in the diagnosis of cerebral venous sinus thrombosis. Radiol Oncol 2016;50(3):263–8.
15. Perry JJ, Stiell IG, Sivilotti ML, et al. Sensitivity of computed tomography performed within six hours of onset of headache for diagnosis of subarachnoid haemorrhage: prospective cohort study. BMJ 2011;343:d4277.

16. Dubosh NM, Bellolio MF, Rabinstein AA, et al. Sensitivity of early brain computed tomography to exclude aneurysmal subarachnoid hemorrhage: a systematic review and meta-analysis. Stroke 2016;47(3):750–5 [Review].

17. Long B, Koyfman A, Runyon MS. Subarachnoid hemorrhage: updates in diagnosis and management. Emerg Med Clin North Am 2017;35(4):803–24 [Review].

18. Long B, Koyfman A. Controversies in the diagnosis of subarachnoid hemorrhage. J Emerg Med 2016;50(6):839–47.

19. Brunell A, Ridefelt P, Zelano J. Differential diagnostic yield of lumbar puncture in investigation of suspected subarachnoid haemorrhage: a retrospective study. J Neurol 2013;260(6):1631–6.

20. Pope JV, Edlow JA. Avoiding misdiagnosis in patients with neurological emergencies. Emerg Med Int 2012;2012:949275.

21. Edlow JA, Selim MH. Atypical presentations of acute cerebrovascular syndromes. Lancet Neurol 2011;10(6):550–60 [Review].

22. Dubosh NM, Edlow JA. Diagnosis of subarachnoid hemorrhage: time for a paradigm shift? Acad Emerg Med 2017;24(12):1514–6.

23. Sandvei MS, Mathiesen EB, Vatten LJ, et al. Incidence and mortality of aneurysmal subarachnoid hemorrhage in two Norwegian cohorts, 1984-2007. Neurology 2011;77(20):1833–9.

24. Vermeulen MJ, Schull MJ. Missed diagnosis of subarachnoid hemorrhage in the emergency department. Stroke 2007;38(4):1216–21.

25. Kowalski RG, Claassen J, Kreiter KT, et al. Initial misdiagnosis and outcome after subarachnoid hemorrhage. JAMA 2004;291(7):866–9.

26. Dubosh NM, Edlow JA, Lefton M, et al. Types of diagnostic errors in neurological emergencies in the emergency department. Diagnosis (Berl) 2015;2(1):21–8.

27. Brown TW, McCarthy ML, Kelen GD, et al. An epidemiologic study of closed emergency department malpractice claims in a national database of physician malpractice insurers. Acad Emerg Med 2010;17(5):553–60.

28. Tinetti ME, Williams CS, Gill TM. Health, functional, and psychological outcomes among older persons with chronic dizziness. J Am Geriatr Soc 2000;48(4):417–21.

29. Newman-Toker DE, Cannon LM, Stofferahn ME, et al. Imprecision in patient reports of dizziness symptom quality: a cross-sectional study conducted in an acute care setting. Mayo Clin Proc 2007;82(11):1329–40.

30. Edlow JA. The timing-and-triggers approach to the patient with acute dizziness. Emerg Med Pract 2019;21(12):1–24.

31. Edlow JA. A new approach to the diagnosis of acute dizziness in adult patients. Emerg Med Clin North Am 2016;34(4):717–42 [Review].

32. Kattah JC, Talkad AV, Wang DZ, et al. HINTS to diagnose stroke in the acute vestibular syndrome: three-step bedside oculomotor examination more sensitive than early MRI diffusion-weighted imaging. Stroke 2009;40(11):3504–10.

33. Kerber KA, Brown DL, Lisabeth LD, et al. Stroke among patients with dizziness, vertigo, and imbalance in the emergency department: a population-based study. Stroke 2006;37(10):2484–7.

34. Newman-Toker DE. Missed stroke in acute vertigo and dizziness: it is time for action, not debate. Ann Neurol 2016;79(1):27–31.

35. Arch AE, Weisman DC, Coca S, et al. Missed ischemic stroke diagnosis in the emergency department by emergency medicine and neurology services. Stroke 2016;47(3):668–73 [Erratum appears in Stroke 2016;47(3):e59].

36. Nakajima M, Hirano T, Uchino M. Patients with acute stroke admitted on the second visit. J Stroke Cerebrovasc Dis 2008;17(6):382–7.

37. Tarnutzer AA, Lee SH, Robinson KA, et al. ED misdiagnosis of cerebrovascular events in the era of modern neuroimaging: a meta-analysis. Neurology 2017; 88(15):1468–77 [Review].
38. Westerberg BD, Lea J, Cameron AF. Post-traumatic dizziness: clinical and medicolegal aspects. Adv Otorhinolaryngol 2019;82:111–8 [Review].
39. Edwards J, Hayden J, Asbridge M, et al. Prevalence of low back pain in emergency settings: a systematic review and meta-analysis. BMC Musculoskelet Disord 2017;18:143.
40. Borczuk P. An evidence-based approach to the evaluation and treatment of low back pain in the emergency department. Emerg Med Pract 2013;15(7):1–24.
41. Ma VY, Chan L, Carruthers KJ. The incidence, prevalence, costs, and impact on disability of common conditions requiring rehabilitation in the US: stroke, spinal cord injury, traumatic brain injury, multiple sclerosis, osteoarthritis, rheumatoid arthritis, limb loss, and back pain. Arch Phys Med Rehabil 2014;95(5):986–95.e1.
42. Chao D, Nanda A. Spinal epidural abscess: a diagnostic challenge. Am Fam Physician 2002;65(7):1341–6.
43. Kachalia A, Gandhi TK, Puopolo AL, et al. Missed and delayed diagnoses in the emergency department: a study of closed malpractice claims from 4 liability insurers. Ann Emerg Med 2007;49(2):196–205.
44. Casazza BA. Diagnosis and treatment of acute low back pain. Am Fam Physician 2012;85(4):343–50.
45. Friedman BW, Chilstrom M, Bijur PE, et al. Diagnostic testing and treatment of low back pain in United States emergency departments: a national perspective. Spine (Phila Pa 1976) 2010;35(24):E1406–11.
46. Mackenzie AR, Laing RB, Smith CC, et al. Spinal epidural abscess: the importance of early diagnosis and treatment. J Neurol Neurosurg Psychiatry 1998; 65(2):209–12.
47. Jalloh I, Minhas P. Delays in the treatment of cauda equina syndrome due to its variable clinical features in patients presenting to the emergency department. Emerg Med J 2007;24(1):33–4.
48. Gardner A, Gardner E, Morley T. Cauda equina syndrome: a review of the current clinical and medico-legal position. Eur Spine J 2011;20(5):690–7.
49. Thakur JD, Storey C, Kalakoti P, et al. Early intervention in cauda equina syndrome associated with better outcomes: a myth or reality? Insights from the Nationwide Inpatient Sample database (2005-2011). Spine J 2017;17(10): 1435–48.
50. Chau AM, Xu LL, Pelzer NR, et al. Timing of surgical intervention in cauda equina syndrome: a systematic critical review. World Neurosurg 2014;81(3–4):640–50.
51. French KL, Daniels EW, Ahn UM, et al. Medicolegal cases for spinal epidural hematoma and spinal epidural abscess. Orthopedics 2013;36(1):48–53.
52. Alerhand S, Wood S, Long B, et al. The time-sensitive challenge of diagnosing spinal epidural abscess in the emergency department. Intern Emerg Med 2017;12(8):1179–83.
53. Davis DP, Salazar A, Chan TC, et al. Prospective evaluation of a clinical decision guideline to diagnose spinal epidural abscess in patients who present to the emergency department with spine pain. J Neurosurg Spine 2011;14(6):765–70.
54. Chima-Melton C, Pearl M, Scheiner M. Diagnosis of spinal epidural abscess: a case report and literature review. Spinal Cord Ser Cases 2017;3:17013.
55. DePasse JM, Ruttiman R, Eltorai AEM, et al. Assessment of malpractice claims due to spinal epidural abscess. J Neurosurg Spine 2017;27(4):476–80.

56. Babu JM, Patel SA, Palumbo MA, et al. Spinal emergencies in primary care practice. Am J Med 2019;132(3):300–6 [Review].
57. Nickel CH, Nemec M, Bingisser R. Weakness as presenting symptom in the emergency department. Swiss Med Wkly 2009;139(17–18):271–2.
58. Lees KR, Bluhmki E, von Kummer R, et al. Time to treatment with intravenous alteplase and outcome in stroke: an updated pooled analysis of ECASS, ATLANTIS, NINDS, and EPITHET trials. Lancet 2010;375(9727):1695–703.
59. Lopez AD, Mathers CD, Ezzati M, et al. Measuring the global burden of disease and risk factors 1990-2001. Global burden of disease and risk factors. New York: Oxford University Press; 2006. Chapter 1.
60. Ganti L, Rastogi V. Acute generalized weakness. Emerg Med Clin North Am 2016; 34(4):795–809.
61. Krishnan C, Kerr DA. Idiopathic transverse myelitis. Arch Neurol 2005;62(6): 1011–3.
62. Willison HJ, Jacobs BC, van Doorn PA. Guillain-Barré syndrome. Lancet 2016; 388(10045):717–27.
63. McGillicuddy DC, Walker O, Shapiro NI, et al. Guillain-Barré syndrome in the emergency department. Ann Emerg Med 2006;47(4):390–3.
64. van den Berg B, Bunschoten C, van Doorn PA, et al. Mortality in Guillain-Barre syndrome. Neurology 2013;80(18):1650–4.
65. van Doorn PA. Diagnosis, treatment and prognosis of Guillain-Barré syndrome (GBS). Presse Med 2013;42(6 Pt 2):e193–201.
66. Smulowitz PB, Zeller J, Sanchez LD, et al. Myasthenia gravis: lessons for the emergency physician. Eur J Emerg Med 2005;12(6):324–6.
67. Frohman EM, Wingerchuk DM. Clinical practice. Transverse myelitis. N Engl J Med 2010;363(6):564–72.
68. Bhat A, Naguwa S, Cheema G, et al. The epidemiology of transverse myelitis. Autoimmun Rev 2010;9(5):A395–9.
69. Edlow JA, McGillicuddy DC. Tick paralysis. Infect Dis Clin North Am 2008;22(3): 397–413, vii.
70. Edlow JA. Tick paralysis. Curr Treat Options Neurol 2010;12(3):167–77.
71. Diaz JH. A 60-year meta-analysis of tick paralysis in the United States: a predictable, preventable, and often misdiagnosed poisoning. J Med Toxicol 2010;6(1): 15–21.
72. Newman-Toker DE, Moy E, Valente E, et al. Missed diagnosis of stroke in the emergency department: a cross-sectional analysis of a large population-based sample. Diagnosis (Berl) 2014;1(2):155–66.
73. Lever NM, Nyström KV, Schindler JL, et al. Missed opportunities for recognition of ischemic stroke in the emergency department. J Emerg Nurs 2013;39(5):434–9.
74. Brandler ES, Sharma M, McCullough F, et al. Prehospital stroke identification: factors associated with diagnostic accuracy. J Stroke Cerebrovasc Dis 2015;24(9): 2161–6.
75. Kuruvilla A, Bhattacharya P, Rajamani K, et al. Factors associated with misdiagnosis of acute stroke in young adults. J Stroke Cerebrovasc Dis 2011;20(6): 523–7.
76. Whiteley WN, Wardlaw JM, Dennis MS, et al. Clinical scores for the identification of stroke and transient ischaemic attack in the emergency department: a cross-sectional study. J Neurol Neurosurg Psychiatry 2011;82(9):1006–10.
77. Byrne B, O'Halloran P, Cardwell C. Accuracy of stroke diagnosis by registered nurses using the ROSIER tool compared to doctors using neurological assessment on a stroke unit: a prospective audit. Int J Nurs Stud 2011;48(8):979–85.

78. Xin Y, Han FG. Diagnostic accuracy of computed tomography perfusion in patients with acute stroke: a meta-analysis. J Neurol Sci 2016;360:125–30.
79. Bruce NT, Neil WP, Zivin JA. Medico-legal aspects of using tissue plasminogen activator in acute ischemic stroke. Curr Treat Options Cardiovasc Med 2011; 13(3):233–9.
80. Weintraub MI. Thrombolysis (tissue plasminogen activator) in stroke: a medicolegal quagmire. Stroke 2006;37(7):1917–22.
81. Bhatt A, Safdar A, Chaudhari D, et al. Medicolegal considerations with intravenous tissue plasminogen activator in stroke: a systematic review. Stroke Res Treat 2013;2013:562564.
82. Liang BA, Zivin JA. Empirical characteristics of litigation involving tissue plasminogen activator and ischemic stroke. Ann Emerg Med 2008;52(2):160–4.
83. Powers WJ, Rabinstein AA, Ackerson T, et al, American Heart Association Stroke Council. 2018 Guidelines for the Early Management of Patients with Acute Ischemic Stroke: a guideline for healthcare professionals from the American Heart Association/American Stroke Association. Stroke 2018;49(3):e46–110 [Review]. [Erratum appears in Stroke 2018;49(3):e138].
84. Miller JB, Merck LH, Wira CR, et al. The advanced reperfusion era: implications for emergency systems of ischemic stroke care. Ann Emerg Med 2017;69(2): 192–201 [Review].
85. Johnston SC, Gress DR, Browner WS, et al. Short-term prognosis after emergency department diagnosis of TIA. JAMA 2000;284(22):2901–6.
86. Chandratheva A, Mehta Z, Geraghty OC, et al, Oxford Vascular Study. Population-based study of risk and predictors of stroke in the first few hours after a TIA. Neurology 2009;72(22):1941–7.
87. American College of Emergency Physicians Clinical Policies Subcommittee (Writing Committee) on Suspected Transient Ischemic Attack, Lo BM, Carpenter CR, Hatten BW, et al. Clinical policy: critical issues in the evaluation of adult patients with suspected transient ischemic attack in the emergency department. Ann Emerg Med 2016;68(3):354–70.e29 [Review]. [Erratum appears in Ann Emerg Med 2017;70(5):758].
88. Jagoda A, Gupta K. The emergency department evaluation of the adult patient who presents with a first-time seizure. Emerg Med Clin North Am 2011; 29(1):41–9.
89. Khoujah D, Abraham MK. Status epilepticus: what's new? Emerg Med Clin North Am 2016;34(4):759–76 [Review].
90. Aranda A, Foucart G, Ducassé JL, et al. Generalized convulsive status epilepticus management in adults: a cohort study with evaluation of professional practice. Epilepsia 2010;51(10):2159–67.
91. Treiman DM, Meyers PD, Walton NY, et al. A comparison of four treatments for generalized convulsive status epilepticus. Veterans Affairs Status Epilepticus Cooperative Study Group. N Engl J Med 1998;339(12):792–8.
92. Kass JS, Rose RV. Driving and epilepsy: ethical, legal, and health care policy challenges. Continuum (Minneap Minn) 2019;25(2):537–42.
93. Huff JS, Melnick ER, Tomaszewski CA, et al, American College of Emergency Physicians. Clinical policy: critical issues in the evaluation and management of adult patients presenting to the emergency department with seizures. Ann Emerg Med 2014;63(4):437–47.e15 [Erratum appears in Ann Emerg Med 2017;70(5):758].

Surviving a Medical Malpractice Lawsuit

Kelly Bookman, MD, Richard D. Zane, MD*

KEYWORDS

- Lawsuit • Malpractice • Expert witness • Tort reform • Negligence • Claim
- Litigation

KEY POINTS

- A medical malpractice case is extremely stressful.
- There are many steps in a medical malpractice lawsuit.
- These steps go from being served, to the disposition, to a trial, and appeals if one loses.
- There are strategies that may be used to defend these cases.

INTRODUCTION

Medical malpractice litigation is pervasive in the United States, with 7.4% of physicians having an annual claim and 75% to 99% of all physicians facing a claim by age 65 years.[1] Emergency physicians (EPs) are at particular risk because the patients typically present to an emergency department (ED) with high-acuity illness[2] and the delivery of emergency care is complex.[3] Also, EPs rarely have an ongoing relationship with their patients, and care is frequently transitioned from one provider to another.[4] ED and hospital crowding further contribute to the high-risk environment of the ED.[5]

Although tort reform has had some effect on the current malpractice crisis, with total and paid claims decreasing over time, the effect has been variable and dependent on jurisdiction.[6] Thirty states have passed legislation to cap noneconomic damages in medical liability cases, but setting limits in other states and at the federal level has been challenging.[7] By understanding the legal system and the medical litigation process, physicians can potentially avoid litigation and, when they are inevitably named in a lawsuit, may better participate in their defense.

Before examining the specifics of the system and process, it is important to understand the intended societal goals of malpractice litigation, which include deterring unsafe practices, compensating persons injured through negligence, and exacting corrective justice.[8] Although these admirable goals form the basis of the current system, they may be difficult to recognize when monetary reward for attorneys and

Department of Emergency Medicine, University of Colorado School of Medicine, Mail Stop B215, 12401 East 17th Avenue, Aurora, CO 80045, USA
* Corresponding author.
E-mail address: richard.zane@ucdenver.edu

Emerg Med Clin N Am 38 (2020) 539–548
https://doi.org/10.1016/j.emc.2020.01.006
0733-8627/20/© 2020 Elsevier Inc. All rights reserved.

patients seems paramount. Equally important to recognize are the similarities and differences in the relationships between the physician and patient and between the attorney and client. Both relationships require professionalism, ethical conduct, extensive skill and training, and confidentiality, but they are practiced in diametrically dissimilar fashions.[9] In the simplest terms, in the physician-patient relationship, the physician's job is to collaborate with the patient to prevent, diagnose, discover, and (if possible) remedy an illness and alleviate suffering. In contradistinction, the legal system represents an adversarial process in which the lawyer has an ethical duty to fervently represent and advocate for a client while attempting to win the case,[10] and winning may not be synonymous with truth or justice. This process requires that a patient or client enters into a situation in which a former physician is now an adversary. Also, contrast the way in which physicians and lawyers are compensated. Although doctors get paid for services rendered, in most medical malpractice cases, attorneys representing patients are paid on contingency, collecting an agreed portion of the settlement after expenses only if they are successful. If the lawsuit is unsuccessful, the attorney not only is uncompensated for time and advocacy but also is likely to have incurred much expense in bringing the case to litigation, which can amount to hundreds of thousands of dollars.[11] Even though an argument could be made that neither relationship nor system of compensation is ideal or even just, it is defining that they are so different.

THE BASICS

The legal system is based on the premise of trial advocacy, which relies on the adversarial arrangement of opposing parties, a judge, and potentially a jury. The jury serves as the decider of fact, whereas the judge decides all questions of law. Some of the questions of law on which a judge may be asked to rule are which statutes apply in a certain situation; what evidence is germane and allowable; and who is permitted to testify, and what they may testify to, in front of the jury. Although all of these issues can affect the outcome of a trial, the jury decides the facts, including whether a physician was negligent or committed malpractice, whether there was any injury related to said malpractice, and whether that injury warrants monetary award. The jury decides the amount of any award, and the judge is only involved if the decision of the jury is unreasonable.[12]

Medical malpractice is defined as the "failure of a physician or health care provider to deliver proper services, either intentionally or through negligence, or without obtaining informed consent."[13] Most medical malpractice litigation in the United States revolves around the concept of negligence[14] and liability, making this type of litigation part of tort law. The word tort comes from the Latin term torquere, which means twisted or wrong.[14] Tort law, as defined by West's *Encyclopedia of American Law*, is:

> a body of rights, obligations, and remedies that is applied by courts in civil proceedings to provide relief for persons who have suffered harm from the wrongful acts of others. The person who sustains injury or suffers pecuniary damage as the result of tortious conduct is known as the plaintiff, and the person who is responsible for inflicting the injury and incurs liability for the damage is known as the defendant or tortfeasor.

Tort law is a combination of legislative enactments and common-law principles. These laws may vary substantially from state to state because they are often based on the precedents from previous rulings. In contrast with legal actions for breach of contract, tort actions do not depend on a previous contract or agreement between the disputing parties. Also, unlike criminal cases in which the government serves as the plaintiff, tort actions are brought by private individuals. The tortfeasor or defendant is not subject to incarceration or fines in civil court.

In a malpractice suit, the plaintiff is usually the patient or someone acting on behalf of the patient, and the defendant is any medical provider, which may include a hospital or health center. A plaintiff can bring a successful medical malpractice claim if 4 essential elements are demonstrated (**Box 1**):

1. There was a duty owed to the plaintiff by the defendant.
   - If a physician or health care provider treated the plaintiff as a patient, this element is usually clear. It is less clear when an EP speaks to a specialist regarding the care and treatment of a patient, but the specialist has not agreed to care for or has not yet cared for that patient. This element may be complicated in situations in which a specialist is said to be curb-sided and does not have a relationship with the patient or an obligation to care for the patient because of being on call.
2. The duty was breached; that is, the health care provider deviated from the prevailing standard of care in treating the patient.
   - Although different from one state to another, the definition of standard of care is usually described as what a reasonably prudent health care provider would do under similar circumstances.[15] Most states describe the standard of care as a national standard, although some specify that the standard is local with specific geographic boundaries. Most deviations in standard of care are proved using expert testimony or the doctrine of res ipsa loquitur, meaning that the thing speaks for itself. The doctrine of res ipsa loquitur signifies that further details are unnecessary and that the facts of the case are self-evident. This doctrine applies to cases in which there has been clear medical error that does not require an expert. An example would be wrong-side surgery, an egregious medication error, or a surgical instrument left in a patient.
3. The breach in the standard of care caused injury.
4. The injury resulted in damage.[16]
   - With no damage, there is no cause for action, regardless of the presence of negligence.

Unlike criminal law, which requires that the defendant be proved guilty beyond reasonable doubt, in a tort claim involving monetary damages, the defendant needs to be proved liable based on a preponderance of the evidence.[17] This definition may vary slightly from one state to another and may include being proved to a reasonable degree of medical certainty, more likely than not, or greater than 50% probability.

Box 1
Four essential elements of a malpractice case

1. A duty is owed to the plaintiff by the defendant

2. The duty was breached; that is, provider deviated from the prevailing standard of care

3. The breach in the standard of care caused injury

4. The injury resulted in damage

Data from Black HC. Editor. Black's law dictionary. 5th edition. St. Paul (MN): West Publishing Co; 1981 and Danzon PM. Medical malpractice- theory, evidence and public policy. Cambridge (MA): Harvard University Press; 1985.

THE PROCESS
Claims and Suits

If a patient or a patient's estate suspects that the patient was a victim of medical negligence, the patient typically consults with an attorney. The attorney interviews the patient and decides whether to proceed with investigating the case. Either the patient has the pertinent medical records or the attorney writes a letter to the care provider requesting medical records. Most letters from attorneys requesting medical records are for insurance purposes. However, if an attorney requests medical records from a hospital and either the law firm is known to specialize in medical malpractice or the patient has been previously identified as a potential litigant by the risk management department, the hospital may initiate an internal investigation.[16]

Having received the medical records, the attorney usually has them assessed by a medical reviewer. Some large law firms have in-house employees who are general practice nurses or physicians and screen cases. For those firms that do not, there is an entire industry dedicated to performing these types of record reviews. When the screeners believe there may be medical negligence, the attorney usually sends the records to an expert in the specific field related to the alleged malpractice to determine whether there was negligence and whether said negligence resulted in harm. Based on the opinions of the experts, the attorney may decline or engage in representing the plaintiff in a formal action. Attorneys may decline participation for multiple reasons other than lack of evidence of negligence or causation. Because most malpractice lawyers are compensated based on contingency, they may decline a case if the potential damages do not warrant the time and expense involved. In contrast, an attorney may pursue a case, despite scant evidence of malpractice or causation, if the potential awards are large. There is much discussion regarding the prevalence of frivolous lawsuits; namely, those that lack evidence of damage and/or deviation in standard of care. A recent closed-case analysis showed that 3% of claims had no demonstrable injury associated with the alleged negligence and 37% were not associated with error. However, most of these cases were denied compensation.[11]

If the attorney believes that the case is meritorious, an allegation of malpractice is formally issued. The types of allegations vary by jurisdiction but they are generally in the form of either a claim or a suit. Formal claims are demands for payment or compensation by claimants who convey their intent to pursue a demand. This formal claim is made directly to the physician, group, hospital, or health care institution and may be communicated in writing, in person, or by phone. The claim usually includes details of the case and rationale for the claim. After a claim is received by a physician or hospital, it is investigated in conjunction with the health care provider's insurance carrier. Based on this investigation a decision is made to defend the claim or to negotiate a settlement. A negotiated settlement takes into account the allegations, the costs associated with litigation, the likelihood of a verdict in favor of the plaintiff, and the potential award for the plaintiff. Physicians may or may not have the right to decline settlement, depending on their specific type of malpractice insurance policy. If the demand is denied, the claimant may either drop the claim or proceed to a suit.[17,18]

In most states, a claim becomes a suit when a plaintiff files a formal complaint with the court, specifically seeking compensatory damages. Every state is slightly different in the way in which a claim becomes a suit, but most require that some proof of evidence is offered that a suit is meritorious and should proceed. The formal filing with the court usually includes a structured description of the case, naming the providers and institutions, explaining why each had a duty to the patient and failed to meet the standard of care, and showing that this deviation contributed to an injury that is due compensatory damages. Many states also require an expert physician who has reviewed the records to swear, in the form of an affidavit, that each of these defendants failed to meet the standard of care. Depending on the state, this may be all that is required to move forward to a formal suit.

In efforts to screen for frivolous lawsuits, some states have added steps that involve a preliminary review by a physician, or expert member panel, to determine whether there is sufficient proof to move the suit forward. In Massachusetts, for example, the state legislature established a medical malpractice tribunal made up of a licensed physician, a justice of the Superior Court, and an attorney.[19] The tribunal is charged with determining:

> if the evidence presented if properly substantiated is sufficient to raise a legitimate question of liability appropriate for judicial inquiry or whether the plaintiff's case is merely an unfortunate medical result.[20]

To date the tribunal has rejected 16% of cases; however, even if the tribunal denies the suit, the plaintiff may override the rejection by posting a $6000 bond, which is returned if the plaintiff wins.[21]

The time between the alleged malpractice occurring and a claim or suit being filed may be several years, and it depends on the specific statute of limitations for that state. Most states define the statute of limitations as taking effect when a plaintiff has become aware of the alleged act of malpractice.[17] For example, if the allegation is a failure to interpret a chest radiograph and recognize an abnormal nodule that is eventually diagnosed as cancer, then the statute of limitations takes effect from the day that the cancer was diagnosed and the previous chest radiograph was determined to have been improperly interpreted. Most states have different statutes of limitations for pediatric and birth injury cases, which may remain in effect until the child is an adult. Consequently, the time between a physician committing an alleged negligent act and being able to present a defense in a court of law may be long. Because of the statutes of limitations, plaintiff attorneys may initially name any medical provider who may have had any role in the alleged malpractice. The rationale behind this practice is that if they have failed to name a specific individual, who may later be implicated in the alleged negligence, before the statute of limitations has passed, then it provides an opportunity for other defendants to assign blame to the unnamed clinician. Ironically, failing to name providers has led to attorneys being named in legal malpractice suits. Although potential claims are not reported to any regulatory agencies, if a physician is named in a formal suit, that physician is usually required to report this on hospital credentialing forms and, depending on the state, medical license applications. Any payment made to a claimant on behalf of a health care provider must be reported to the National Practitioner Data Bank.[17]

After a complaint has been officially filed with the court, the named parties are formally notified that they have been named and what their alleged role was. In most states, the notification is accomplished in the form of a subpoena, which is served on the health care provider. Some hospitals have arrangements with the court that allow them to accept the subpoena on behalf of a provider and guarantee delivery, in the absence of which, an officer of the court personally hand-delivers the subpoena to the health care provider. This experience can be harrowing because it may be unexpected and the person hand-delivering the notice is unknown, may be in uniform, identifies the health care provider by name, hands them the document, and says, "Dr. Smith, you have been served." This event may occur anywhere, including the provider's place of employment or home. Once physicians have been notified of a pending complaint, they should immediately notify both their risk management department and insurance carrier. The risk management department and carrier do an internal investigation if they have not already done so. The carrier generally assigns an attorney or instructs the provider on how to arrange for attorney representation.

At this point, the suit is in the discovery period. During this time, which may last months to years depending on the state, the plaintiff and defense begin to obtain facts relevant to the case.[22] In addition to more medical records, hospital policies and procedures may be collected and a list of witnesses developed, including factual witnesses, such as coworkers and family members, and expert witnesses. During this phase of the suit, factual witnesses and the plaintiff are likely to be deposed. In many states, the defendants are requested to answer interrogatories, which are specific written questions used to establish the facts of the case.[17] Before being deposed, defendants may also have their unsworn statements taken. An unsworn statement is similar to a deposition except that the statement is not evidence and may not be used in a court of law. Expert witnesses review the case and communicate their opinions to the attorneys as to whether or not standard of care was breached and whether that breach contributed to the alleged damage. Initially, the experts review the medical records but may or may not have had an opportunity to review the depositions of the defendant and factual witnesses. After they have reviewed the evidence available, they are asked for their final opinions. The defendants and the plaintiff are required to disclose their respective experts to each other and are given the opportunity to investigate the opinions held by the experts. The manner in which this is done varies by state. In many states, experts must disclose their opinions in a written document that is submitted to the court; the opposing side is then given an opportunity to depose the experts to determine the details and basis of their opinions. Attorneys are not required to disclose expert witnesses whose opinions were sought and found not to have been favorable to their case. This situation occasionally results in an attorney "shopping" a case to multiple experts until a favorable opinion is found.

After the discovery phase is complete, the opposing parties may meet to discuss the possibility of resolving the case before it goes to trial. Physicians' insurance policies may or may not allow them to refuse to settle a case before going to trial. These settlement meetings may happen based on the desires of either of the parties or the carrier, or they may be required by some states before proceeding to trial. These meetings may involve an arbitrator, who serves as an impartial third party, attempting to negotiate a settlement. Most arbitration meetings are nonbinding, neither party being required to accept the position of the arbitrator or to settle the action. In some states, the opposing parties may choose binding arbitration in lieu of a trial. In binding arbitration cases, there is usually more than 1 arbitrator who hears the case and decides the issues of law and fact. There is a decision, on whether there was deviation in the standard of care and whether that deviation caused harm. Damages are assigned and binding arbitration decisions are final.

If the case goes to trial, depending on the state and the agreement of the parties, the defendant physician may opt for a bench trial instead of a jury trial. In a bench trial, the judge serves as judge and jury. At trial, each party is represented by an attorney, including the hospital if it is party to the suit. The plaintiff and defendant have the opportunity to make opening statements to the jury and then the plaintiff presents evidence to the jury, usually in the form of factual and expert witnesses. When experts are first called, they are asked a series of questions by the attorney who has retained their services; this is called direct testimony. The attorney representing the opposing party is then able to question (ie, cross-examine) that expert. After the plaintiff rests the case, the defense has an opportunity to present evidence and witnesses to counter the plaintiff's evidence.

At any point during the trial, the parties may agree to settle the case; they may also consent to certain stipulations before the trial to mitigate potential losses. For instance, the parties may agree to a high-low agreement, meaning that, no matter what the outcome, the plaintiff is guaranteed a minimum amount and the defense a maximum.[23] After closing statements by both parties, the jury deliberates, and assigns a verdict and any compensatory damages.

In certain circumstances, physicians may consider retaining their own counsel, separate from counsels approved by their carriers. For instance, a physician may be provided counsel who is also assigned to represent codefendants, including physicians from other specialties or the hospital. Although it may seem as if all of these parties should be aligned in their defense, attorneys representing multiple parties may be conflicted and not be able to vigorously represent one client when also representing another. For example, adequate representation of 2 EPs by 1 attorney may be difficult if both cared for a patient during the same visit, the first transferring the case to the second after initial evaluation and testing, but not contributing to the medical decision making, and the second discharging the patient. Another instance in which a physician may consider hiring separate counsel is when a plaintiff has made an offer to settle a matter for less than the physician's coverage limits, but the carrier wishes to proceed to trial. This counsel may make an arrangement with the carrier so that:

1. The physician is not held liable should a verdict be returned with an award that is greater than the policy limits
2. The physician is not personally responsible for the amount of the verdict in excess of policy limits

Expert Witnesses

The role of the expert witness is a matter of continually evolving national discussion. A medical expert is required to establish the standard of care and whether there was a breach of that standard. Most physicians bring a tremendous amount of professionalism to the process and play an important role in explaining this complicated concept to a lay jury.[9] Regardless of whether they are testifying on behalf of the physician or the patient, experts have a duty to independently examine the facts, formulate an opinion, and be able to interpret and present complex medical issues in a cogent way that a layperson may understand.

In general, most states have minimum requirements for experts, including that they are licensed to practice medicine and possess sufficient experience, education, and training to opine on the standard of care. In addition, some states have specific requirements, such as having a minimum percentage of time spent in clinical practice in the specific field, having board certification in that specialty, and practicing in a similar setting as the defendant. The required qualifications to be an expert are not universal; there remain states where a physician need only be licensed to qualify as an expert and testify for or against any physician, regardless of the expert's training, experience, board certification status, or practice setting. In some states, it is still possible for a physician who is not specialty trained or board certified to opine on the standard of care for a specialty physician.

Attorneys present witnesses whose opinions favor their side in the case. The system is adversarial, and therefore both sides offer evidence to further their arguments,[9,16] including often diametrically divergent opinions from experts. Because neither side is obligated to show evidence that is not supportive of their argument, the jury, which is impartial, may not be exposed to the entirety of the evidence. After an attorney has introduced an expert, the opposing counsel has the opportunity to cross-examine the expert, which may serve to discredit that expert's medical opinions and motivation for testifying. It is routine for experts to be questioned about how much of their income is derived from expert testimony, how often they are employed by the same firm, and how often they testify on behalf of patients versus health care providers.[12]

Expert witnesses have been the focus of much scrutiny regarding their motivation and the lack of impartiality of their testimony. It is common for a witness to have testified in one manner for a defense attorney and in a contradictory manner for a plaintiff's attorney in a similar case. There have also been occasions in which a physician reviews the same case for both sides. A simple Internet search for expert witness services yields thousands of experts who advertise their services as well as companies who specialize in locating medical experts. This situation has led many specialty societies to issue position statements regarding the responsibilities and expectations of the expert witness in malpractice cases; some societies and colleges have sanctioned members and even revoked membership because of questionable testimony.[24]

Although there is no governing body that oversees expert testimony, specialty societies have attempted to begin the process of oversight. The American Academy of Emergency Medicine (AAEM) published a *Position Statement on Ethical Expert Conduct and Testimony*[25] and the American College of Emergency Physicians (ACEP) issued *Expert Witness Guidelines*[26] in an attempt to address the issue of unethical expert testimony. Both include guidelines for testimony and descriptions of the minimum requirements to qualify as an expert. Some investigators and specialty societies have endorsed the obligations of experts and admonished them to be available to both plaintiff and defendant to preserve their independence from undue influence and to uphold their responsibility to the truth.

AAEM has a link on its Web site for "remarkable" testimony. The Web site allows physicians to submit testimony that "seems farfetched, unbelievable, or just plain wrong." The case and the testimony are then reviewed by the AAEM malpractice task force to determine whether the testimony is remarkable. The expert is then given an opportunity to respond to the accusation that the testimony was remarkable. The testimony, the letter to the expert, and the expert's response to AAEM are then posted.

Tort Reform

The case for tort reform has waxed and waned for years, depending on the political will at the time, most recently becoming a cause célèbre because of the federal government's response to rapidly increasing malpractice insurance premiums. To physicians who have been dealing with escalating insurance premiums and decreasing reimbursement, and the perception of a more litigious work environment, tort reform has come to symbolize a way to possibly relieve these pressures.[27] When speaking of tort reform, physicians are most commonly speaking of efforts to change the current medical malpractice system, which may include limits on damages, altering the ways plaintiff attorneys may be compensated, and creating special malpractice courts in which a panel of experts substitutes for a lay jury, among other ideas. However, tort reform is broader than an isolated theory and it could be applied to many subjects[28] in addition to medical malpractice, such as tobacco liability, construction, and the automobile industry.

The United States is not alone in attempting to use tort reform to stem a malpractice crisis; Canada, Australia, New Zealand, and Sweden have changed laws to limit medical liability. The California Medical Injury Compensation Reform Act of 1975 was one of the earliest models of tort reform aimed squarely at medical malpractice.[27] It addressed attorney fees, created time limits on suits, capped noneconomic damages, and introduced binding arbitration. Although malpractice premiums did decrease and stabilize, there remains much debate over the value of tort reform versus insurance regulation in reducing premiums.[29] Given the highly political nature of tort reform, national health care quality experts have advocated that efforts should be focused on injury prevention and insurance regulation restructuring, rather than on tort reform.[30]

SUMMARY

Being named in a malpractice case may be one of the most stressful events in a physician's career, and participating in a trial is likely to be remembered for a lifetime. Despite the climate of tort reform and the reported lack of real justice in the current system, it is a system that is unlikely to change anytime soon. By understanding and knowing the system and proactively participating in the defense, the traumatic experience of being named in a malpractice case can be mitigated.

DISCLOSURE

The authors have nothing to disclose.

REFERENCES

1. Jena AB, Seabury S, Lakdawalla D, et al. Malpractice risk according to physician specialty. N Engl J Med 2011;365(7):629–36.
2. Fordyce J, Blank FSJ, Pekow P, et al. Errors in a busy emergency department. Ann Emerg Med 2003;42:324–33.
3. Kachalia A, Gandhi TK, Puopolo AL, et al. Missed and delayed diagnoses in the emergency department: a study of closed malpractice claims from 4 liability insurers. Ann Emerg Med 2007;49:196–205.
4. Kuhn G. Circadian rhythm, shift work, and emergency medicine. Ann Emerg Med 2001;37:88–98.
5. Moskop JC, Geiderman JM, Marshall KD, et al. Another look at the persistent moral problem of emergency department crowding. Ann Emerg Med 2018. https://doi.org/10.1016/j.annemergmed.2018.11.029.
6. Terrence W, Brown MD, Kelen GD, et al. An epidemiologic study of closed emergency department malpractice claims in a national database of physician malpractice insurers. Acad Emerg Med 2010;17(5):553–60.
7. States exploring innovative medical liability reforms. Available at: https://www.ama-assn.org/practice-management/sustainability/states-exploring-innovative-medical-liability-reforms. Accessed June 20, 2019.
8. Keeton WP, Dobbs DB, Keeton RE, et al. Prosser and Keeton on the law of torts. 5th edition. St Paul (MN): West Publishing; 1984.
9. Amon E. Expert witness testimony. Clin Perinatol 2007;34:473–88.
10. Wecht CH, Koehler SA. Book review. J Leg Med 2005;26:529–34.
11. Studdert DM, Mello MM, Gawande AA, et al. Claims, errors and compensation payments in medical malpractice litigation. N Engl J Med 2006;354:2024–33.
12. Jerrold L. The role of the expert witness. Surg Clin North Am 2007;87:889–901.
13. Luce JM. Medical malpractice and the chest physician. Chest 2008;134(5):1044–50.
14. Sage WM, Kersh R. Medical malpractice and the U.S. health care system. New York: Cambridge University Press; 2006. p. 11–2.

15. Black HC, editor. Black's law dictionary. 5th edition. St Paul (MN): West Publishing Co; 1981.
16. Danzon PM. Medical malpractice- theory, evidence and public policy. Cambridge (MA): Harvard University Press; 1985.
17. Claims management and the legal process. Risk management foundation of the Harvard Medical Institutions. Cambridge (MA): Risk Management Foundation; 1994.
18. Sanbar SS. Legal medicine. 6th edition. Philadelphia: Mosby; 2004.
19. Norris DM. A medical malpractice tribunal experience. J Am Acad Psychiatry Law 2007;35(3):286–9.
20. Massachusetts General Law Annotated, Chapter 231: Section 60B. Malpractice actions against providers of health care; tribunal, 2007. Available at: http://www.mass.gov/legis/laws/mgl/231-60b.htm.
21. About the medical malpractice tribunal. Massachusetts Medical Society. Available at: http://www.massmed.org/tribunal/about/#.XQgcC9NKiRs. Accessed June 20, 2019.
22. Szalados JE. Legal issues in the practice of critical care medicine: a practical approach. Crit Care Med 2007;35(2 Suppl):S44–58.
23. Teichman PG. How high-low agreements work in a malpractice case. Fam Pract Manag 2007;14(5):43–5.
24. Blackett WB. AANS testimony rules rewritten: new rules for neurosurgical medical/legal expert opinion service. AANS Bulletin 2005;13(1):33.
25. Available at: https://www.aaem.org/resources/statements/position/ethical-expert-conduct-and-testimony.
26. Available at: https://www.acep.org/patient-care/policy-statements/expert-witness-guidelines-for-the-specialty-of-emergency-medicine/.
27. Millard WB. Elephants, blind sharpshooters, golddiggers, and beyond: the prospects for constructive tort reform (Part 1 of A 2-Part series). Ann Emerg Med 2007;50(1):59–63.
28. Studdert DM, Mello MM, Brennan TA. Medical malpractice. N Engl J Med 2004; 350:283–92.
29. How insurance reform lowered doctors' medical malpractice rates in California: and how malpractice caps failed. Presented by the Foundation for Taxpayer and Consumer Rights a nonprofit, nonpartisan organization. Santa Monica (CA), March 7, 2003.
30. Sage WM. Putting the patient in patient safety: linking patient complaints and malpractice risk. JAMA 2002;287:3003–5.

Moving?

Make sure your subscription moves with you!

To notify us of your new address, find your **Clinics Account Number** (located on your mailing label above your name), and contact customer service at:

Email: journalscustomerservice-usa@elsevier.com

800-654-2452 (subscribers in the U.S. & Canada)
314-447-8871 (subscribers outside of the U.S. & Canada)

Fax number: 314-447-8029

Elsevier Health Sciences Division
Subscription Customer Service
3251 Riverport Lane
Maryland Heights, MO 63043

*To ensure uninterrupted delivery of your subscription, please notify us at least 4 weeks in advance of move.

Printed and bound by CPI Group (UK) Ltd, Croydon, CR0 4YY

03/10/2024

01040402-0013